HEAD AND NECK ANATOMY
A CLINICAL REFERENCE

HEAD AND NECK ANATOMY
A CLINICAL REFERENCE

Barry KB Berkovitz

Reader in Special Dental Anatomy
Division of Anatomy, Cell and Human Biology
King's College, London, UK

Bernard J Moxham

Professor and Head of Anatomy Unit
School of Molecular and Medical Sciences
University of Wales, Cardiff, UK

MARTIN DUNITZ

© 2002 Martin Dunitz Ltd, a member of the Taylor & Francis group

First published in the United Kingdom in 2002
by Martin Dunitz Ltd, The Livery House, 7–9 Pratt Street, London NW1 0AE

Tel.:   +44 (0) 20 74822202
Fax.:   +44 (0) 20 72670159
E-mail: info@dunitz.co.uk
Website: http://www.dunitz.co.uk

A CIP record for this book is available from the British Library.

ISBN 1-899066-75-6

Distributed in the USA by
Fulfilment Center
Taylor & Francis
7625 Empire Drive
Florence, KY 41042, USA
Toll Free Tel.:   +1 800 634 7064
E-mail: cserve@routledge_ny.com

Distributed in Canada by
Taylor & Francis
74 Rolark Drive
Scarborough, Ontario M1R 4G2, Canada
Toll Free Tel.:   +1 877 226 2237
E-mail: tal_fran@istar.ca

Distributed in the rest of the world by
ITPS Limited
Cheriton House
North Way
Andover, Hampshire SP10 5BE, UK
Tel.:   +44 (0)1264 332424
E-mail: reception@itps.co.uk

Project management: Top Draw Design
Medical illustrators: Philip Wilson FMAA, RMIP
                       Debbie Maizels CBiol, MIBiol

Printed in China by Imago

CONTENTS

ACKNOWLEDGEMENTS

We are grateful to the following whose generosity in providing us with appropriate specimens to photograph have made this book possible.

Professors KE Webster, M Berry and S Standring, Division of Anatomy, Cell and Human Biology, GKT School of Biomedical Sciences, London: figures 2.1, 2.15, 3.28a, 3.30, 3.31, 3.38, 5.4, 5.15, 5.16, 5.24, 5.29, 5.31, 5.33, 5.35, 6.6, 6.7, 6.9, 6.17, 6.19, 6.26, 6.27, 7.5, 7.10, 7.17, 7.18, 7.21, 7.22, 7.29, 8.3, 8.5, 8.7, 8.8, 8.10, 8.14, 9.5, 9.12, 9.16, 10.2, 10.8b, 10.11, 10.12, 10.21, 10.22, 10.25, 10.33, 10.39, 10.41, 10.42, 10.47, 10.48, 10.49, 10.51, 10.52b, 10.57, 10.59, 10.63, 10.65, 10.66, 10.67, 10.69, 10.70, 10.71, 11.1, 11.6, 12.1, 12.3, 12.9, 12.10, 12.18, 13.4-13.13. For photographing these specimens we are grateful to Ms S Smith and Mr L Kelberman.

Professors CM Dean and P O'Higgins, Anatomy and Developmental Biology, University College London, London: figures 2.14, 2.20, 2.21, 3.35, 3.36, 5.10, 5.11, 5.14, 5.17, 5.22, 5.23, 5.25, 6.3b, 6.10, 7.19, 7.20b, 7.23, 7.28, 7.31, 7.32, 7.35, 8.4, 8.13, 8.15, 9.4, 9.19, 10.5, 10.6, 10,26, 10.8a, 10.9, 10.10, 10.12, 10.29, 10.31, 10.37, 10.46, 10.50, 10.52a, 10.53, 10.54, 10.60, 10.62, 11.7, 12.15, 12.19. For photographing these specimens, we are grateful to Mrs J Pendjiky.

Professor L Garey, Anatomy Department, Imperial College Medical School, London: figures 2.22, 2.23, 3.9, 3.17, 3.31, 3.32, 3.34, 5.18, 6.14, 6.30, 6.31, 7.20a, 7.30, 7.37, 8.9, 10.22, 10.32, 10.45, 10.64, 10.68, 11.2, 11.8, 11.9, 11.15, 12.2, 12.6, 12.16

The Royal College of Surgeons of England, London: figures 3.40, 3.41, 5.19, 5.27, 5.28, 5.30, 5.34, 6.3a, 6.11a, 6.25, 6.29, 7.33, 10.28, 11.10, 11.13, 11.14, 12.4, 12.5, 12.7, 12.14. For photographing these specimens, we are grateful to Mr F Sambrook.

Dr JH Musgrave, School of Medical Sciences, University of Bristol, Bristol: figures 5.12, 6.16, 6.20, 11.3.

Also to Mr SA Hickey for figure 12.12.

For technical assistance, we are grateful to Mr D Farr and Mr G Bridgeman, Division of Anatomy, Cell and Human Biology, GKT School of Biomedical Sciences, London; Ms W Birch, Mr D Dudley and Mr J Norton, Anatomy and Developmental Biology, University College London, London; Mr D Gunner and Mr L Aldridge, Anatomy Department, Imperial College Medical School, London.

PREFACE

In recent years, and in many countries of the world, the undergraduate medical curriculum and the provisions made for postgraduate medical training have changed markedly. Such changes have occurred for both educational and political reasons. As a result, subject disciplines have been redefined, new teaching methods and philosophies have been introduced, new subject-matter has been incorporated alongside the traditional disciplines, and examinations and standards have been altered. In consequence, anatomy teaching has had to change radically in many medical schools and this is reflected in some modern textbooks which sacrifice detail to provide a simplified and general account of the structure of the human body. Paradoxically, all this change is taking place against a background of increasing specialisation and, at the postgraduate level, there is a need for textbooks which give detailed coverage of specific regions of the body. A volume dealing with head and neck anatomy should be welcome for two reasons. First, this region is especially complex. Second, the head and neck is the concern of a variety of specialists, for example, neurologists, neurosurgeons, ear nose and throat surgeons, ophthalmologists, maxillofacial surgeons and oral and dental surgeons.

A proper appreciation of anatomy relies not merely upon the assimilation of a mass of facts, but upon an awareness of the spatial relationships of structures, thus making anatomy essentially a 'visual' subject. However, a number of textbooks do not sufficiently emphasise the illustrations. Our textbook, however, incorporates a sufficiently large number of colour photographs of dissections of the head and neck to make it serve as both an atlas and a textbook. Line drawings are also included to complement the colour illustrations, both to aid the understanding of certain topics and to illustrate areas not readily amenable to dissection.

We hope that the clinicians who use the book to further their specialist interests will find it of benefit in guiding them through this complicated subject. We would also be grateful to hear from readers about ways to improve our book.

BKB Berkovitz
BJ Moxham

chapter 1
THE SKULL

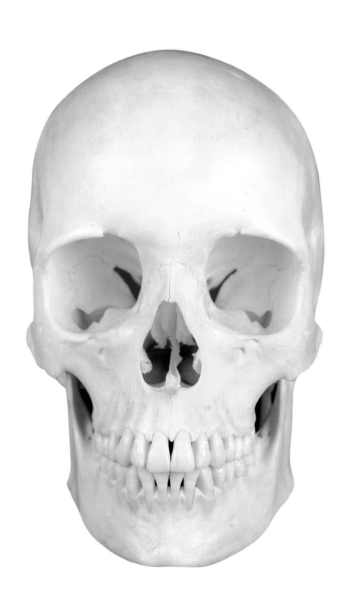

Chapter 1 THE SKULL

The skull is the bony skeleton of the head and is the most complex osseous structure in the body. It protects the brain, the organs of special sense and the cranial parts of the respiratory and digestive systems. The skull also provides attachments for many of the muscles of the head and neck.

Although often thought of as a single bone, the skull is composed of twenty-eight separate bones (see Table 1.1). Many of these bones are flat bones, consisting of two thin plates of compact bone enclosing a narrow layer of cancellous bone. In terms of shape, however, the bones are far from flat and can show pronounced curvatures. The term diploe is used to describe the cancellous bone within the flat bones of the skull.

In order to make the skull easier to understand, several subdivisions have been proposed. Firstly, one can subdivide the skull into cranium and mandible. This subdivision is based upon the fact that, whereas most of the bones of the skull articulate by relatively fixed joints, the mandible is easily detached. The cranium may then itself be subdivided into a number of regions (see below).

Secondly, one can subdivide the skull into neurocranium and viscerocranium. The neurocranium is defined as that part of the skull which houses and protects the brain and the organs of special sense. The viscerocranium is that region associated with the cranial parts of the respiratory and digestive tracts.

The cranial vault	The upper, dome-like part of the skull (including the skullcap or calvaria)
The cranial base	The inferior surface of the skull extracranially and the floor of the cranial cavity intracranially
The facial skeleton	The face (including the orbital cavities and the nasal fossae)
The jaws	The tooth-bearing bones
The acoustic cavities	The ear
The cranial cavity	The interior of the skull housing the brain

THE EXTRACRANIAL APPEARANCE OF THE SKULL

The following views of the exterior of the skull will be described:

The norma verticalis	The skull seen from above
The norma occipitalis	The skull seen from behind
The norma frontalis	The skull seen from in front
The norma lateralis	The skull seen from the side
The norma basalis	The skull seen from below

They are described in this order so that the less complex regions are considered first.

Table 1.1 The bones of the skull.

Name	Number	Primary location	Short description
Ethmoid	1	Nasal and orbital cavities of face	T-shaped. Processes form superior and middle conchae of lateral wall of nasal cavities
Frontal	1	Cranial vault	Forms forehead and roof of orbital cavities
Inferior concha	2	Nasal cavity of face	Projects from lateral wall of nasal cavity
Incus	2	Acoustic cavity	Shaped like an anvil
Lacrimal	2	Orbital cavity of face	Situated on medial wall of orbital cavity. Related to lacrimal sac
Malleus	2	Acoustic cavity	Shaped like a hammer
Mandible	1	Jaws	Forms lower jaw
Maxilla	2	Jaws	Forms upper jaw. Also contributes to nasal and orbital cavities
Nasal	2	Face	Forms bridge of nose
Occipital	1	Cranial vault	Forms back of head. Also contributes to cranial base
Palatine	2	Nasal cavity of face	L-shaped. Contributes to lateral wall of nose and hard palate
Parietal	2	Cranial vault	Forms mid-portion of cranial vault
Sphenoid	1	Cranial base	Butterfly-shaped. Also contributes to orbital and nasal cavities and lateral sides of skull
Stapes	2	Acoustic cavity	Stirrup-shaped
Temporal	2	Cranial base	Also contributes to lateral sides of skull
Vomer	1	Nasal cavity of face	Contributes to nasal septum
Zygomatic	2	Face	Forms cheek bone

THE NORMA VERTICALIS (1.1)

This view is so named because the most superior point of the skull is termed the vertex. The region observed is the skullcap or calvaria.

The calvaria is approximately oval in shape, the anteroposterior dimension being the greater. It is usually wider posteriorly than anteriorly. It is comprised of four bones separated by three prominent sutures. Anteriorly is found the squamous part of the frontal bone. Posteriorly is the squamous part of the occipital bone. Between the frontal and occipital bones lie the two parietal bones. The suture between the frontal bone and the parietal bones is termed the coronal suture. It is this suture which gives name to the coronal plane of the body. The midline suture between the parietal bones is the sagittal suture and this gives name to the sagittal plane. The junction of the coronal and sagittal sutures is termed the breg-

ma. The bregma corresponds to the anterior fontanelle ('soft spot') on the fetal skull. The suture dividing the occipital bone from the parietal bones is the lambdoid suture. The point of meeting of the lambdoid and sagittal sutures is called the lambda. This site marks the position of the posterior fontanelle on the fetal skull.

The calvaria is otherwise rather featureless. The region of maximum convexity of the parietal bone is called the parietal tuberosity. Close to the tuberosity run the superior and inferior temporal lines, though these lines are best seen in the norma lateralis. Parietal foramina may be found on either side of the sagittal suture. They transmit emissary veins (veins which link the intracranial and extracranial venous systems) from the superior sagittal sinus within the cranium. Sometimes terminal branches of the occipital arteries also pass through the parietal foramina.

1.1 The external surface of the calvaria

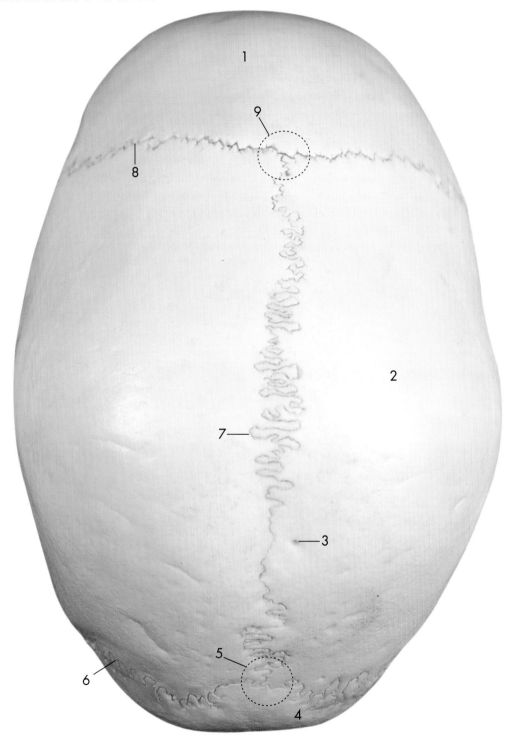

1 Frontal bone (squamous part)	6 Lambdoid suture
2 Parietal bone	7 Sagittal suture
3 Parietal foramen	8 Coronal suture
4 Occipital bone (squamous part)	9 Bregma
5 Lambda	

THE NORMA OCCIPITALIS (1.2)

Viewed from behind, the occipital bone is prominent. Thus is derived the term norma occipitalis. The lambdoid suture is also conspicuous, being seen in its entirety. A common variation is the presence of islands of bone within the suture. These sutural bones arise from separate centres of ossification but they have no clinical significance. Inferiorly, the lambdoid suture meets the occipitomastoid and the parietomastoid sutures. These sutures lie above and behind the mastoid process of the temporal bone. The temporal bones, though most clearly seen on the lateral sides of the skull, just appear as the mastoid processes to form the inferolateral parts of the back of the skull. The superolateral parts are formed by the parietal bones.

A marked feature at the back of the skull is the external occipital protuberance. It appears on the occipital bone in the midline as either a ridge or a distinct process. Extending laterally from the protuberance are two ridges called the superior nuchal lines. These lines finish above the mastoid processes. Inferior nuchal lines run parallel to, and below the superior nuchal lines. Above the superior nuchal lines may be seen the supreme nuchal lines. The external occipital protuberance and the nuchal lines are associated with muscle attachments. The supreme nuchal lines afford attachment to the epicranial aponeurosis of the scalp (see page 150). The roughened appearance of the occipital bone between the nuchal lines is also due to muscle attachments.

The muscles attached to the skull in the occipital region are:

Longissimus capitis	Superior nuchal line
Occipital belly of occipitofrontalis	Superior nuchal line
Semispinalis capitis	Between superior and inferior nuchal lines
Splenius capitis	Superior nuchal line
Sternocleidomastoid	Mastoid process and superior nuchal line
Superior oblique	Between superior and inferior nuchal lines
Trapezius	External occipital protuberance and superior nuchal line

The attachments of these muscles are described with the norma basalis.

1.2 The occipital view of the skull

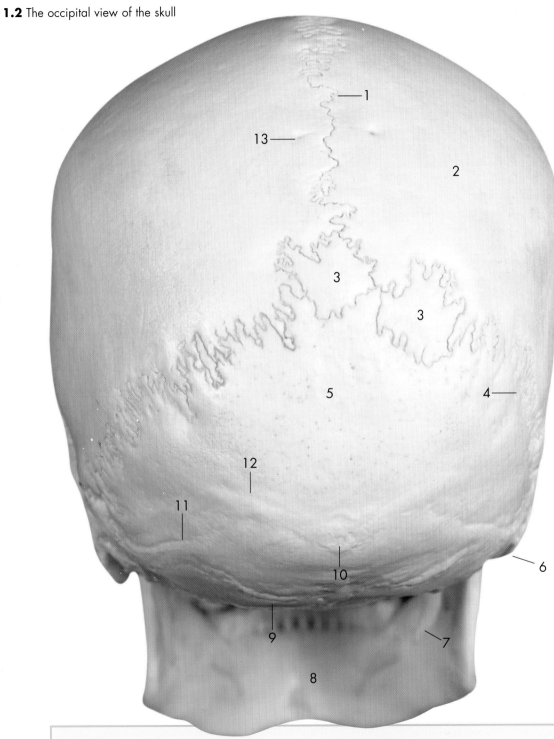

1 Sagittal suture	8 Mandible
2 Parietal bone	9 Inferior nuchal line
3 Sutural bones in region of lambda	10 External occipital protuberance
4 Lambdoid suture	11 Superior nuchal line
5 Occipital bone (squamous part)	12 Supreme nuchal line
6 Mastoid process of temporal bone	13 Parietal foramen
7 Styloid process	

THE NORMA FRONTALIS (1.3)

Most of the features seen on the front of the skull relate to the face. In particular, there are four apertures associated with the facial skeleton: the two orbital apertures, the anterior nasal aperture (the piriform aperture) and the oral aperture between the jaws. The osteology of the orbital and nasal apertures and of the orbital cavity and the nasal fossa are considered with the skull articulations.

The upper part of the facial skeleton is formed by the frontal bone and is related to the forehead. Above the bridge of the nose lies a slight elevation termed the glabella. This part of the frontal bone joins the nasal bones and the frontal processes of the maxillary bones at the frontonasal and frontomaxillary sutures. At the superior rim of each orbit are found the supra-orbital foramen (or notch) and the frontal notch. These transmit the supra-orbital and supra-trochlear nerves (and accompanying vessels) from the orbit onto the forehead. Laterally, the zygomatic processes of the frontal bone join the cheek bones (zygomatic bones) at the frontozygomatic sutures.

The central part of the face is occupied by the maxillary bones. Each bone not only contributes to the upper jaw but also to the nasal aperture, the bridge of the nose, the floor of an orbital cavity and the bones of the cheek. Beneath the inferior rim of each orbit lies the infra-orbital foramen. Through this foramen the infra-orbital nerve (from the maxillary division of the trigeminal nerve) and accompanying vessels pass onto the face. At the inferior margin of the nasal aperture in the midline lies a projection termed the anterior nasal spine. The two maxillary bones meet at the intermaxillary suture.

The lower part of the face is formed by the body of the mandible. In the midline is the prominence of the chin, the mental protuberance. In line with the supra-orbital and infra-orbital foramina lies the mental foramen. The mental nerve (from the mandibular division of the trigeminal nerve) and accompanying vessels pass through this foramen.

1 Frontal bone	15 Alveolus of mandible (lower jaw)
2 Glabella	16 Body of mandible
3 Zygomatic process of frontal bone	17 Mental protuberance
4 Greater wing of sphenoid bone	18 Mental foramen
5 Frontal process of maxilla	19 Intermaxillary suture
6 Lacrimal bone	20 Anterior nasal aperture
7 Nasal bone	21 Nasal conchae
8 Zygomatic bone	22 Infra-orbital foramen
9 Nasal septum	23 Zygomaticofacial foramen
10 Body of maxilla	24 Inferior orbital fissure
11 Anterior nasal spine	25 Superior orbital fissure
12 Alveolus of maxilla (upper jaw)	26 Frontal notch
13 Ramus of mandible	27 Supra-orbital notch
14 Angle of mandible	28 Zygomatic process of maxilla

1.3 The frontal view of the skull

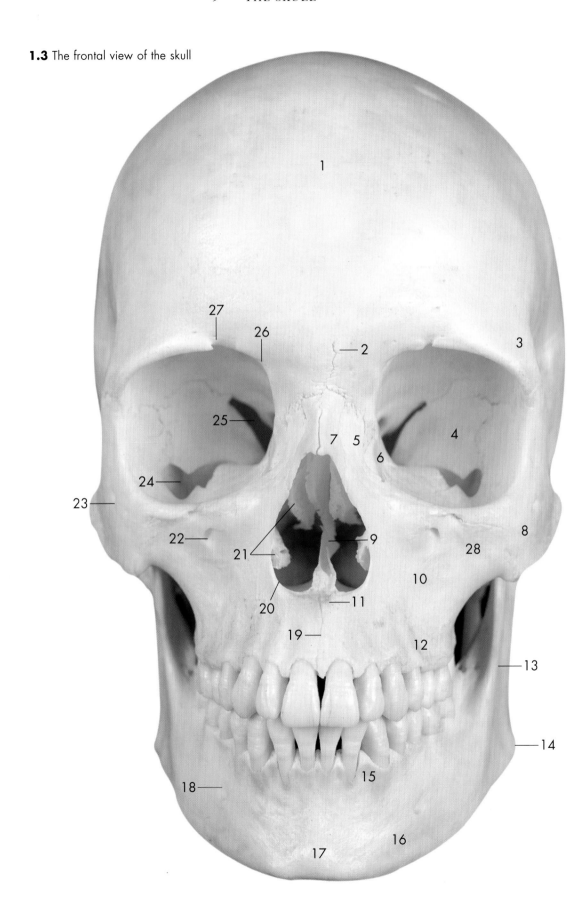

The muscles attached to the front of the skull (1.4) are:

Buccinator	Maxillary and mandibular buccal alveolar plates in region of molars
Corrugator supercilii	Frontal bone
Depressor anguli oris	Mandible below mental foramen
Depressor labii inferioris	Mandible between chin and mental foramen
Depressor septi	Maxilla below nasal aperture
Levator anguli oris	Maxilla below the infra-orbital foramen
Levator labii superioris	Inferior rim of orbit above infra-orbital foramen
Levator labii superioris alaeque nasi	Frontal process of maxilla
Masseter	Zygomatic arch and lateral surface of ramus of mandible
Mentalis	Incisive fossa of mandible
Nasalis	Maxilla close to nasal aperture
Orbicularis oculi	Nasal part of the frontal bone, frontal process of maxilla and crest of lacrimal bone
Platysma	Inferior border of body of mandible
Procerus	Nasal bone
Temporalis	Temporal fossa and coronoid process and anterior border of ramus
Zygomaticus major	Zygomatic bone
Zygomaticus minor	Zygomatic bone

1 Corrugator supercilii
2 Orbicularis oculi
3 Medial palpebral ligament
4 Procerus
5 Levator labii superioris alaeque nasi
6 Levator labii superioris
7 Zygomaticus minor
8 Zygomaticus major
9 Levator anguli oris
10 Compressor naris
11 Dilator naris
12 Depressor septi
13 Buccinator
14 Depressor labii inferioris
15 Depressor anguli oris
16 Platysma
17 Mentalis
18 Masseter
19 Temporalis

1.4 The frontal view of the skull showing areas for muscle attachments

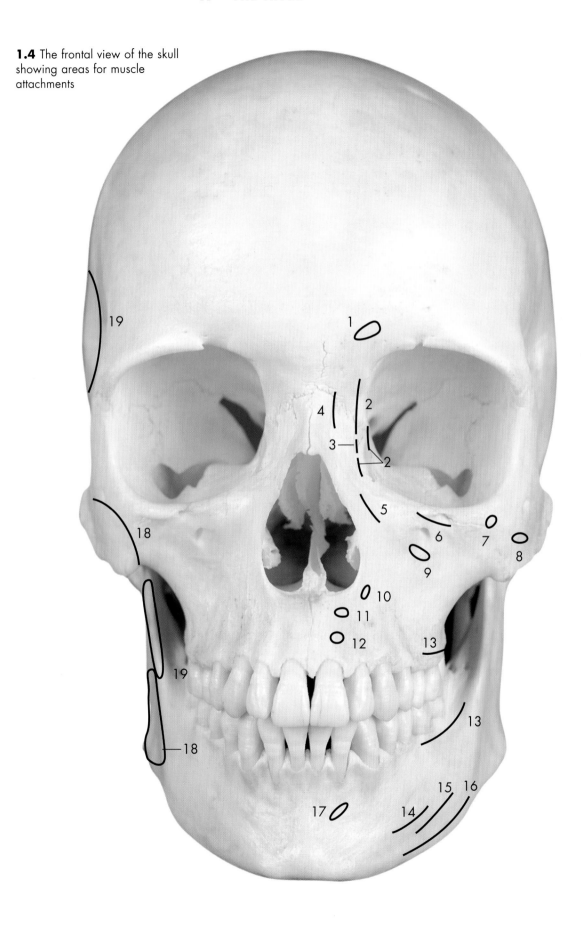

THE NORMA LATERALIS (1.5)

The skull, viewed from the side, can be subdivided into three zones. Anteriorly is the face and posteriorly is the occipital region. These have already been described. The intermediate zone shows two fossae, the temporal and infratemporal fossae. The boundary between the fossae is the zygomatic arch. The calvaria superiorly has been described with the norma verticalis.

The temporal fossa is so named because it is related to the temple of the head. The fossa is bounded inferiorly by the zygomatic arch, superiorly and posteriorly by the temporal lines on the calvaria and anteriorly by the frontal process of the zygomatic bone. It continues beneath the zygomatic arch into the infratemporal fossa. The temporal lines often present anteriorly as distinct ridges but become much less prominent as they arch across the parietal bone. Indeed, the superior line usually disappears posteriorly. On the other hand, the inferior temporal line becomes distinct once more as it curves down the squamous part of the temporal bone, forming a supramastoid crest at the base of the mastoid process. The superior temporal line gives attachment to the temporal fascia (see page 128). The inferior temporal line provides attachment for the temporalis muscle (see page 128).

The floor of the temporal fossa is formed by the frontal, sphenoid (greater wing), parietal and temporal (squamous part) bones. These four bones meet at an area termed the pterion where there is an H-shaped junction of sutures. This is an important landmark on the side of the skull. It overlies the middle meningeal vessels intracranially and corresponds to the sphenoidal fontanelle on the neonatal skull.

The suture between the temporal and parietal bones is called the squamosal suture. The sphenosquamosal suture lies between the greater wing of the sphenoid and the squamous part of the temporal bone.

The lateral surface of the ramus of the mandible should also be briefly described at this point. The ramus is a plate of bone projecting upwards from the back of the body of the mandible. Most of its lateral surface provides attachment for the masseter muscle. Two prominent processes are seen superiorly, the coronoid and condylar processes. The coronoid process is the site for the insertion of the temporalis muscle. The condylar process articulates with the mandibular fossa of the temporal bone at the temporomandibular synovial joint. Between the two processes is the mandibular notch. The angle of the mandible is the region where the inferior and posterior borders of the ramus meet.

The zygomatic arch stands clear of the rest of the skull, the gap being where the temporal and infratemporal fossae communicate. Whereas the bones of the cheek comprise the zygomatic bone and the zygomatic processes of the frontal, maxillary and temporal bones, the zygomatic arch is a term restricted to that part formed by the temporal process of the zygomatic bone and the zygomatic process of the temporal bone. These processes meet at the zygomaticotemporal suture. The suture between the frontal process of the zygomatic bone and the zygomatic process of the temporal bone is termed the frontozygomatic suture. The zygomatico-maxillary suture marks the union of the maxillary margin of the zygomatic bone and the zygomatic process of the maxillary bone. The zygomatic bone also joins the sphenoid bone, at the sphenozygomatic suture. As the zygomatic process of the temporal bone passes posteriorly, it becomes associated with the mandibular fossa and the supramastoid crest.

1.5 The lateral view of the skull

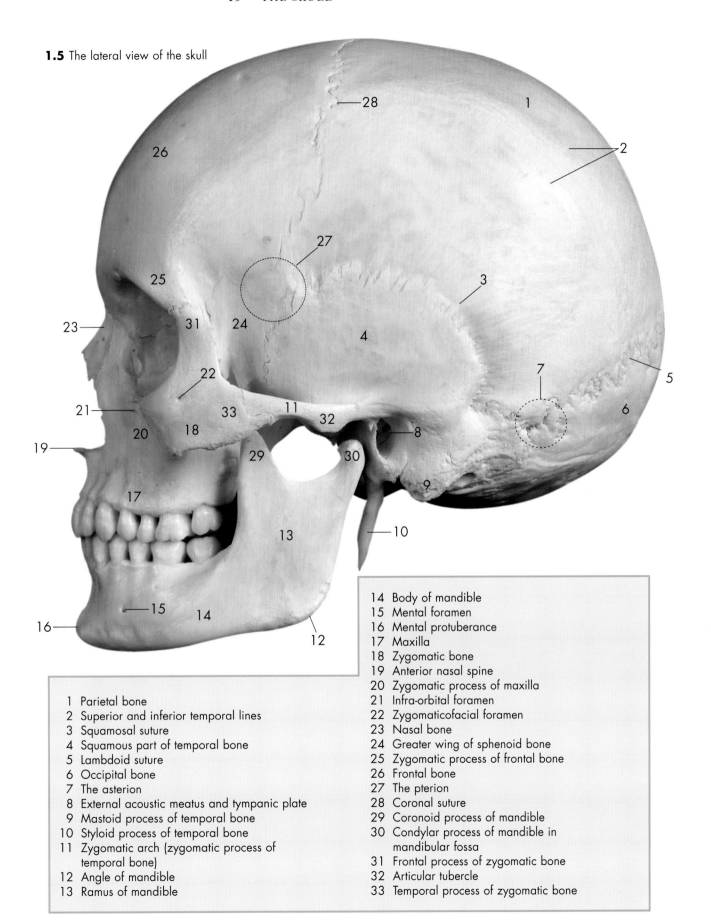

1   Parietal bone
2   Superior and inferior temporal lines
3   Squamosal suture
4   Squamous part of temporal bone
5   Lambdoid suture
6   Occipital bone
7   The asterion
8   External acoustic meatus and tympanic plate
9   Mastoid process of temporal bone
10 Styloid process of temporal bone
11 Zygomatic arch (zygomatic process of temporal bone)
12 Angle of mandible
13 Ramus of mandible
14 Body of mandible
15 Mental foramen
16 Mental protuberance
17 Maxilla
18 Zygomatic bone
19 Anterior nasal spine
20 Zygomatic process of maxilla
21 Infra-orbital foramen
22 Zygomaticofacial foramen
23 Nasal bone
24 Greater wing of sphenoid bone
25 Zygomatic process of frontal bone
26 Frontal bone
27 The pterion
28 Coronal suture
29 Coronoid process of mandible
30 Condylar process of mandible in mandibular fossa
31 Frontal process of zygomatic bone
32 Articular tubercle
33 Temporal process of zygomatic bone

The upper border of the zygomatic arch serves as an attachment for the temporal fascia. The inferior border and the deep surface provide attachment for the masseter muscle. A small foramen, the zygomaticofacial foramen, lies on the outer surface of the zygomatic bone. Another foramen, the zygomaticotemporal foramen, is situated on the inner surface. These foramina transmit nerves and vessels of the same name onto the face.

The temporal bone is a prominent structure on the lateral aspect of the skull. As mentioned, its squamous part lies in the floor of the temporal fossa and its zygomatic process contributes to the bones of the cheek. Additional features found are the mandibular fossa and its articular tubercle, the tympanic plate and external acoustic meatus, and the mastoid and styloid processes.

The mandibular fossa has also been called the glenoid fossa. It is the part of the temporomandibular joint into which the condylar process of the mandible articulates. It is bounded in front by the articular tubercle and behind by the tympanic plate. Occasionally, there is a postglenoid tubercle. The articular tubercle is important functionally as it provides a surface down which the mandibular condyle glides during mandibular movements. The tubercle also marks the site of attachment of the lateral ligament of the temporomandibular joint (see page 132).

The tympanic part of the temporal bone contributes most of the margin of the external acoustic meatus, the squamous part forming the upper margin and the upper part of the posterior margin. The margin is roughened to provide an attachment for the cartilaginous part of the meatus. Above and behind the meatus lies a small depression, the suprameatal triangle, which is related to the lateral wall of the mastoid antrum (see page 300).

The mastoid process is the large prominence located immediately behind the external acoustic meatus. It is the site of attachment of a prominent muscle of the neck, the sternocleidomastoid muscle. Above the process lies the supramastoid crest which is continuous with the inferior temporal line. The mastoid process articulates with the parietal and occipital bones at the parietomastoid and occipitomastoid sutures. The junction of these sutures with the lambdoid suture is termed the asterion. This corresponds to the mastoid fontanelle in the newborn skull. A mastoid foramen may be found near the occipitomastoid suture. This foramen transmits an emissary vein from the sigmoid sinus.

The styloid process is a long, slender process which emerges from the base of the skull in front of the mastoid process. It projects downwards and forwards towards the mandible. The base of the styloid process is formed by the tympanic part of the temporal bone. The process gives attachment to several muscles and ligaments.

The infratemporal fossa has the following bony boundaries: the ramus of the mandible laterally, the lateral pterygoid plate of the sphenoid bone medially, the infratemporal surface of the greater wing of the sphenoid superiorly, and the maxilla anteriorly. Beneath the zygomatic arch, the infratemporal fossa communicates with the temporal fossa. Between the lateral pterygoid plate and the maxilla lies the pterygomaxillary fissure. This fissure marks the site where the infratemporal fossa communicates with the pterygopalatine fossa (1.6) (for the osteology of this fossa, see page 210).

1.6 View of skull demonstrating some of the bony boundaries associated with the infratemporal fossa

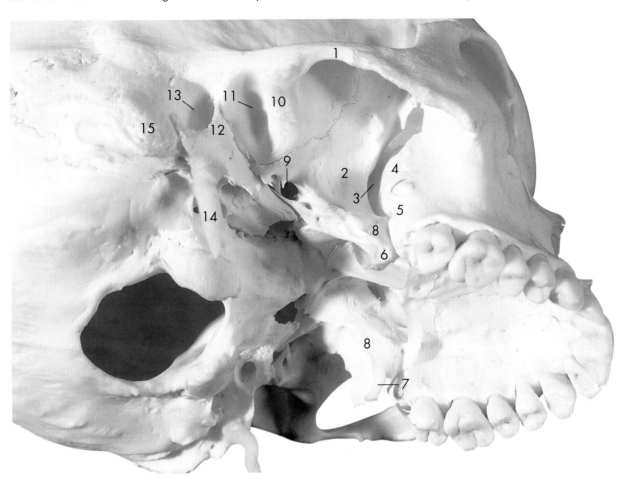

1 Zygomatic arch
2 Lateral pterygoid plate
3 Pterygomaxillary fissure
4 Infratemporal surface of maxilla
5 Tuberosity of maxilla
6 Pyramidal process of palatine bone
7 Pterygoid hamulus
8 Medial pterygoid plate
9 Foramen ovale
10 Articular tubercle
11 Mandibular fossa
12 Tympanic part of temporal bone
13 External acoustic meatus
14 Styloid process
15 Mastoid process

The muscles attached to the lateral side of the skull (1.7) are:

Buccinator	Maxillary and mandibular buccal alveolar plates in region of molars
Corrugator supercilii	Frontal bone
Depressor anguli oris	Mandible below mental foramen
Depressor labii inferioris	Mandible between chin and mental foramen
Depressor septi	Maxilla below nasal aperture
Levator anguli oris	Maxilla below infra-orbital foramen
Levator labii superioris	Inferior rim of orbit above infra-orbital foramen
Levator labii superioris alaeque nasi	Frontal process of maxilla
Masseter	Zygomatic arch, lateral surface of mandibular ramus
Mentalis	Incisive fossa of mandible
Nasalis	Maxilla close to nasal aperture
Occipital belly of occipitofrontalis	Superior nuchal line
Orbicularis oculi	Nasal part of frontal bone, frontal process of maxilla, crest of lacrimal bone
Platysma	Inferior border of body of mandible
Procerus	Nasal bone
Sternocleidomastoid	Mastoid process, superior nuchal line
Temporalis	Temporal fossa, coronoid process of mandible and anterior border of ramus
Zygomaticus major	Zygomatic bone
Zygomaticus minor	Zygomatic bone

1.7 The lateral view of the skull showing muscle attachments

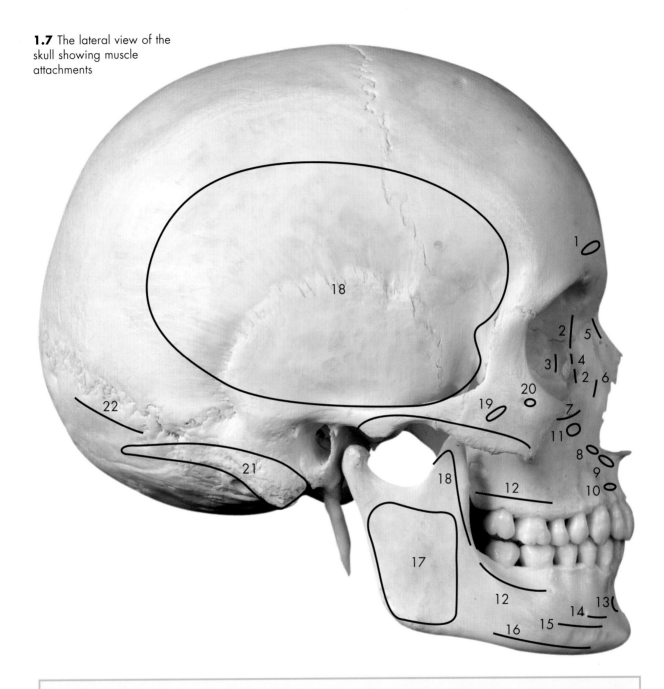

1 Corrugator supercilii
2 Orbicularis oculi (orbital and palpebral parts)
3 Orbicularis oculi (lacrimal part)
4 Medial palpebral ligament
5 Procerus
6 Levator labii superioris alaeque nasi
7 Levator labii superioris
8 Compressor naris
9 Dilator naris
10 Depressor septi
11 Levator anguli oris

12 Buccinator
13 Mentalis
14 Depressor labii inferioris
15 Depressor anguli oris
16 Platysma
17 Masseter
18 Temporalis
19 Zygomaticus major
20 Zygomaticus minor
21 Sternocleidomastoid
22 Occipital belly of occipitofrontalis

THE NORMA BASALIS (1.8, 1.9)

The inferior surface of the cranium is very irregular and presents the most complex of the surfaces of the skull. This complexity is increased by the fact that this region has many of the foramina through which structures enter and exit the cranial cavity. The region can be simplified by subdividing it into three zones. The anterior zone is comprised of the hard palate and the dentition of the upper jaw. The posterior zone lies behind a transverse plane drawn just in front of the foramen magnum. The intermediate zone is occupied mainly by the base of the sphenoid bone, the petrous processes of the temporal bones and the basilar part of the occipital bone. Whereas the intermediate and posterior zones are directly related to the cranial cavity (the middle and posterior cranial fossae), the anterior zone is related to the roof of the mouth and is some distance from the anterior cranial fossa.

The hard palate is formed by the two palatine processes of the maxillary bones and the two horizontal plates of the palatine bones. It is bounded anteriorly and laterally by the alveolus of the upper jaw which supports the teeth.

A cross-shaped set of sutures traverse the palate. Running anteroposteriorly and dividing the palate into right and left halves is the median palatine suture. This suture is continuous with the intermaxillary suture between the maxillary central incisor teeth. Behind the central incisors, the junction between the palatine processes of the maxillary bones is incomplete, thus forming the incisive fossa. Incisive foramina (two lateral or one anterior and one posterior) pass into this fossa and transmit the nasopalatine nerves and the terminal parts of the greater palatine vessels. Running transversely across the palate between the maxillary and the palatine bones is the transverse palatine suture. This suture is incomplete on each side and forms the greater palatine foramina. Through the greater palatine foramen pass the greater palatine nerve and vessels. Behind the foramen lie one or more lesser palatine foramina, through which pass the lesser palatine nerves and vessels.

The posterior borders of the horizontal plates of the palatine bones are concave and in the midline form a sharp ridge of bone, the posterior nasal spine. To the posterior edge of the hard palate is attached the fibrous aponeurosis of the soft palate which is formed by the tendons of the tensor veli palatini muscles.

The shape of the hard palate varies but is often dome-shaped. The arching of the palate occurs both anteroposteriorly and from side to side.

Above the hard palate are the nasal fossae, separated in the midline by the nasal septum. The posterior part of the septum is formed by the vomer. This bone lies on the body of the sphenoid. The two posterior nasal apertures (choanae) are located where the nasal fossae end. The lateral walls of the apertures beneath the hard palate are formed by the perpendicular plates of the palatine bones. A small canal called the palatovaginal canal is found in this region which transmits a nerve and an artery to the nasopharynx (the pharyngeal branch of the pterygo-palatine ganglion and an accompanying branch from the maxillary artery). Another canal, the vomero-vaginal canal, may sometimes be found which leads into the anterior end of the palatovaginal canal. It transmits a small artery (the pharyngeal branch of the sphenopalatine artery).

1.8 Osteology of the hard palate

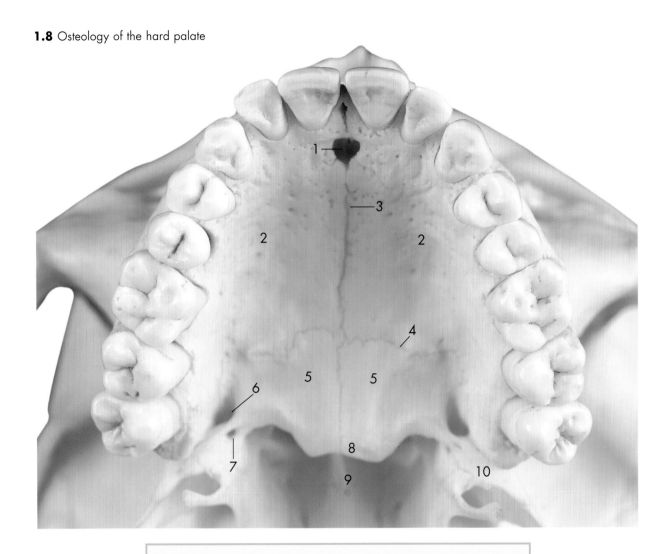

1 Incisive fossa
2 Palatine processes of the maxillae
3 Median palatine suture
4 Transverse palatine suture
5 Horizontal plates of the palatine bones
6 Greater palatine foramen
7 Lesser palatine foramen
8 Position of posterior nasal spine
9 Vomer
10 Pyramidal process of palatine bone

A prominent feature of the posterior zone of the cranial base is the foramen magnum. Associated with this foramen are the occipital condyles, the hypoglossal canals (anterior condylar canals) and the condylar canals (posterior condylar canals). Lateral to the foramen magnum are the jugular foramina. Other features of this part of the skull are the mastoid and styloid processes of the temporal bone, the stylomastoid foramina, the mastoid notches and the squamous part of the occipital bone up to the external occipital protuberance and the superior nuchal lines.

The foramen magnum is the largest foramen of the skull. Through it the cranial cavity (the posterior cranial fossa) and the vertebral canal communicate. The major structures passing through the foramen are the medulla oblongata of the brain stem, the vertebral arteries and the spinal accessory nerves. Anteriorly lies the apical ligament of the dens (an upwardly directed bony process from the second cervical vertebra) and the membrana tectoria of the atlanto-occipital joint (see page 92). Behind is the medulla oblongata and its covering meninges. Structures which pass through the foramen magnum with the medulla are: the vertebral arteries, the anterior and posterior spinal arteries, the spinal parts of the accessory nerves, and the meningeal branches of upper cervical nerves. The anterior margin of foramen magnum provides attachment for the anterior atlanto-occipital membrane and the posterior margin provides attachment for the posterior atlanto-occipital membrane (see page 92).

The occipital condyles lie near the anterior margin of the foramen magnum. They are facets for articulation with the vertebral column at the atlanto-occipital joints. They display marked curvatures in all planes. Within each condyle is the hypoglossal canal. This communicates with the posterior cranial fossa and transmits the hypoglossal nerve. It also transmits the meningeal branch of the ascending pharyngeal artery (a branch of the external carotid artery) and an emissary vein (from the basilar plexus). Behind each condyle is a depression termed the condylar fossa. The condylar canal passes into this fossa and transmits an emissary vein from the sigmoid sinus.

The jugular foramen is an irregular foramen situated lateral to the occipital condyle. It is really a large fissure formed between the jugular process of the occipital bone and the jugular fossa of the petrous part of the temporal bone. Anteriorly, the inferior petrosal sinus passes through the foramen. Midway, the foramen transmits the glossopharyngeal, vagus and accessory nerves. Posteriorly lies the internal jugular vein. A mastoid canaliculus runs through the lateral wall of the jugular fossa. This transmits the auricular branch of the vagus nerve. On the ridge between the jugular fossa and the opening of the carotid canal is the canaliculus for the tympanic nerve (a branch of the glossopharyngeal nerve to the cavity of the middle ear).

Between the mastoid process and the root of the styloid process is the stylomastoid foramen. Through this foramen emerges the facial nerve before it enters the parotid gland. Also passing through is an artery, the stylomastoid branch of the posterior auricular artery (a branch of the external carotid). Medial to the mastoid process is the mastoid notch. This is the site of attachment of the posterior belly of the digastric muscle. Medial to the notch is a groove in which runs the occipital artery (a branch of the external carotid).

1 Palatine process of maxilla	14 Occipital condyle
2 Median palatine suture	15 Mastoid process of temporal bone
3 Transverse palatine suture	16 Mastoid notch
4 Horizontal plate of palatine bone	17 Groove for occipital artery
5 Zygomatic arch	18 External occipital crest
6 Greater wing of sphenoid	19 Inferior nuchal line
7 Pterygoid hamulus	20 Superior nuchal line
8 Medial and lateral pterygoid plates of sphenoid bone	21 Squamous part of occipital bone
9 Opening of pterygoid canal	22 External occipital protuberance
10 Foramen lacerum	23 Foramen magnum
11 Mandibular fossa	24 Condylar canal
12 External acoustic meatus	25 Stylomastoid foramen
13 Styloid process of temporal bone	26 Jugular foramen
	27 Carotid canal

1.9 The external surface of the base of the skull

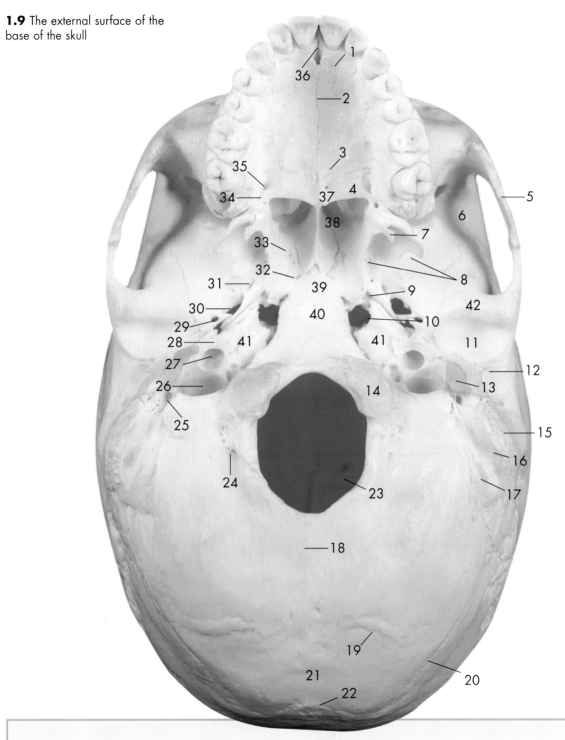

28 Spine of sphenoid	
29 Foramen spinosum	36 Incisive fossa
30 Foramen ovale	37 Posterior nasal spine
31 Sphenoidal foramen	38 Vomer contributing to nasal septum
32 Vomerovaginal canal	39 Body of sphenoid
33 Palatovaginal canal	40 Basilar part of occipital bone
34 Lesser palatine foramen	41 Petrous processes of temporal bones
35 Greater palatine foramen	42 Articular tubercle of temporal bone

The intermediate zone of the cranial base is essentially comprised of four osseous structures. Anteriorly lies the body of the sphenoid bone and posteriorly the basilar part of the occipital bone. Where these meet is a primary cartilaginous joint termed the spheno-occipital synchondrosis. This joint is important for growth of the skull in an anteroposterior direction and it does not ossify until about 20 years of age. The intermediate zone is completed by the petrous processes of the two temporal bones. These are found passing from the lateral sides of the base of the skull towards the spheno-occipital synchondrosis. A petrous process meets the basilar part of the occipital bone at the petro-occipital suture. This suture is deficient posteriorly where the jugular foramen is situated. Between the petrous process and the infratemporal surface of the greater wing of the sphenoid is the sphenopetrosal synchondrosis and the groove for the auditory tube. The apex of the petrous process does not meet the spheno-occipital joint. Consequently, a large fissure is present which is called the foramen lacerum. The intermediate zone is related to the middle cranial fossa and the anterior wall of the posterior cranial fossa.

The intermediate zone displays a considerable number of fissures and foramina. Already mentioned is the foramen lacerum. Despite its size, the foramen does not transmit any large structures. Its upper part is related to the internal opening of the carotid canal. Thus, the internal carotid artery and its accompanying venous and sympathetic plexuses cross over the foramen lacerum on its intracranial aspect. The lower part of the foramen lacerum is filled with cartilage. Within the foramen, the greater petrosal branch of the facial nerve and the deep petrosal nerve from the carotid sympathetic plexus join to form the nerve of the pterygoid canal (see page 216). Indeed, the pterygoid canal can be seen on the base of the skull at the anterior margin of the foramen lacerum above and between the pterygoid plates of the sphenoid bone. The pterygoid canal leads into the pterygopalatine fossa and contains not only the nerve of the pterygoid canal but also accompanying blood vessels.

Lateral to the foramen lacerum and passing through the infratemporal surface of the greater wing of the sphenoid are the foramen ovale and the foramen spinosum. The foramen ovale communicates with the middle cranial fossa and contains the mandibular division of the trigeminal nerve (and also the accessory meningeal artery from the maxillary artery). The foramen spinosum lies anterior to the spine of the sphenoid (hence its name) and posterior to the foramen ovale. It also communicates with the middle cranial fossa. It transmits the middle meningeal vessels and the meningeal branch of the mandibular nerve (nervus spinosus).

Anterior to the foramen ovale a small foramen is sometimes found, the sphenoidal emissary foramen (of Vesalius). This contains an emissary vein linking the pterygoid venous plexus in the infratemporal fossa with the cavernous sinus in the middle cranial fossa.

Behind the foramen lacerum and within the petrous part of the temporal bone is the carotid canal through which passes the internal carotid artery.

Other features of the intermediate zone are the pterygoid plates, pterygoid hamulus and scaphoid fossa, the mandibular fossa and its articular tubercle, the petrosquamous, petrotympanic and squamotympanic fissures, the spine of the sphenoid, and the pharyngeal tubercle on the basilar part of the occipital bone.

The pterygoid plates are processes of the sphenoid bone. There are two plates, the lateral and the medial pterygoid plates. They are located immediately behind the maxillary third molar tooth and are important for the attachment of muscles. The space between the plates is called the pterygoid fossa. At its base is a depression for the attachment of the tensor veli palatini muscle which is called the scaphoid fossa. Anteriorly, the two plates are fused, except for a narrow gap (the pterygoid notch) which is filled by the pyramidal process of the palatine bone. The medial pterygoid plate has a hook-shaped process called the pterygoid hamulus which projects behind the posterior border of the hard palate. The tensor veli palatini muscle twists around the hamulus before inserting into the soft palate. Also attached to the hamulus is a fibrous band termed the pterygomandibular raphe. The other attachment of the raphe is the mandible. The raphe is important for providing the origins of two muscles (the buccinator in the cheek and the superior constrictor of the pharynx).

The mandibular fossa was briefly described with the norma lateralis (see page 12). When viewed on the cranial base, the fossa appears as a thin-walled depression and the articular tubercle is now seen as a distinct ridge anterior to the fossa. Three fissures can be distinguished behind the mandibular fossa. The squamotympanic fissure extends from the spine of the sphenoid, between the mandibular fossa and the tympanic plate of the temporal bone, and up the anterior margin of the external acoustic meatus. Within this fissure can be seen a thin wedge of bone which is the inferior margin of the tegmen tympani (part of the petrous part of the temporal bone, see page 298). This divides the squamotympanic fissure into two, the petrotympanic and petrosquamous fissures. The petrotympanic fissure transmits the chorda tympani branch of the facial nerve from the skull into the infratemporal fossa.

The spine of the sphenoid is located medial to the mandibular fossa and posterior to the foramen spinosum. It varies considerably in size. The spine is the site of attachment of the sphenomandibular ligament.

The pharyngeal tubercle is found centrally on the basilar part of the occipital bone. It marks the site of attachment of the highest fibres of the superior constrictor muscle of the pharynx and of the pharyngeal raphe. The muscles attached to the base of the cranium extracranially (1.10) are:

Digastric	Mastoid notch
Lateral pterygoid	Lateral side of lateral pterygoid plate and infratemporal surface of greater wing of sphenoid
Levator veli palatini	Petrous part of temporal bone
Longissimus capitis	Superior nuchal line
Longus capitis	Basilar part of occipital bone
Medial pterygoid	Medial side of lateral pterygoid plate, tuberosity of maxilla
Musculus uvulae	Posterior margin of hard palate in midline
Occipital belly of occipitofrontalis	Superior nuchal line
Palatopharyngeus	Posterior margin of hard palate laterally
Rectus capitis anterior	Basilar part of occipital bone
Rectus capitis lateralis	Jugular process of occipital bone
Rectus capitis posterior major and minor	Below inferior nuchal line
Semispinalis capitis	Between superior and inferior nuchal lines
Splenius capitis	Superior nuchal line
Sternocleidomastoid	Mastoid process, superior nuchal line
Styloglossus	Styloid process
Stylohyoid	Styloid process
Stylopharyngeus	Styloid process
Superior constrictor	Medial pterygoid plate and pharyngeal tubercle
Superior oblique	Between superior and inferior nuchal lines
Tensor veli palatini	Scaphoid fossa, spine of sphenoid
Trapezius	External occipital protuberance, superior nuchal line

---

1 Musculus uvulae
2 Palatopharyngeus
3 Superior constrictor of pharynx
4 Medial pterygoid (deep head)
5 Medial pterygoid (superficial head)
6 Lateral pterygoid (upper head)
7 Masseter
8 Styloglossus
9 Stylohyoid
10 Stylopharyngeus
11 Pharyngeal raphe
12 Longus capitis
13 Rectus capitis anterior
14 Rectus capitis lateralis
15 Posterior belly of digastric

16 Longissimus capitis
17 Splenius capitis
18 Sternocleidomastoid
19 Occipital belly of occipitofrontalis
20 Trapezius
21 Semispinalis capitis
22 Superior oblique
23 Rectus capitis posterior minor
24 Rectus capitis posterior major
25 Capsule of atlanto-occipital joint
26 Capsule of temporomandibular joint
27 Levator veli palatini
28 Tensor veli palatini
29 Cartilaginous part of auditory tube

1.10 The external surface of the base of the skull showing muscle attachments

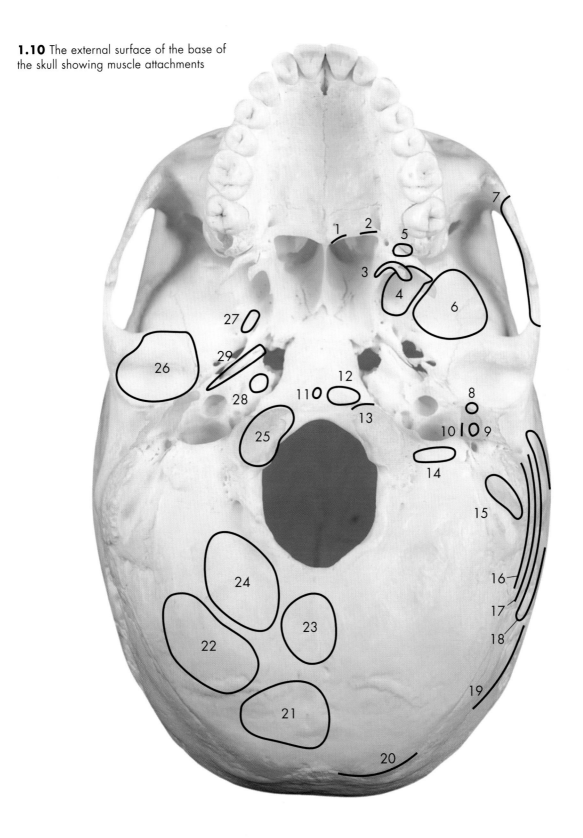

THE INTRACRANIAL APPEARANCE OF THE SKULL (1.11)

The cranial cavity of the skull accommodates the brain and associated structures. A detailed description of the contents of the cranial cavity is presented in Chapter 8.

The internal surface of the calvaria shows many of the features already described for the norma verticalis. However, the sutures tend to be less distinct because their gradual obliteration with age commences on the intracranial surface. Additional features seen intracranially include the frontal crest, some grooves for vascular structures and some depressions associated with arachnoid granulations.

The frontal crest is a prominent projection into the cranial cavity anteriorly. It provides attachment for a sheet of meninges, the falx cerebri, which passes between the two cerebral hemispheres of the brain. Running from the frontal crest and across the calvaria in the midline is a groove for the superior sagittal venous sinus. On each side of this groove may be found the depressions for the arachnoid granulations (see page 272). Deep grooves for middle meningeal vessels are often found on the parietal bones.

A median sagittal section of the skull highlights the division of the cranial cavity into three distinct fossae, the anterior, middle and posterior cranial fossae. The three fossae have a marked step-like appearance, such that the floor of the anterior cranial fossa is at the highest level and the floor of the posterior fossa at the lowest.

1.11 The internal surface
of the calvaria

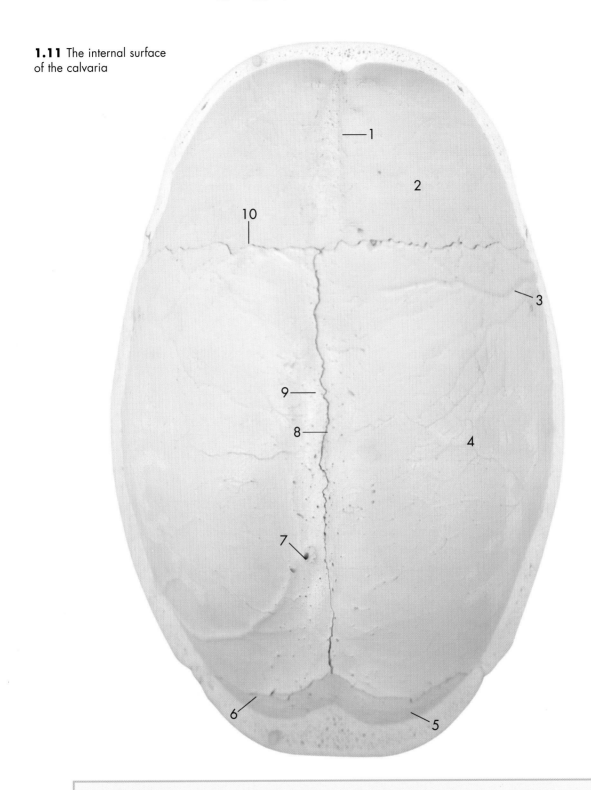

1 Frontal crest	6 Lambdoid suture
2 Frontal bone	7 Parietal foramen
3 Groove for middle meningeal vessels	8 Sagittal suture
4 Parietal bone	9 Groove for superior sagittal sinus
5 Occipital bone	10 Coronal suture

THE ANTERIOR CRANIAL FOSSA (1.12)

The floor of the anterior cranial fossa is formed by the frontal bone (orbital plates), the ethmoid bone (cribriform plates and crista galli) and the sphenoid bone (lesser wings and jugum). Unlike the other cranial fossae, it does not directly communicate with the inferior surface of the cranium but instead is related to the roofs of the orbits and the nasal fossae. Two sutures divide the sphenoid from the other bones, the frontosphenoid suture and the spheno-ethmoidal suture. The cribriform plate of the ethmoid bone fills a gap (the ethmoidal notch) between the medial ends of the orbital parts of the frontal bone and is depressed below the level of the rest of the floor. Extending upwards from the cribriform plate is a process termed the crista galli. This serves as a point of attachment of the falx cerebri.

There are three openings in the floor of the anterior cranial fossa, two cribriform plates and a foramen caecum. The cribriform plates transmit olfactory nerves into the roof of the nose. The foramen caecum lies immediately in front of the crista galli. It occasionally allows the passage of an emissary vein linking the superior sagittal venous sinus to the veins in the nose. The anterior ethmoidal nerve (a branch of the ophthalmic division of the trigeminal nerve from the orbit) enters the cranial cavity where the cribriform plate meets the orbital part of the frontal bone and passes into the roof of the nose via a small foramen to the side of the crista galli. Indeed, the nerve grooves the crista galli. Accompanying the nerve are the anterior ethmoidal vessels. Posterior ethmoidal vessels also run through the cribriform plate.

THE MIDDLE CRANIAL FOSSA (1.12)

The floor of the middle cranial fossa is formed by the body of the sphenoid bone centrally and the greater wings of the sphenoid and the squamous and petrous parts of the temporal bones laterally. The middle cranial fossa is directly related extracranially to the intermediate zone of the cranial base.

In the midline, the prominent structure is the pituitary fossa (sella turcica). This fossa is situated in the upper surface of the body of the sphenoid bone and lies above the sphenoidal sinuses. The anterior slope of the pituitary fossa has an elevation called the tuberculum sellae. In front of the tuberculum sellae is the prechiasmatic groove which is associated with the optic chiasma (see page 258) and leads into the optic canals. The pituitary fossa is bounded posteriorly by a plate of bone termed the dorsum sellae. Lateral to the pituitary fossa is a groove (the carotid groove) for the internal carotid artery. Anterior and posterior clinoid processes occupy the 'four corners' of the pituitary fossa. These provide sites of attachment for a sheet of the meninges called the diaphragma sellae which roofs over the pituitary fossa.

The regions lateral to the pituitary fossa provide deep depressions for the temporal lobes of the brain. Each region is related to the apex of the orbit anteriorly, the temporal fossa laterally and the infratemporal fossa inferiorly. With the exception of the optic canals, the lateral regions of the middle cranial fossa have all the foramina.

The openings of the middle cranial fossa on each side are: the optic canal, superior orbital fissure, foramen rotundum, foramen ovale, foramen spinosum, emissary sphenoidal foramen (of Vesalius), and the foramen lacerum.

The optic canal links the central area of the middle cranial fossa with the apex of the orbit. It transmits the optic nerve and the ophthalmic artery (a branch of the internal carotid artery).

The superior orbital fissure lies between the greater and lesser wings of the sphenoid bone. It is located on the anterior wall of the middle cranial fossa and links the fossa with the apex of the orbit. The fissure transmits many structures. The nerves passing through it are the oculomotor, trochlear and abducent nerves, the lacrimal, frontal and nasociliary branches of the ophthalmic division of the trigeminal nerve, and filaments from the internal carotid plexus (sympathetic). It also transmits the ophthalmic veins, and the orbital branch of the middle meningeal artery and the recurrent branch of the lacrimal artery.

1.12 The floor of the cranial cavity

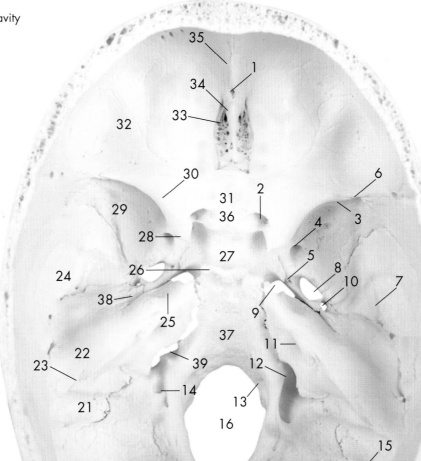

1 Foramen caecum
2 Optic canal
3 Superior orbital fissure
4 Foramen rotundum
5 Sphenoidal foramen
6 Openings of canal for middle
  meningeal vessels
7 Groove associated with middle
  meningeal vessels
8 Foramen ovale
9 Foramen lacerum
10 Foramen spinosum
11 Internal acoustic meatus
12 Jugular foramen
13 Hypoglossal canal
14 Condylar canal
15 Mastoid foramen
16 Foramen magnum
17 Internal occipital protuberance
18 Internal occipital crest
19 Groove associated with transverse sinus
20 Squamous part of occipital bone
21 Groove associated with sigmoid sinus
22 Petrous part of temporal bone
23 Groove associated with superior petrosal sinus
24 Squamous part of temporal bone

25 Trigeminal impression
26 Posterior clinoid process on dorsum sellae
27 Pituitary fossa in body of sphenoid
28 Anterior clinoid process
29 Greater wing of sphenoid
30 Lesser wing of sphenoid
31 Jugum of sphenoid bone
32 Orbital part of frontal bone
33 Cribriform plate of ethmoid
34 Crista galli
35 Frontal crest
36 Prechiasmatic groove
37 Basilar part of occipital bone
38 Hiatus and groove for greater petrosal nerve
39 Petro-occipital fissure

The foramen rotundum lies within the greater wing of the sphenoid. It allows communication between the lateral part of the middle cranial fossa and the pterygopalatine fossa. Passing through it is the maxillary division of the trigeminal nerve. The foramen ovale is also present in the greater wing of the sphenoid, but it links the middle cranial fossa to the infratemporal fossa. The major structure passing through it is the mandibular division of the trigeminal nerve. In addition, there is the lesser petrosal branch of the glossopharyngeal nerve, the accessory meningeal branch of the maxillary artery, and an emissary vein from the cavernous venous sinus to the pterygoid venous plexus in the infratemporal fossa.

The foramen spinosum lies just behind the foramen ovale. It transmits the meningeal branch of the mandibular division of the trigeminal nerve and the middle meningeal vessels. In front of, and medial to, the foramen ovale is the sphenoidal emissary foramen (of Vesalius). Both the sphenoidal emissary foramen and foramen spinosum link the middle cranial fossa and the infratemporal fossa. The sphenoidal emissary foramen is often absent but, when present, it transmits an emissary vein from the cavernous sinus to the pterygoid plexus.

The foramen lacerum lies at the junction between the apex of the petrous process, the sphenoid bone and the basilar part of the occipital bone. Structures associated with the foramen are the internal carotid artery (entering from behind and emerging above), the greater petrosal nerve and the deep petrosal nerve which join to form the nerve of the pterygoid canal, a meningeal branch of the ascending pharyngeal artery (a branch of the external carotid artery), and emissary veins linking the cavernous sinus and pterygoid venous plexus.

Other features seen on the floor of the middle cranial fossa are the trigeminal impression, hiatuses and grooves for the greater and lesser petrosal nerves, the petrous ridge and arcuate eminence, and grooves for the middle meningeal vessels and the superior petrosal venous sinuses. With the exception of the grooves for the middle meningeal vessels, these features are associated with the petrous part of the temporal bone.

The trigeminal impression is a shallow fossa situated behind the foramen lacerum. It indicates the site of the ganglion of the trigeminal nerve.

The greater and lesser petrosal nerves arise within the temporal bone in the region of the middle ear. They emerge onto the floor of the middle cranial fossa through hiatuses, the hiatus for the lesser petrosal nerve lying lateral to that of the greater petrosal nerve. The groove for the greater petrosal nerve runs forwards from the hiatus to the foramen lacerum. The groove for the lesser petrosal nerve runs forwards from the hiatus towards the foramen ovale.

The petrous ridge marks the boundary between the middle and posterior cranial fossae. A distinct bulge termed the arcuate eminence lies on the petrous ridge. This indicates the position of the anterior (superior) semicircular canal of the internal ear. Running along the ridge is the groove for the superior petrosal venous sinus. This sinus links the cavernous and the sigmoid sinuses. There is a conspicuous groove for the middle meningeal vessels. This groove runs across the floor of the middle cranial fossa, from the foramen spinosum, and up onto the lateral wall of the fossa where it may divide into a groove for the frontal branches of the vessels and a groove for the parietal branches.

THE POSTERIOR CRANIAL FOSSA (1.12)

The posterior cranial fossa is the largest of the cranial fossae. It contains the brain stem (the cerebellum posteriorly and the pons and medulla oblongata anteriorly). The floor and posterior wall of the posterior cranial fossa are formed mainly by the occipital bone (lateral and lower squamous parts). The anterior wall of the fossa leading up to the middle cranial fossa is formed by the basilar part of the occipital bone, the temporal bones (petrous and mastoid parts) and the sphenoid bone (dorsum sellae and posterior part of the body). The region corresponds extracranially with the posterior zone of the cranial base.

The foramen magnum is the most prominent structure in the floor of the posterior cranial fossa. Passing through the foramen are the medulla oblongata, the apical ligament of the dens of the second cervical vertebra, the membrana tectoria of the atlanto-occipital joint, the vertebral and spinal arteries, the spinal parts of the accessory nerves, and the meningeal branches of the cervical spinal nerves. The hypoglossal canals (anterior condylar canals) and condylar canals (posterior condylar canals) lie close to the foramen magnum. The hypoglossal canal transmits the hypoglossal nerve (and its recurrent branch), the meningeal branch of the ascending pharyngeal artery and an emissary vein linking the basilar plexus intracranially with the internal jugular vein extracranially. The condylar canal carries an emissary vein between the sigmoid sinus and the occipital veins, and a meningeal branch of the occipital artery.

Other features found in the floor of the fossa are the internal occipital protuberance and crest, and grooves for some of the dural venous sinuses. The internal occipital protuberance lies at the confluence of some venous sinuses. Extending down from the protuberance to the foramen magnum is the internal occipital crest. This crest gives attachment to the falx cerebelli (a layer of meninges passing between the two hemispheres of the cerebellum of the brain). Grooves which are often very prominent are found for the transverse, sigmoid, and superior sagittal sinuses. The occipital sinus may groove the internal occipital crest. The margins of the grooves for the transverse sinuses provide attachment for the tentorium cerebelli (a layer of meninges which passes between the occipital lobes and the cerebellum of the brain).

That part of the fossa in front of the foramen magnum formed by the basilar part of the occipital bone and the sphenoid bone is termed the clivus. Between the clivus and each petrous process of a temporal bone is the petro-occipital fissure. This fissure is occupied in life by a sliver of cartilage. The posterior end of the fissure is widened to form the jugular foramen. Passing through the jugular foramen is the internal jugular vein as it continues from the sigmoid sinus. In addition, it transmits the glossopharyngeal, vagus and accessory nerves, the inferior petrosal sinus and a meningeal branch of the occipital artery. The inferior petrosal sinus runs from the cavernous sinus to the jugular foramen in a groove closely related to the petro-occipital fissure. The posterior surface of the petrous part of the temporal bone shows an internal acoustic meatus for the passage of the facial and vestibulocochlear nerves into the ear. Labyrinthine vessels also pass through this meatus. Behind the opening of the internal acoustic meatus is the opening for the aqueduct of the vestibule of the ear (see page 308).

THE BONES OF THE SKULL

The 28 bones of the skull are categorised into the following groups:

- The bones of the vault of the skull
- The bones of the base of the skull
- The bones of the face
- The bones of the jaws
- The bones of the ear

The bones in each of these categories are listed in Table 1.1 (see page 3).

The bones of the ear are described with the rest of the anatomy of the ear (see pages 302–304).

THE BONES OF THE VAULT OF THE SKULL

The frontal bone, the two parietal bones and the occipital bone comprise the vault of the skull.

The frontal bone (1.13, 1.14)

The frontal bone is a single bone located at the front of the vault of the skull. It has three parts, squamous, nasal and orbital parts. Within the bone are found two cavities termed the frontal air sinuses.

The squamous part of the frontal bone forms the major portion of the bone. Externally, it is related to the forehead and is considerably convex. Indeed, the most prominent bulges are termed the frontal tuberosities. The tuberosities are most apparent on skulls of the young. The posterior border of the squamous part is markedly serrated for articulation with the parietal bones at the coronal suture. The squamous part inferiorly forms the supra-orbital margins where it meets the orbital parts of the frontal bone. Just above the supra-orbital margins are the curved ridges of the superciliary arches. These meet above the nose to form another ridge called the glabella. The superciliary arches are larger in the male.

The lateral two-thirds of each supra-orbital margin is sharp whereas the medial third is rounded. At the junction is found the supra-orbital notch or foramen which transmits the supra-orbital nerve and vessels from the orbit onto the forehead. A small frontal notch or foramen may be found just medial to the supra-orbital notch and, when present, transmits the supratrochlear nerve and vessels onto the forehead.

The supra-orbital margin projects laterally as the zygomatic process of the frontal bone. This process articulates with the frontal process of the zygomatic bone. A ridge extends backwards from the zygomatic process to divide into the anterior parts of the superior and inferior temporal lines. The area of the frontal bone below the temporal lines is the temporal surface. This surface forms the anterosuperior portion of the temporal fossa.

The nasal part of the frontal bone forms a small portion of the roof of the nose. It lies in the midline between the supra-orbital margins. The serrated free margin of the nasal part articulates with the nasal bones, the frontal processes of the maxillary bones, and the lacrimal bones. A small, thin plate of bone projects downwards in the midline as the nasal spine. This spine makes a minor contribution to the nasal septum, articulating in front with the nasal bone and behind with the perpendicular plate of the ethmoid bone.

1.13 The frontal view of the skull to show the external surface of the frontal bone

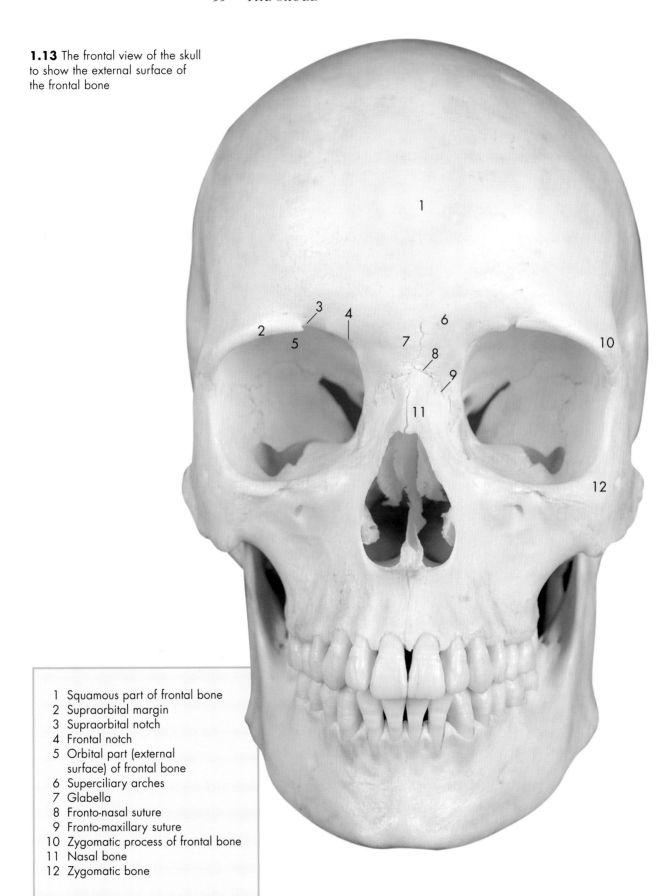

1 Squamous part of frontal bone
2 Supraorbital margin
3 Supraorbital notch
4 Frontal notch
5 Orbital part (external surface) of frontal bone
6 Superciliary arches
7 Glabella
8 Fronto-nasal suture
9 Fronto-maxillary suture
10 Zygomatic process of frontal bone
11 Nasal bone
12 Zygomatic bone

The orbital parts of the frontal bone consist of two plates which lie horizontally to form the roofs of the orbits. They also contribute to the floor of the anterior cranial fossa. Each plate meets the squamous part of the frontal bone at the supra-orbital margin. The orbital plates are separated from each other by the ethmoidal notch, and only occasionally are they joined posteriorly. The ethmoidal notch houses the cribriform plate of the ethmoid.

Each orbital plate presents two surfaces, the orbital (external) surface and the cranial (internal) surface. The orbital surface is concave. In the anterolateral corner is a fossa in which lies the lacrimal gland. In the anteromedial corner may be found a depression or tubercle, the trochlear fovea (or tubercle). This marks the site of attachment of the fibrocartilaginous pulley (trochlea) through which passes the superior oblique muscle of the eye. The posterior margin of the orbital plate is serrated for articulation with the lesser wing of the sphenoid bone.

The margins of the ethmoidal notch articulate with the lateral masses (labyrinths) of the ethmoid bone and thereby complete the roofs of the ethmoidal air cells. Impressions of the air cells may therefore be seen on this margin. In addition, grooves related to the anterior and posterior ethmoidal nerves and vessels can be seen on this margin. These grooves become canals with articulation of the ethmoidal labyrinth. The frontal sinuses can be visualised around the anterior portion of the ethmoidal notch.

The internal surface of the frontal bone shows relatively few features. The squamous part is concave and laterally shows grooves related to the middle meningeal vessels. In the midline, just above the front end of the ethmoidal notch, is a ridge termed the frontal crest. At the base of this crest is a groove which becomes the foramen caecum on articulation with the cribriform plate of the ethmoid. The foramen caecum may be blind-ended or may contain an emissary vein passing between the roof of the nose and the superior sagittal sinus. On following the frontal crest as it passes upwards and backwards, it gives way to a groove for the superior sagittal sinus. This sinus lies within the attached margins of the falx cerebri. Small depressions on each side of groove for the superior sagittal sinus are related to arachnoid granulations.

The muscles which gain attachment to the frontal bone are:

- Corrugator supercilii

- Orbital part of orbicularis oculi

- Temporalis

The parietal bones (1.15, 1.16)

The two parietal bones form the bulk of the vault of the skull behind the frontal bone.

Each bone is quadrilateral in shape and presents as a curved plate. The four corners of the bone are referred to as the angles and each is named after the bone with which it articulates. Thus, there are frontal (anterosuperior), occipital (posterosuperior), sphenoidal (antero-inferior) and mastoid (postero-inferior) angles. The frontal angle relates to the bregma, the occipital angle to the lambda, the sphenoidal angle to the pterion and the mastoid angle to the asterion.

All the margins of the parietal bone are serrated. The sagittal (superior) margin is the longest and shows the deepest serrations. Here, the two parietal bones meet to form the sagittal suture. A small foramen, the parietal foramen, is sometimes found close to the sagittal margin. It transmits an emissary vein (joining veins on the scalp with the superior sagittal sinus) and sometimes a terminal branch of the occipital artery (a branch of the external carotid). The frontal (anterior) margin meets the frontal bone at the coronal suture. The occipital (posterior) margin articulates with the occipital bone to form the lambdoid suture. The squamous (inferior) margin is the shortest margin of the parietal bone. It can be subdivided into three parts. Its central portion is concave and bevelled (at the expense of its external surface) where it meets the squamous part of the temporal bone. There is a short, thin anterior portion (also bevelled at the expense of the external surface) which articulates with the greater wing of the sphenoid. The posterior part of the squamous margin is thicker and unites with the mastoid process of the temporal bone.

1.14 The floor of the cranial cavity to show the internal surface of the frontal bone

1 Frontal crest
2 Foramen caecum
3 Crista galli
4 Cribriform plate
5 Orbital part (internal surface)
6 Lesser wing of sphenoid bone

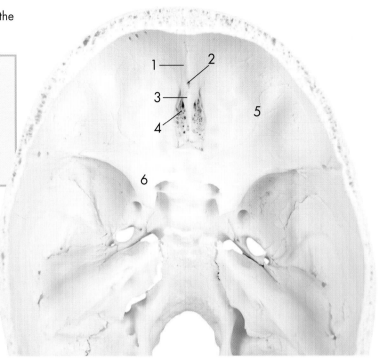

1.15 The lateral surface of the skull to show the external surface of the parietal bone

1 Frontal (antero-superior) angle
2 Sagittal margin
3 Occipital (postero-superior) angle
4 Occipital margin
5 Mastoid (postero-inferior) angle
6 Squamous margin
7 Sphenoidal (antero-inferior) angle
8 Frontal margin
9 Superior temporal line
10 Inferior temporal line
11 Frontal bone
12 Occipital bone
13 Temporal bone
14 Sphenoid bone

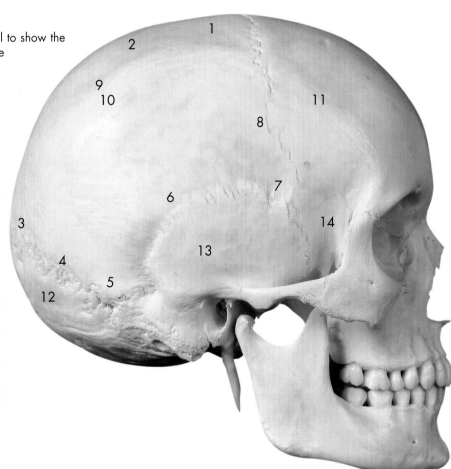

The external surface of the parietal bone is essentially featureless. It is convex and shows a protuberance near its centre termed the parietal tuberosity. The superior and inferior temporal lines curve in an anteroposterior direction along its middle.

The concave internal surface of the parietal bone shows grooves related to the middle meningeal vessels, which pass upwards and backwards. A groove is present along the sagittal margin which is for the superior sagittal sinus. Small depressions may be seen near the groove for the sagittal sinus which are related to arachnoid granulations. A groove is also found in the region of the mastoid angle for the transverse sinus as it bends downwards to become the sigmoid sinus.

The parietal bone gives attachment to the temporalis muscle at and below the inferior temporal line. The superior temporal line gives attachment to the temporal fascia.

The occipital bone (1.17–1.19)

This is a single bone which lies at the back of the vault of the skull. Its inferior portion curves forwards and contains the foramen magnum and the occipital condyles for articulation with the atlas (first cervical vertebra). The occipital bone is divided into four parts according to their relationship with the foramen magnum. The greater part of the bone lies above the foramen magnum and is termed the squamous part. The part lying in front of the foramen magnum is termed the basilar part. On each side of the foramen magnum are the lateral (or condylar) parts.

The squamous part of the occipital bone articulates with the parietal and temporal bones. The upper portion of the squamous part has the most serrated margin and articulates with the parietal bones at the lambdoid suture. The lower portion of the squamous part unites with the mastoid process of the temporal bone at the occipitomastoid suture. The region which lies at the lambda is termed the superior angle. That part which lies at the asterion is termed the lateral angle.

The external surface of the squamous part of the occipital bone is convex and is divided into two regions. The upper half is relatively smooth and the lower half presents a roughened appearance due to the attachment of muscles. In the midline, partly delineating these two areas, is a projection termed the external occipital protuberance. The central point of this protuberance is the inion. From this protuberance, a thin ridge called the external occipital crest passes downwards to the foramen magnum. This crest gives attachment to the ligamentum nuchae, a fibro-elastic band which runs up the back of the cervical vertebral column (see page 90). Three lines may be seen running across the roughened region of the squamous part. Two lines originate from the external occipital protuberance. The upper line is the supreme nuchal line which gives attachment to the epicranial aponeurosis of the scalp (see page 150). The lower line is the superior nuchal line. Running from the external occipital crest, parallel and below the superior nuchal line, is the inferior nuchal line.

The internal surface of the squamous part is concave and is divided into four fossae by a cross-shaped pattern of ridges and grooves. At the centre of the cross lies the internal occipital protuberance. A groove housing the superior sagittal sinus passes upwards from this protuberance. Passing laterally from the internal occipital protuberance are grooves related to the transverse sinuses. The right transverse groove is usually continuous with the groove for the superior petrosal sinus whereas the left transverse sinus is continuous with the straight sinus (see page 276). Finally, the internal occipital crest runs vertically downwards from the internal occipital protuberance before bifurcating near the foramen magnum. The upper fossae delineated by this system of ridges and grooves are termed the cerebral fossae. They are approximately triangular in shape and are related to the occipital lobes of the brain. The lower fossae are the cerebellar fossae. They are related to the inferior surface of the cerebellum of the brain stem. They are larger than the cerebral fossae and are rectangular in shape.

1.16 The internal surface of the calvaria to show the internal surface of the parietal bone

1 Parietal bone
2 Groove for middle meningeal vessels
3 Coronal suture
4 Sagittal suture
5 Parietal foramen
6 Lambdoid suture

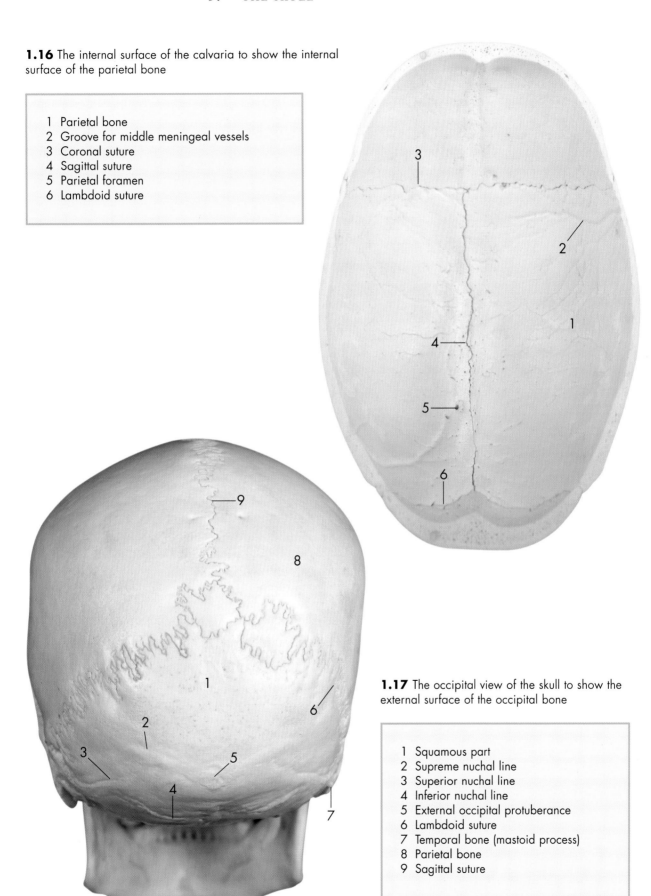

1.17 The occipital view of the skull to show the external surface of the occipital bone

1 Squamous part
2 Supreme nuchal line
3 Superior nuchal line
4 Inferior nuchal line
5 External occipital protuberance
6 Lambdoid suture
7 Temporal bone (mastoid process)
8 Parietal bone
9 Sagittal suture

The ridges and grooves on the internal surface of the squamous part of the occipital bone also give attachment to layers of the meninges of the brain. To the margins of the groove containing the superior sagittal sinus is attached the falx cerebri which separates the cerebral hemispheres of the brain. To the margins of the grooves for the transverse sinuses is attached the tentorium cerebelli which lies between the cerebral hemispheres and the cerebellum of the brain. The internal occipital crest affords attachment to the falx cerebelli which lies between the two hemispheres of the cerebellum.

The basilar part of the occipital bone lies in front of the foramen magnum. It is fused anteriorly with the body of the sphenoid, though up until about the age of 20 years this is the site of the spheno-occipital synchondrosis. At its sides, the basilar part articulates with the petrous part of the temporal bone at the petro-occipital suture. Externally, the basilar part exhibits a small pharyngeal tubercle. To this tubercle is attached the pharyngeal raphe and the uppermost fibres of the superior constrictor muscle of the pharynx. The internal surface of the bone is grooved, forming the clivus. Against the clivus lies part of the brain stem (the lower part of the pons and the medulla oblongata). Laterally, a groove for the inferior petrosal sinus may be seen.

The lateral parts of the occipital bone are also called the condylar parts because they have the occipital condyles which articulate with the vertebral column at the atlanto-occipital joints. Each lateral part articulates with the mastoid part of a temporal bone at the occipitomastoid suture.

The external surface of the lateral part shows the following features: an occipital condyle, a condylar fossa with a condylar canal (posterior condylar canal), and a jugular process.

Each occipital condyle articulates with a superior articular facet on the atlas vertebra. It is oval in outline and is convex in all planes. The long axis of the condyle is directed anteroposteriorly and slightly medially while the articular surface faces laterally. Each condyle contains the hypoglossal canal (anterior condylar canal). The main structure passing through this canal is the hypoglossal nerve. In addition, the canal transmits the recurrent meningeal branch of the nerve and sometimes a meningeal branch of the ascending pharyngeal artery (a branch of the external carotid), and an emissary vein linking the basilar plexus to the internal jugular vein.

Immediately behind each condyle is a small depression which is named the condylar fossa. The superior articular facet of the atlas slides backwards into this fossa when the head is fully extended. The condylar fossa may be traversed by the condylar canal (posterior condylar canal) which allows passage of an emissary vein (linking the sigmoid sinus with the occipital veins) and a meningeal branch of the occipital artery (a branch of the external carotid).

Lateral to the posterior part of the occipital condyle is a projection termed the jugular process. This process is indented at the jugular notch and forms the posterior boundary of the jugular foramen.

A bulge on the internal surface of the lateral part of the occipital bone, the jugular tubercle, lies above the hypoglossal canal. The tubercle may be grooved by the inferior petrosal sinus. Behind this is another groove, the groove for the sigmoid sinus. This marks the site where the sigmoid sinus passes through the jugular foramen to become the internal jugular vein.

1.18 The base of the skull to show the external surface of the occipital bone

1 Pharyngeal tubercle
2 Basilar part
3 Occipital condyle
4 Jugular process
5 Condylar canal
6 Foramen magnum
7 External occipital crest
8 Inferior nuchal line
9 Superior nuchal line
10 Squamous part
11 External occipital protuberance
12 Jugular foramen
13 Temporal bone (petrous part)
14 Temporal bone (mastoid process)

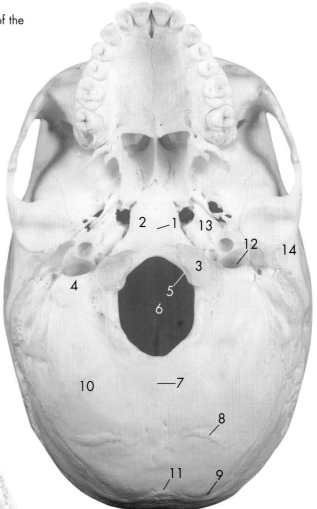

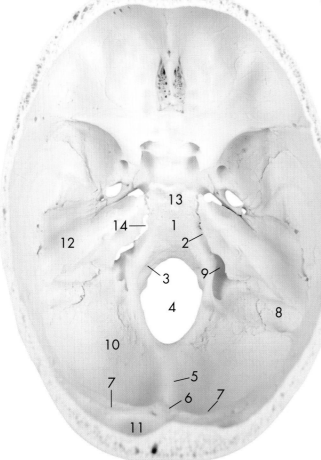

1.19 The floor of the cranial cavity to show the internal surface of the occipital bone

1 Basilar part
2 Groove for inferior petrosal sinus
3 Hypoglossal canal
4 Foramen magnum
5 Internal occipital crest
6 Internal occipital protuberance
7 Groove for transverse sinus
8 Groove for sigmoid sinus
9 Jugular foramen
10 Squamous part (cerebellar fossa)
11 Squamous part (cerebral fossa)
12 Temporal bone (petrous part)
13 Sphenoid bone (dorsum sellae)
14 Petro-occipital fissure

The foramen magnum is the largest foramen in the skull. The major structures passing through it are the medulla oblongata of the brain stem, the vertebral arteries and the spinal accessory nerves. Around the margins of the foramen are ligaments associated with the joints connecting the vertebral column to the base of the skull (see pages 92).

The following muscles are attached to the occipital bone:

- Longus capitis

- Occipital belly of occipitofrontalis

- Rectus capitis anterior

- Rectus capitis lateralis

- Rectus capitis posterior major and minor

- Splenius capitis

- Sternocleidomastoid

- Superior constrictor

- Superior oblique

- Trapezius

THE BONES OF THE BASE OF THE SKULL

The bones comprising the floor of the cranial cavity are the ethmoid, frontal, sphenoid, temporal, and occipital bones. The occipital and frontal bones have already been described in connection with the bones of the vault of the skull. The ethmoid bone is considered with the face, as it contributes significantly to the orbital and nasal cavities.

The sphenoid bone (1.20, 1.22)
This single bone forms much of the anterior part of the intermediate zone of the cranial base and most of the floor of the middle cranial fossa.

The sphenoid bone is often described as being butterfly-shaped. It consists of a central body and three paired processes. Extending laterally from the body are the lesser wings in front and the greater wings behind. Extending downwards from the junction of the body and greater wings are the pterygoid processes.

Anteriorly, the sphenoid bone articulates with the frontal and ethmoid bones above, and the vomer and palatine bones below. Laterally, it meets the zygomatic, parietal and temporal bones. Posteriorly, it joins the occipital bone.

There are usually two air sinuses within the body of the sphenoid bone.

The body of the sphenoid bone occupies a central position within the middle cranial fossa. The superior surface is smooth and saddle-shaped, hence the term sella turcica (Turkish saddle). The depression of the sella turcica is the pituitary fossa. The pituitary fossa is delineated anteriorly by a horizontal ridge termed the tuberculum sellae. The lateral margins of the ridge are sometimes elevated to form middle clinoid processes. Above the tuberculum sellae lies the prechiasmatic groove. This leads laterally into the optic canal. The chiasma of the optic nerves is related to this surface. In front of the prechiasmatic groove is the jugum which is related to the gyri recti of the frontal lobe of the brain and to the olfactory tracts. A vertical plate of bone called the dorsum sellae forms the posterior boundary of the pituitary fossa. The free lateral margins of the dorsum sella project as the posterior clinoid processes. The posterior surface of the dorsum sellae is concave and forms part of the clivus on which is situated the upper part of the pons.

1.20 Isolated sphenoid bone viewed from the front

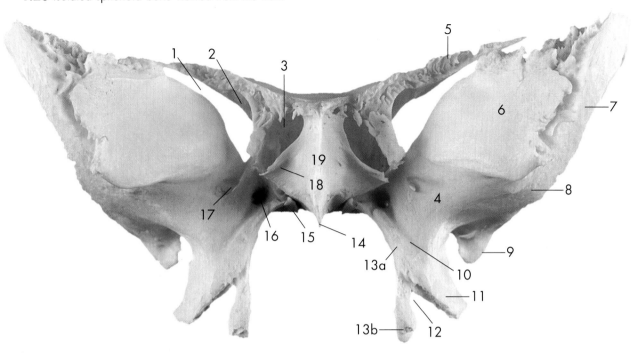

1 Superior orbital fissure	11 Lateral pterygoid plate
2 Optic canal	12 Pterygoid notch
3 Sphenoidal air sinus in body of sphenoid	13 Medial pterygoid plate (a) surmounted by pterygoid hamulus (b)
4 Maxillary surface of greater wing	14 Rostrum
5 Frontal margin of lesser wing	15 Vaginal process
6 Orbital surface of greater wing	16 Pterygoid canal
7 Temporal surface of greater wing	17 Foramen rotundum
8 Infratemporal crest of greater wing	18 Concha
9 Spine	19 Crest
10 Pterygoid process	

The inferior surface of the body of the sphenoid presents a midline ridge termed the rostrum. This ridge fits into a groove on the upper border of the vomer bone.

The anterior surface of the body of the sphenoid contains the apertures of the sphenoidal sinuses which drain into the spheno-ethmoidal recesses in the nose. The sphenoidal sinuses are partitioned by a thin bony septum. The sinuses are bounded antero-inferiorly by two curved plates of bone, the sphenoidal conchae. These project inferiorly to form the sphenoidal crest which articulates with the perpendicular plate of the ethmoid. The conchae also overlap on to the inferior surface of the body of the sphenoid to articulate medially with the alae of the vomer. The superolateral corner of the anterior surface meets the back of the labyrinth of the ethmoid bone and completes the posterior ethmoidal air cells.

Before the age of 20 years, the posterior surface of the body of the sphenoid is separated from the basilar part of the occipital bone by the spheno-occipital synchondrosis. This primary cartilaginous joint is a main contributor to forward growth of the face. After the age of twenty years, the synchondrosis disappears and there is then complete bony union.

The side of the body of the sphenoid is related to the cavernous sinus. At the posterolateral region of the body (where the greater wing is attached) is located the carotid groove. In this groove runs the internal carotid artery. The groove is bounded laterally by a sharp projection called the sphenoid lingula.

The lesser wings of the sphenoid bone are two thin, triangular plates of bone projecting from the anterolateral corner of the superior surface of the body of the sphenoid. They are separated from the greater wings below by the superior orbital fissures.

The main structures passing through the fissure are the oculomotor, trochlear, ophthalmic and abducent nerves and the ophthalmic veins.

The base of each lesser wing is attached to the body by two roots which pass on either side of the optic canal. Through this canal run the optic nerve and ophthalmic artery. The anterior (frontal) margin of the lesser wing is serrated for articulation with the frontal bone. The posterior margin delineates the anterior and middle cranial fossae. It is smooth and projects medially as the anterior clinoid process. The upper surface of the lesser wing contributes to the anterior cranial fossa, the lower surface to the posterior part of the roof of the orbit.

Two folds of meninges are attached to the anterior and posterior clinoid processes. The diaphragma sellae roofs over the pituitary fossa with an opening in its centre for the pituitary stalk. The tentorium cerebelli has its free border attached to the anterior clinoid processes and the attached border fixed to the posterior clinoid processes.

The greater wings of the sphenoid bone extend outwards and forwards from the sides of the posterior part of the body. The anteroposterior dimensions are greater than the mediolateral ones.

The anterior margin shows a roughened triangular portion medially (the frontal margin) for articulation with the frontal bone, and a smooth concave surface laterally (parietal margin) where it meets the parietal bone at the pterion. The lateral margin (squamous margin) is serrated for articulation with the squamous part of the petrous bone. The posterior margin articulates with the petrous part of the temporal bone.

The external surface of the greater wing can be subdivided into lateral and anterior surfaces.

1.21 The floor of the cranial cavity to show the sphenoid bone

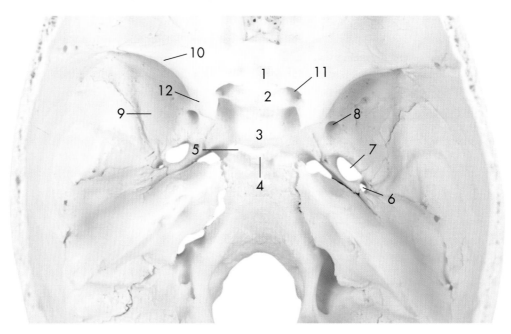

1	Jugum
2	Prechiasmatic groove
3	Pituitary fossa
4	Dorsum sellae
5	Posterior clinoid process
6	Foramen spinosum
7	Foramen ovale
8	Foramen rotundum
9	Greater wing
10	Lesser wing
11	Optic canal
12	Anterior clinoid process

The lateral surface is further subdivided into upper and lower parts by a horizontal ridge termed the infratemporal crest. The upper part is seen in the floor of the temporal fossa and is called the temporal surface. It is concave from front to back and contributes to the anterior part of the temporal fossa. There is a vertical crest anteriorly which forms its zygomatic margin. This margin articulates with the zygomatic bone. The lower part below the infratemporal crest is almost horizontal and forms the roof of the infratemporal fossa. The foramen ovale and the foramen spinosum lie towards the back of this surface. Behind the foramen spinosum, the bone is raised to form the spine of the sphenoid (to which is attached the sphenomandibular ligament). The posterior margin here is grooved and is related to the cartilaginous component of the auditory tube running from the middle ear to the nasopharynx.

The anterior part of the greater wing is mainly formed by the orbital surface of the sphenoid. This part presents as a flat plate which is quadrilateral and which comprises the posterior half of the lateral wall of the orbit. The orbital surface faces forwards and inwards. Its sloping posterior margin is a boundary of the superior orbital fissure. It may exhibit a small tubercle which gives attachment to the common tendinous ring associated with the recti muscles of the eye (see page 242). The inferior margin of the orbital surface is smooth and bounds the inferior orbital fissure posterolaterally. The region immediately below the superior orbital fissure is termed the maxillary surface. This surface faces the maxillary bone and forms part of the posterior wall of the pterygopalatine fossa. Emerging onto the maxillary surface is the foramen rotundum.

The internal (cerebral) surface of each greater wing is concave and contributes to the floor of the middle cranial fossa. It is related to the temporal lobe of the brain.

There are three foramina in the greater wing of the sphenoid bone. The foramen rotundum is, as its name suggests, round in outline. It transmits the maxillary division of the trigeminal nerve from the middle cranial fossa into the pterygopalatine fossa. Just in front of the posterior margin of the greater wing is an oval-shaped opening termed appropriately the foramen ovale. It allows the passage between the middle cranial fossa and the infratemporal fossa of the mandibular division of the trigeminal nerve, the lesser petrosal branch of the glossopharyngeal nerve, the accessory meningeal branch of the maxillary artery, and some emissary veins. Behind the foramen ovale lies the foramen spinosum which transmits the middle meningeal vessels and the meningeal branch of the mandibular division of the trigeminal nerve.

Two additional foramina may be found in the greater wing. The sphenoidal emissary foramen (of Vesalius) is present in about 40% of skulls. It is situated medial to the foramen ovale and it allows the passage of emissary veins linking the cavernous sinus and the pterygoid venous plexus in the infratemporal fossa. An occasional petrosal (innominate) foramen lies medial to the foramen spinosum and transmits the lesser petrosal nerve when this does not pass through the foramen ovale.

The pterygoid processes of the sphenoid bone arise from the inferior surface of the body where the greater wings are attached. Each process consists of two vertically aligned plates, the medial and lateral pterygoid plates. The plates are joined along their anterior margins except inferiorly where there is a small notch, the pterygoid notch. This notch receives the pyramidal process of the palatine bone. Posteriorly, the pterygoid plates diverge and enclose a space called the pterygoid fossa.

The lateral surface of the lateral pterygoid plate forms part of the medial boundary of the infratemporal fossa. Its anterior margin bounds the pterygomaxillary fissure. The medial surface of the medial pterygoid plate bounds the lateral wall of the posterior nasal aperture (choana).

The medial pterygoid plate ends in a small, curved process called the pterygoid hamulus. At the base of the hamulus is a groove which is related to the tendon of the tensor veli palatini muscle.

1.22 The base of the skull to show the sphenoid bone

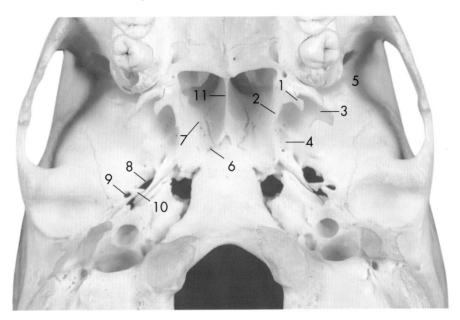

1 Pterygoid hamulus
2 Medial pterygoid process
3 Lateral pterygoid process
4 Scaphoid fossa
5 Greater wing
6 Vomerovaginal canal
7 Palatovaginal canal
8 Foramen ovale
9 Foramen spinosum
10 Spine of sphenoid bone
11 Vomer bone

The base of the pterygoid process is traversed by the pterygoid canal. The opening of the canal lies at the base of the medial pterygoid plate, just below the carotid sulcus. The pterygoid canal emerges below and medial to the foramen rotundum. Like the foramen rotundum, the pterygoid canal opens into the pterygopalatine fossa through its posterior wall. Through this canal pass the nerve and artery of the pterygoid canal.

From the base of the pterygoid process, a small plate of bone projects medially over the inferior surface of the body of the sphenoid bone to articulate with the ala of the vomer. This is the vaginal process. A groove on the undersurface of the vaginal process is converted into the palatovaginal canal by articulation with the upper surface of the sphenoidal process of the palatine bone. The pharyngeal branch of the pterygopalatine ganglion and the pharyngeal branch of the sphenopalatine artery pass through this canal.

Sometimes a canal is present between the upper surface of the vaginal process of the sphenoid bone and the ala of the vomer. This canal is called the vomerovaginal canal and anteriorly joins the palatovaginal canal. It transmits the pharyngeal branch of the sphenopalatine artery.

The scaphoid fossa is present between the pterygoid plates at their base.

The following muscles are attached to the sphenoid bone:

- Lateral pterygoid

- Medial pterygoid

- Superior constrictor

- Temporalis

- Tensor veli palatini

The temporal bones (1.23–1.26)

There are two temporal bones. Each bone contributes to the base and to the lower lateral aspect of the skull. It consists of four parts, the squamous, tympanic and petrous parts, and the styloid process. The mastoid process is here considered to be a component of the petrous part. The temporal bone also contains the auditory and vestibular systems (these are considered with the ear, see Chapter 9). The mastoid part has a variable number of air cells which open into the tympanic cavity.

The squamous part of the temporal bone can be divided into three regions : a temporal portion, a zygomatic process and a mandibular fossa (glenoid fossa).

The temporal portion consists of a thin, vertical plate of bone. Its external surface is gently convex and forms part of the temporal fossa. Posteriorly, the external surface shows a groove related to the middle temporal branch of the superficial temporal artery (a branch of the external carotid). The internal (cerebral) surface of the temporal portion is concave. It shows ridges related to the temporal lobe of the brain and grooves related to middle meningeal vessels. At the junction of the temporal portion of the squamous part of the temporal bone with the petrous portion of the bone there is usually evidence of a petrosquamous fissure. Rarely, a more conspicuous groove is present at this site and indicates the position of a petrosquamous venous sinus which opens posteriorly into the transverse sinus. The petrosquamous sinus communicates by an emissary vein with the external jugular vein. The upper margin of the temporal portion is bevelled (at the expense of the cerebral surface) for articulation with the parietal bone. Antero-inferiorly, the margin is thicker for articulation with the greater wing of the sphenoid.

1.23 The lateral view of the skull to show the external surface of the temporal bone

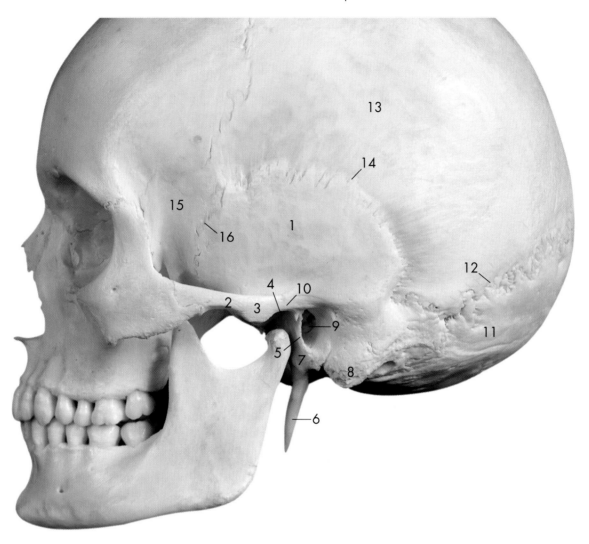

1 Squamous part	9 External acoustic meatus
2 Zygomatic process	10 Postglenoid tubercle
3 Articular tubercle	11 Occipital bone
4 Mandibular fossa	12 Lambdoid suture
5 Tympanic part	13 Parietal bone
6 Styloid process	14 Squamosal suture
7 Sheath of styloid process	15 Sphenoid bone (greater wing)
8 Mastoid process	16 Sphenosquamosal suture

The zygomatic process projects outwards and forwards from the lowermost part of the external surface of the temporal portion. In front, it articulates with the temporal process of the zygomatic bone to complete the zygomatic arch. Posteriorly, the upper border of the zygomatic process continues above and behind the external acoustic meatus as a ridge. This ridge passes above the mastoid process and is termed the supramastoid crest. The crest gives attachment to the temporal fascia. Between the crest and the upper border of the external acoustic meatus is often found a triangular depression termed the suprameatal pit or triangle (a landmark for operative procedures on the mastoid antrum). The anterior part of the pit may bear a small projection, the suprameatal spine. The inferior surface of the zygomatic process shows a ridge called the articular tubercle. Behind the tubercle, the zygomatic process is concave where it forms the lateral margin of the mandibular fossa. In front of the external acoustic meatus, the zygomatic process terminates inferiorly as the postglenoid tubercle. This tubercle is however not always present.

The mandibular fossa is situated at the cranial base. It lies beneath and medial to the zygomatic process and immediately anterior to the external acoustic meatus. It articulates with the head of the condyle to form the temporomandibular joint. The mandibular fossa is an oval depression. It is bounded anteriorly by the articular tubercle. Posteriorly, the fossa is separated from the tympanic part of the temporal bone by the squamotympanic fissure. Medially, a projection from the petrous part of the temporal bone comes to lie within this fissure to divide it into the petrosquamous and the petrotympanic fissures.

The tympanic part of the temporal bone is a semicircular plate of bone which forms the anterior, inferior and posterior boundaries of the bony part of the external acoustic meatus. It is demarcated from the mastoid process behind by the tympanomastoid fissure. The anterior wall of the tympanic part bounds the mandibular fossa posteriorly. The inferior border of the tympanic part is sharp and is called the tympanic crest. The tympanic crest overlaps the styloid process and thus forms the sheath of the styloid process. The lateral margin of the tympanic part is roughened for attachment of the cartilaginous part of the external acoustic meatus.

The petrous part of the temporal bone is the solid wedge of bone which forms most of the posterior and inferior portions of the temporal bone. Internally, it lies at the boundary between the middle and posterior cranial fossae. It can be subdivided into the petrous part proper and the mastoid part. An alternative term is the petromastoid part of the temporal bone.

The petrous part proper is pyramidal in shape with an apex, a base, two internal surfaces (anterior and posterior) and an external surface (inferior). The apex has a broad flattened surface which articulates with the posterolateral corner of the body of the sphenoid and forms a margin for the foramen lacerum. The apex has the opening for the carotid canal which allows the passage of the internal carotid artery towards the cavernous sinus. The base of the petrous part proper is continuous with the mastoid and squamous parts of the temporal bone, the union with the squamous part being marked by the petrosquamous fissure.

1.24 The temporal bone, as seen from the base of the skull

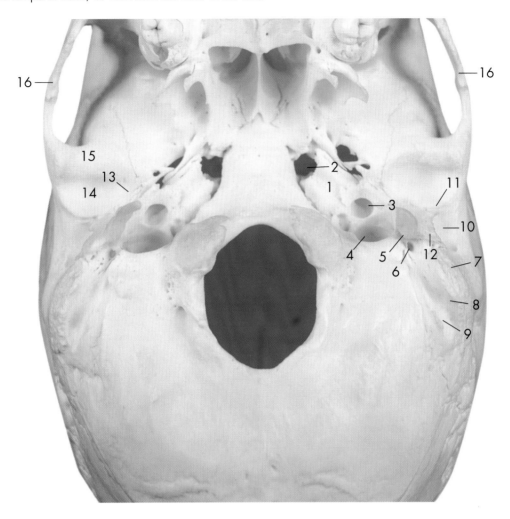

1 Petrous process of the temporal bone
2 Foramen lacerum
3 Carotid canal
4 Jugular foramen
5 Styloid process
6 Stylomastoid foramen
7 Mastoid process
8 Mastoid notch
9 Groove for occipital artery
10 External acoustic meatus
11 Squamotympanic fissure
12 Tympanic part of temporal bone
13 Tegmen tympani separating petro-squamous and petrotympanic fissures
14 Mandibular fossa
15 Articular tubercle
16 Zygomatic arch

The internal (cerebral) aspect of the petrous part proper has a ridge running along the superior margin on which is a groove for the superior petrosal sinus. The ridge subdivides the internal surface into anterior and posterior surfaces. In front of the ridge is the anterior surface which forms the posterior boundary of the middle cranial fossa and is related to the temporal lobe of the brain. Behind the ridge is the posterior surface which constitutes the anterior portion of the posterior cranial fossa and is related to the cerebellum.

The posterior surface slopes downwards and slightly medially. At its medial end, close to the apex, there is a groove for the inferior petrosal sinus. About halfway along the surface is the opening of the internal acoustic meatus. Just behind this opening, and below the level of the arcuate eminence, is a shallow fossa termed the subarcuate fossa. Behind and below the fossa is a narrow slit which is the external opening of the aqueduct of the vestibule (see page 308). The inferior margin of the posterior surface is separated in part from the occipital bone by the jugular foramen, while the posterolateral margin is related to the groove for the sigmoid sinus.

The anterior surface slopes downwards and outwards. Its medial end, adjacent to the apex, is marked by a depression called the trigeminal impression. The trigeminal ganglion is situated here. Beneath the trigeminal impression is the carotid canal. By the side of the trigeminal impression is a slight concavity overlying the internal acoustic meatus. Beyond this, and about halfway along the length of the anterior surface, is a ridge termed the arcuate eminence. This ridge is produced by the underlying anterior (superior) semicircular canal. Between the arcuate eminence and the petrosquamous fissure is the tegmen tympani. This thin plate of bone forms the roof of the mastoid antrum and the tympanic cavity and also contributes to the auditory tube and the canal for the tensor tympani muscle. A portion of the tegmen tympani is seen between the squamous and tympanic parts of the temporal bone at the mandibular fossa. Two small foramina may be seen in the tegmen tympani near the arcuate eminence. These foramina lead into grooves running forwards and medially towards the sphenoid bone. The medially positioned groove runs to the foramen lacerum and transmits the greater petrosal nerve. The laterally positioned groove runs towards the foramen ovale and transmits the lesser petrosal nerve.

1.25 The temporal bone, as seen intracranially

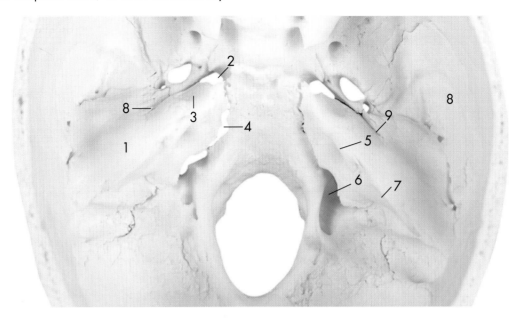

1 Petrous process of temporal bone
2 Foramen lacerum
3 Trigeminal impression
4 Petro-occipital fissure
5 Internal acoustic meatus
6 Jugular foramen
7 Groove associated with superior petrosal sinus
8 Squamous part of temporal bone
9 Hiatus and groove for greater petrosal nerve

The inferior surface of the petrous part proper contributes to the external surface of the cranial base. Its posterior third shows a pronounced depression, the jugular fossa. This fossa is related to the upper part of the internal jugular vein. On the lateral wall of the jugular fossa is found the mastoid canaliculus through which passes the auricular branch of the vagus nerve. Immediately in front of the jugular fossa is the opening of the carotid canal for transmission of the internal carotid artery. The ridge separating the opening of the carotid canal and the jugular fossa shows the tympanic canaliculus for passage of the tympanic branch of the glossopharyngeal nerve (also the inferior tympanic branch of the ascending pharyngeal artery). A triangular depression is seen close to the medial margin of the jugular fossa and directly below the opening of the internal acoustic meatus. In this depression lies the external opening of the cochlear canaliculus (see page 308). The medial margin of the inferior surface of the petrous part proper forms the upper boundary of the jugular foramen. This margin may be notched (the jugular notch) below the level of the internal acoustic meatus. Through the jugular foramen run the internal jugular vein and the glossopharyngeal, vagus and accessory nerves. In front of the carotid canal, the bone is roughened for attachment of the levator veli palatini muscle. The lateral margin of the inferior surface of the petrous part proper gives attachment to the cartilaginous part of the auditory tube.

The mastoid part of the temporal bone lies below the squamous part and behind the tympanic part. Most of it is comprised of the prominent mastoid process. Medial to the process is a deep groove, the mastoid notch. Medial to the mastoid notch is a small groove related to the occipital artery. The lateral surface of the mastoid part of the temporal bone is roughened for muscle attachments. A mastoid foramen is sometimes found near the posterior border. It gives passage to an emissary vein (linking the sigmoid sinus and the occipital veins) and to a meningeal branch from the occipital artery. The main feature on the internal surface of the mastoid is a deep groove related to the sigmoid sinus. The internal opening of the mastoid foramen is seen close to the groove of the sigmoid sinus. The thick upper border of the mastoid articulates with the mastoid angle of the parietal bone. The posterior border articulates with the squamous part of the occipital bone.

The styloid process of the temporal bone is an elongated, narrow projection of bone. It passes downwards and forwards from the base of the temporal bone where it lies between the tympanic part and the posterior border of the jugular foramen. Between the styloid and mastoid processes lies the stylomastoid foramen. The facial nerve and the stylomastoid branch of the posterior auricular artery pass through this foramen.

The following muscles are attached to the temporal bone:

- Digastric (posterior belly)
- Levator veli palatini
- Longissimus capitis
- Masseter
- Occipital belly of occipitofrontalis
- Splenius capitis
- Sternocleidomastoid
- Styloglossus
- Stylohyoid
- Stylopharyngeus
- Temporalis

1.26 The relationships of the temporal bone with other bones comprising the cranial base

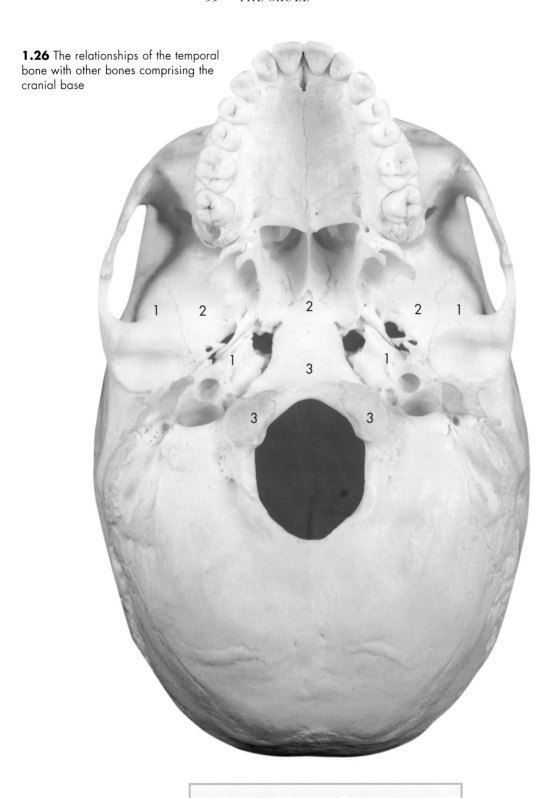

1 Temporal bone
2 Sphenoid bone
3 Occipital bone

THE BONES OF THE FACE

This section includes not only the bones seen on the norma frontalis of the skull, but also some of the bones which contribute to the nasal and orbital cavities. Two of the bones in this region have already been described, the frontal bone with the vault of the skull and the sphenoid bone with the base of the skull. The jaws (maxillary bones and mandible) are considered in the subsequent section.

The zygomatic bones (1.27, 1.28)

The two zygomatic bones form the skeleton of the cheeks. Each consists of a trapezoidal body with two processes projecting from the upper and lower corners of the posterior margin (the frontal and temporal processes respectively). An orbital plate projects inwards from the upper margin.

The lateral surface of the body of the zygomatic bone is smooth and slightly convex. Its medial or maxillary margin articulates with the zygomatic process of the maxillary bone. The inferior border is free and provides attachment for the masseter muscle. The posterior or temporal margin is notched and inferiorly it projects as the temporal process whose serrated margin unites with the zygomatic process of the temporal bone to form the zygomatic arch. Superiorly, the temporal margin continues upwards as the posterior border of the frontal process, giving attachment to the temporal fascia. The frontal process itself articulates with the zygomatic process of the frontal bone. The superior or orbital margin of the zygomatic bone is concave and contributes to both the inferior and lateral margins of the orbit.

Projecting inwards from the orbital margin is a shelf of bone which forms an orbital plate. Its upper or orbital surface is concave and forms the anterior part of the lateral wall of the orbit. The superior margin of the orbital plate at the frontal process articulates with the zygomatic process of the frontal bone. Just below this margin, there is usually a small tubercle. This is known as the marginal tubercle (Whitnall's tubercle) and to it are attached the lateral palpebral raphe from the orbicularis oculi muscle and the lateral palpebral ligament. The orbital plate also articulates with the greater wing of the sphenoid bone at the sphenoidal margin.

The entire surface of the zygomatic bone viewed medially is called the temporal surface. It can be subdivided into two regions. Anteriorly, it shows a roughened area for articulation with the zygomatic process of the maxilla. Posteriorly, the temporal surface includes the lower surface of the orbital plate and the temporal surface of the temporal process. This posterior region is smooth and forms the anterior boundary of the temporal fossa.

The zygomatic bone has three foramina. On the orbital surface of the orbital plate is found the zygomatico-orbital foramen. Through this pass the zygomaticofacial and zygomaticotemporal branches of the maxillary division of the trigeminal nerve. The zygomaticofacial nerve then runs through a canal and emerges onto the face at the zygomaticofacial foramen on the lateral surface of the zygomatic bone. The zygomatico-temporal nerve passes through the zygomaticotemporal foramen on the temporal surface of the bone.

The muscles attached to the zygomatic bone are:

- Levator labii superioris
- Masseter
- Temporalis
- Zygomaticus major
- Zygomaticus minor

1.27 The zygomatic bone, as seen from the front of the skull

1 Zygomatic bone
2 The zygomatic process of the frontal bone
3 The zygomatic process of the maxillary bone
4 The zygomaticofacial foramen

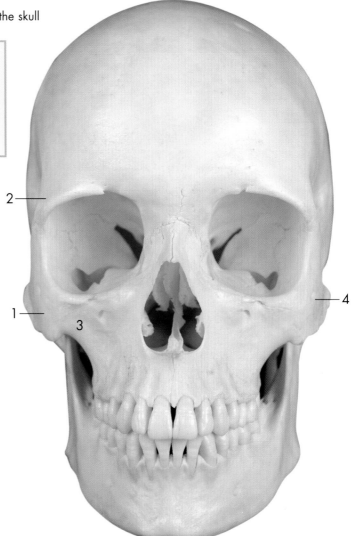

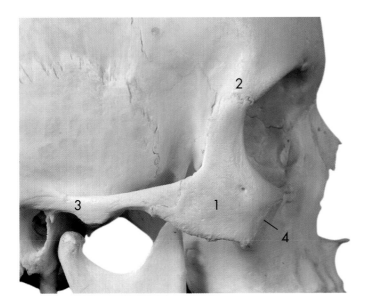

1.28 The zygomatic bone as seen from a lateral view of the skull

1 The zygomatic bone
2 The zygomatic process of frontal bone
3 Zygomatic arch, zygomatic process of temporal bone
4 Zygomatic process of maxillary bone

The ethmoid bone (1.29–1.31)

The ethmoid is a single bone which makes a significant contribution to the middle third of the face. It forms parts of the nasal septum, roof and lateral wall of the nose, and a considerable part of the medial wall of the orbital cavity. In addition, the ethmoid makes a small contribution to the floor of the anterior cranial fossa. Four parts can be distinguished, the perpendicular plate, the cribriform plate and two ethmoidal labyrinths.

The perpendicular plate of the ethmoid is a thin, quadrilateral plate of bone which descends vertically in the midline from the cribriform plate to form the upper part of the nasal septum. In front, it articulates with the nasal bone above and the septal cartilage below. Behind, it meets the sphenoidal crest of the body of the sphenoid. Below and behind, the perpendicular plate joins the vomer bone.

The cribriform plate of the ethmoid forms the upper surface of the ethmoid bone. It lies horizontally, filling the ethmoid notch of the frontal bone. It forms the roof of the nose and derives its name from the fact that it is penetrated by numerous foramina containing branches of the olfactory nerves. Projecting vertically upwards in the midline is a triangular plate of bone, the crista galli. From the anterior border of the crista galli arise two small, wing-like plates of bone called the alae. When articulated with the frontal bone, the alae contribute to an opening termed the foramen caecum. An emissary vein may pass through this opening, linking the superior sagittal sinus with veins in the nose. The falx cerebri is attached to the posterior border of the crista galli. The anterior ethmoidal nerves pass into the nose through slits lying on each side of the crista galli.

The ethmoidal labyrinths (lateral masses) hang vertically downwards from the lateral margins of the cribriform plate. Each labyrinth consists of a network of air cells separated by bony trabeculae and bounded by a lateral plate (orbital plate) and a medial surface (nasal surface). The air cells are however incompletely surrounded by bone and become roofed over by adjacent bones. The upper surface of the ethmoidal labyrinth articulates with the frontal bone, the posterior surface is covered by the sphenoidal concha and the orbital process of the palatine bone.

The orbital plate of the labyrinth is a smooth, quadrilateral plate of bone. Anteriorly, the exposed air cells are covered over by the lacrimal bone and by the frontal process of the maxilla. Below, the orbital plate articulates with the maxillary bone. Above, there are grooves for the anterior and posterior ethmoidal nerves and vessels which are converted into foramina by articulation with the frontal bone. However, the posterior groove and foramen are frequently absent.

The medial surface of the ethmoidal labyrinth forms part of the lateral wall of the nose. Two thin, scroll-like plates of bone hang down from it. The upper plate is the superior nasal concha, the lower is the middle nasal concha. The middle concha is larger and extends more anteriorly. The groove between the conchae is termed the superior meatus. Into this open the posterior ethmoidal air cells. The region below the attached margin of the middle nasal concha curves upwards and forwards to form a channel termed the infundibulum in the middle meatus of the nose. The anterior ethmoidal air cells open here. A swelling of the bone in this region overlies the middle ethmoidal air cells, the ethmoidal bulla. An opening in or over the bulla is the site of drainage for these air cells. A thin, curved plate of bone runs lateral to the anterior part of the middle nasal concha. This is the uncinate process. The region between this process and the ethmoidal bulla above corresponds to the hiatus semilunaris (see page 198).

1.29 The isolated ethmoid bone viewed anteriorly

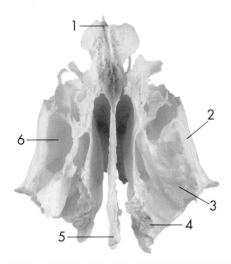

1 Crista galli
2 Orbital plate
3 Uncinate process
4 Middle nasal concha
5 Perpendicular plate
6 Ethmoidal labyrinth and air cells

1.30 The ethmoid bone and the septum of the nose

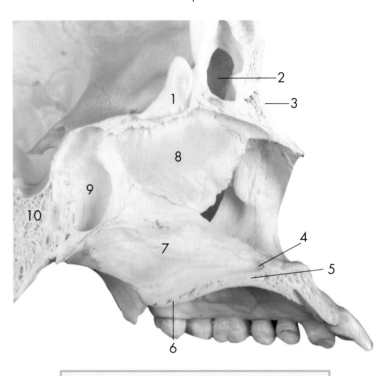

1 Cribriform plate of ethmoid
2 Frontal sinus
3 Nasal bone
4 Opening of incisive canal
5 Palatine process of maxilla
6 Horizontal process of palatine bone
7 Vomer
8 Perpendicular plate of ethmoid
9 Sphenoidal sinus
10 Body of sphenoid

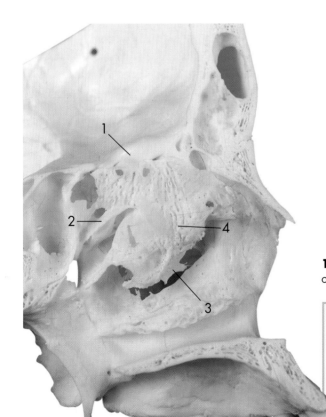

1.31 The ethmoid bone, comprising part of the lateral wall of the nose

1 Cribriform plate of ethmoid
2 Superior concha
3 Uncinate process of ethmoid
4 Middle concha

The palatine bones (1.32–1.34)

Each palatine bone is roughly L-shaped. It has a perpendicular plate which forms part of the lateral wall of the nose, and a horizontal plate which forms the posterior one-third of the hard palate. A pyramidal process arises posteriorly at the junction between the two plates.

The perpendicular plate of the palatine bone is rectangular (the vertical dimension being about twice that of the anteroposterior one). The upper border presents a notch, the sphenopalatine notch. In front of the notch lies the orbital process. Behind the notch is the sphenoidal process. In articulating with the inferior surface of the body of the sphenoid, the notch is converted into the sphenopalatine foramen. This foramen transmits the nasopalatine and posterior superior nasal nerves and the sphenopalatine vessels from the pterygopalatine fossa into the nasal cavity. The remaining part of the perpendicular plate has a lateral (maxillary) surface and a medial (nasal) surface.

The orbital process projects upwards and outwards from the upper border of the perpendicular plate. Its smooth, upper (orbital) surface forms the most posterior portion of the floor of the orbit. Its lateral surface forms part of the medial wall of the pterygopalatine fossa and is closely related to the maxillary nerve. From the medial side, the orbital process is hollowed out to contain an air cell. The air cell may communicate with the posterior ethmoidal air cells or with the sphenoidal sinus. The orbital process articulates with the maxillary, ethmoid and sphenoid bones.

The sphenoidal process projects upwards and inwards from the upper border of the perpendicular plate to articulate with the body of the sphenoid, the medial pterygoid plate, and the ala of the vomer.

The lateral (maxillary) surface of the perpendicular plate is roughened inferiorly for articulation with the maxilla (at the nasal surface behind the opening of the maxillary sinus). The upper part is smooth and contributes to the medial wall of the pterygopalatine fossa. The greater palatine groove is found running down the posterior margin of the lateral surface. The groove is converted into a canal (the greater palatine canal) when the bone is articulated with the maxilla. This canal transmits both greater and lesser palatine nerves and vessels. At the lower end of the anterior border of the perpendicular plate is a projection termed the maxillary process. This covers the postero-inferior portion of the hiatus of the maxillary sinus. The posterior border of the perpendicular plate articulates with the medial pterygoid plate.

The medial (nasal) surface of the perpendicular plate is smooth and shows near its middle a horizontal ridge, the conchal crest. This crest articulates with the inferior nasal concha. The concavity below the conchal crest forms part of the inferior meatus of the lateral wall of the nose. The concavity above the crest contributes to the middle meatus and extends upwards to the region of the sphenopalatine notch where another horizontal ridge, the ethmoid crest, is situated. To this crest is attached the middle nasal concha of the ethmoid bone. The small region lying above the ethmoid crest contributes to the superior meatus of the nose.

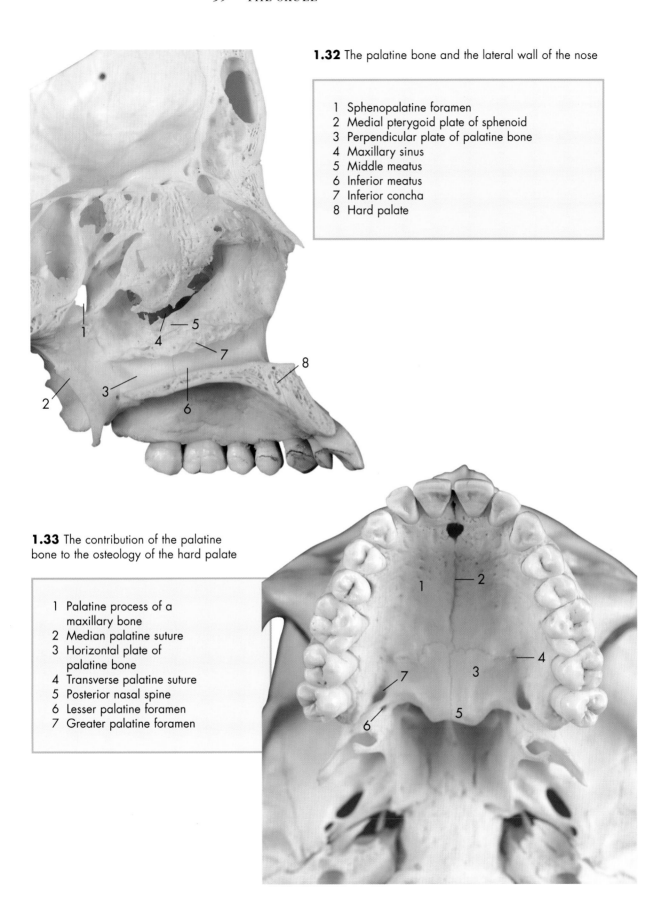

1.32 The palatine bone and the lateral wall of the nose

1 Sphenopalatine foramen
2 Medial pterygoid plate of sphenoid
3 Perpendicular plate of palatine bone
4 Maxillary sinus
5 Middle meatus
6 Inferior meatus
7 Inferior concha
8 Hard palate

1.33 The contribution of the palatine bone to the osteology of the hard palate

1 Palatine process of a maxillary bone
2 Median palatine suture
3 Horizontal plate of palatine bone
4 Transverse palatine suture
5 Posterior nasal spine
6 Lesser palatine foramen
7 Greater palatine foramen

The horizontal plate of the palatine bone is quadrilateral (the mediolateral dimension being greater than the anteroposterior one). The upper (nasal) surface is slightly concave and forms the posterior third of the floor of the nose. The lower (palatal) surface forms the posterior third of the hard palate and, near its posterior border, may exhibit a ridge termed the palatal crest which helps to attach the tendon of the tensor veli palatini muscle. The medial border of the horizontal plate is thickened and articulates with the horizontal process of the opposite side at the median palatine suture. The upper margin of the medial border forms the nasal crest which articulates with the vomer. The anterior border of the horizontal plate articulates with the palatine process of the maxilla at the transverse palatine suture. The posterior border of the horizontal plate is smooth and concave. Medially, it contributes to the posterior nasal spine. To this spine is attached the musculus uvulae. The lateral border of the horizontal plate is attached to the inferior border of the perpendicular plate. At this junction is seen the lower margin of the greater palatine groove.

The pyramidal process of the palatine bone projects backwards, outwards and slightly downwards from the posterior surface of the palatine bone at the junction between the perpendicular and horizontal plates. It articulates in the space between the maxillary tuberosity and the pterygoid notch of the pterygoid process. The inferior surface of the pyramidal process shows one or more openings, the lesser palatine foramina. These are continuous above with the greater palatine groove and transmit the lesser palatine nerves and vessels.

The muscles attached to the palatine bone are:

- Medial pterygoid (superficial head)

- Musculus uvulae

- Palatopharyngeus

- Tensor veli palatini

The vomer bone (1.35)

This single bone is a thin plate shaped like a ploughshare. It forms the postero-inferior portion of the nasal septum. Its superior border shows a groove lying between two wing-like projections or alae. The rostrum of the sphenoid bone fits into this groove. When the ala of the vomer meets the vaginal process and body of the sphenoid, it completes the vomerovaginal canal. Through this occasional canal passes a pharyngeal branch of the sphenopalatine artery. The inferior border of the vomer lies anterior to the superior border and fits into the nasal crest running along the middle of the upper surface of the hard palate. The anterior border of the vomer slopes downwards and forwards. Inferiorly, it is grooved and receives the inferior border of the cartilaginous nasal septum. Superiorly, it joins with the perpendicular plate of the ethmoid. The posterior border of the vomer is free and does not articulate with other structures. It is slightly concave and slopes downwards and forwards to form a prominent midline ridge between the two posterior nasal apertures. Each side of the vomer presents a groove running downwards and forwards which is related to the nasopalatine nerve and vessels.

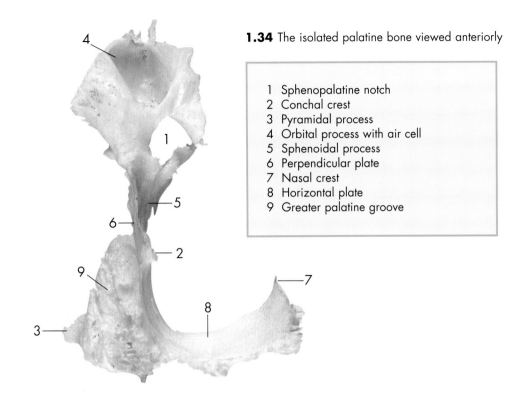

1.34 The isolated palatine bone viewed anteriorly

1 Sphenopalatine notch
2 Conchal crest
3 Pyramidal process
4 Orbital process with air cell
5 Sphenoidal process
6 Perpendicular plate
7 Nasal crest
8 Horizontal plate
9 Greater palatine groove

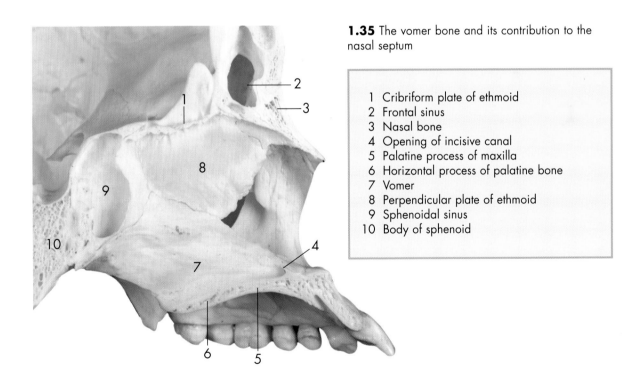

1.35 The vomer bone and its contribution to the nasal septum

1 Cribriform plate of ethmoid
2 Frontal sinus
3 Nasal bone
4 Opening of incisive canal
5 Palatine process of maxilla
6 Horizontal process of palatine bone
7 Vomer
8 Perpendicular plate of ethmoid
9 Sphenoidal sinus
10 Body of sphenoid

The nasal bones (1.36)

The two nasal bones form the upper part of the bridge of the nose. Each nasal bone is quadrilateral (being longer than it is wide). The upper border articulates with the nasal part of the frontal bone. The lower border is sharp and notched and forms the upper boundary of the anterior nasal aperture. The lower border gives attachment to the lateral nasal cartilage. The lateral border of the nasal bone meets the frontal process of the maxilla. The medial border meets its fellow in the midline and is thickened above to form a vertical crest which makes a small contribution to the nasal septum. It therefore articulates with the septal cartilage and with the perpendicular plate of the ethmoid.

The smooth, outer surface of the nasal bone is convex, but is concave near the upper border. The internal surface is concave throughout and in its upper part shows a groove related to the external nasal branch of the anterior ethmoidal nerve.

The procerus muscle is attached to the external surface of the nasal bone.

The inferior nasal conchae (1.37)

Each concha consists of a curved plate of bone which is attached to the lateral wall of the nose. The posterior end of the bone is more pointed than the anterior end. Its longer lower border lies free within the nasal cavity, is thickened and often curves inwards. The upper border serves to attach the bone to the lateral wall of the nose, articulating with four different bones. Its anterior slopes and is attached to the conchal crest of the maxilla. Its posterior slope articulates with the conchal crest of the perpendicular plate of the palatine bone. The middle third of the upper border is more or less horizontal and shows two small processes, a lacrimal process anteriorly and an ethmoid process posteriorly. The lacrimal process meets the descending process of the lacrimal bone and helps to complete the nasolacrimal canal. The ethmoid process articulates with the uncinate process of the ethmoid. From the middle portion of the upper border, a thin, triangular plate of bone (the maxillary process) projects downwards to partially cover the hiatus of the maxillary sinus. The maxillary process articulates with the maxilla and with the maxillary process of the palatine bone. The medial surface of the inferior nasal concha is convex and shows pits and grooves related to blood vessels. The lateral surface is smoother and concave.

The lacrimal bones (1.38)

Each of these two bones is small, thin and rectangular. It lies in the anterior part of the medial wall of the orbit. In front, the lacrimal bone articulates with the frontal process of the maxilla. Behind, it meets the orbital plate of the ethmoid. Above, it joins the frontal bone and below, the maxilla. The lateral surface is divided into two areas by a vertical crest termed the posterior lacrimal crest. This crest ends below in a hook-shaped process termed the lacrimal hamulus. The area in front of the crest is concave and, together with the adjacent area of the frontal process of the maxilla, forms the fossa for the lacrimal sac. The area behind the posterior lacrimal crest forms part of the medial wall of the orbit. The upper part of the medial (nasal) surface of the lacrimal bone covers the anterior ethmoidal air cells. The lower part contributes to the lateral wall of the nose in the middle meatus and narrows the opening of the maxillary sinus. A descending process continues inferiorly to articulate with the inferior nasal concha and adjacent part of the maxilla to complete the nasolacrimal duct.

The lacrimal part of the orbicularis oculi muscle arises from the lateral surface of the lacrimal bone.

1.36 The nasal bones *in situ*

1 Frontal bone
2 Glabella
3 Nasal bone
4 Frontal process
  of maxilla
5 Anterior nasal
  (piriform) aperture

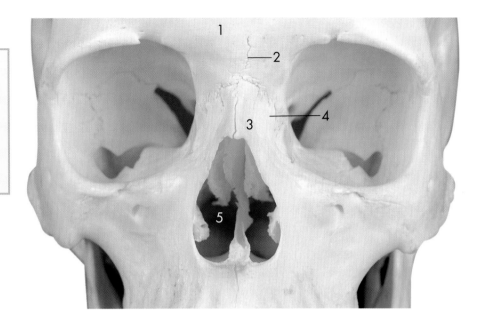

1.37 The inferior nasal concha

1 Medial pterygoid plate of sphenoid
2 Perpendicular plate of palatine bone
3 Opening of maxillary sinus
4 Middle meatus
5 Inferior meatus
6 Inferior concha
7 Hard palate
8 Uncinate process of ethmoid
Arrow indicates position of opening of
nasolacrimal canal

1.38 The lacrimal bone in the medial wall of
the orbit

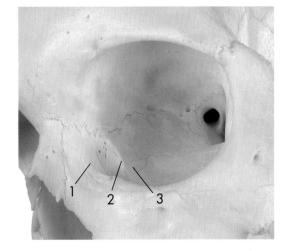

1 Fossa for lacrimal sac
2 Posterior lacrimal crest
3 Lacrimal bone

THE BONES OF THE JAWS

The jaws are the tooth-bearing bones. They are comprised of three bones. The two maxillary bones form the upper jaw whereas the lower jaw is a single bone, the mandible.

The maxillary bones (1.39–1.41)

The maxillary bones support the teeth of the upper jaw and contribute much of the skeleton of the upper face. Each bone consists of a body and four processes, the frontal, zygomatic, alveolar and palatine processes. The body contains the maxillary air sinus.

The maxillary bones show many articulations. On the face, the maxillary bones articulate with each other, and with the nasal bones, the nasal cartilages and the frontal bone. Laterally, they articulate with the zygomatic bones. Each maxillary bone also joins with the vomer, the septal cartilage, the lacrimal bone, the ethmoid bone and the inferior nasal concha to contribute to the skeleton of the nasal fossa and the orbit.

The body of the maxilla is essentially pyramidal in shape. Its base faces the nasal cavity and its apex is located within the zygomatic process. It presents four main surfaces: anterior (facial), posterior (infratemporal), medial (nasal) and superior (orbital).

The anterior surface of the body of the maxilla forms the skeleton of the anterior part of the cheek. The anterior surface is demarcated from the posterior surface by the zygomatic process and by a ridge (the zygomatico-alveolar or jugal crest) running from the zygomatic process to the socket of the first molar tooth. A ridge called the canine eminence overlies the root of the canine tooth. It separates the anterior surface into two concave areas: a shallow, incisive fossa in front and a deeper, canine fossa behind. The anterior surface is delineated from the orbital surface by the infra-orbital margin. Below this margin lies the infra-orbital foramen through which pass the infra-orbital branch of the maxillary nerve and the infra-orbital vessels.

The posterior surface of the body of the maxilla forms the anterior wall of the infratemporal fossa. Its lower, posterior extremity presents a convexity termed the maxillary tuberosity. Immediately above the tuberosity, the surface of the bone is roughened for articulation of the pyramidal process of the palatine bone. In front of the tuberosity may be seen several small foramina associated with the posterior superior alveolar nerves and vessels which supply the posterior maxillary teeth. Above the tuberosity, the posterior surface forms the anterior boundary of the pterygopalatine fossa.

The medial (nasal) surface of the body of the maxilla forms part of the lateral wall of the nose. The upper posterior part of this surface shows the large opening (hiatus) leading into the maxillary sinus. In the natural (*in vivo*) state, the hiatus is reduced in size by the articulation of the palatine bone, the uncinate process of the ethmoid, the inferior nasal concha and the lacrimal bone, and by the overlying mucosa. One or two shallow depressions may be found above and behind the hiatus. These help to complete some of the ethmoidal air cells. Behind and below the maxillary sinus lies the greater palatine groove. This is converted into a canal carrying the greater palatine nerve and vessels by the perpendicular plate of the palatine bone. In front of the maxillary sinus lies a deep vertical groove. This is called the lacrimal groove which, with the lacrimal bone, forms the nasolacrimal canal. Anterior to the nasolacrimal canal is an obliquely-running ridge termed the conchal crest. This articulates with the inferior nasal concha. The concave area above the crest therefore bounds the middle meatus of the nasal cavity, whereas the concave area below bounds the inferior meatus.

1.39 The contribution of the maxillary bones to the facial skeleton

1 Frontal process of maxilla
2 Anterior nasal (piriform) aperture
3 Orbital plate of maxilla
4 Infra-orbital foramen
5 Body of maxilla
6 Zygomatic process of maxilla
7 Alveolus of maxilla (upper jaw)
8 Intermaxillary suture
9 Anterior nasal spine

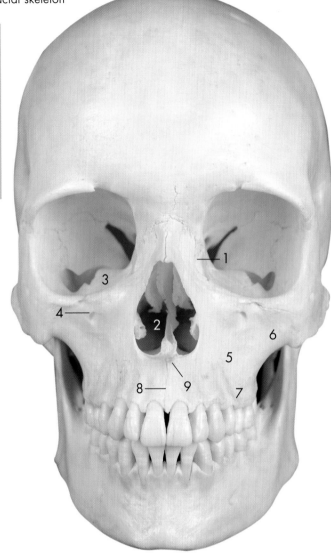

1.40 An oblique–lateral view of the skull demonstrating the maxillary bone and its contribution to the osteology of the hard palate

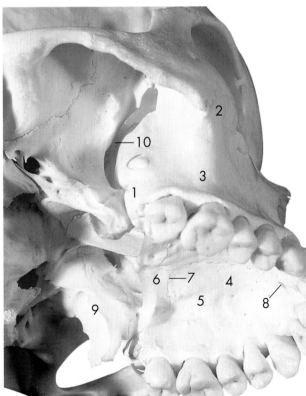

1 Tuberosity of maxilla
2 Zygomatic process of maxilla
3 Alveolus of maxilla
4 Palatine process of maxilla
5 Median palatine suture
6 Horizontal plate of palatine bone
7 Transverse palatine suture
8 Incisive fossa
9 Pterygoid plates of sphenoid bone
10 Pterygomaxillary fissure leading into pterygopalatine fossa

The superior (orbital) surface of the body of the maxilla forms much of the floor of the orbit. It is triangular in shape. A groove, the infra-orbital groove, is present midway along the posterior border of this surface and, running forwards and medially, eventually forms the infra-orbital canal. This canal exits at the infra-orbital foramen and transmits the infra-orbital nerve and vessels. The nerve is a branch of the maxillary division of the trigeminal. The maxillary nerve itself also grooves the bone at the junction between the superior and posterior surfaces of the body of the maxilla. The rounded, posterior border of the orbital surface forms the anterior boundary of the inferior orbital fissure. The medial border of the orbital surface presents anteriorly the lacrimal groove which is bounded in front by the anterior lacrimal crest. The anterior border of the orbital surface forms the medial part of the inferior margin of the orbit.

The frontal process of the maxilla projects upwards from the body and is situated between the nasal bone in front and the lacrimal bone behind. Its lateral surface is divided into two areas by the vertically-running anterior lacrimal crest. Behind the crest, the bone is grooved for the nasolacrimal canal. To the crest itself is attached the medial palpebral ligament (see page 240). The medial surface of the frontal process shows an obliquely-running ethmoidal crest. To this is attached the middle nasal concha. The bone above the crest helps to enclose the anterior ethmoidal air cells.

The zygomatic process of the maxilla projects laterally from the body. It is pyramidal in shape and has a roughened superolateral surface for articulation with the zygomatic bone. Its posterior surface is smooth and concave and forms part of the anterior boundary of the infratemporal fossa.

The palatine process of the maxilla extends horizontally from the medial surface of the maxilla where the body meets the alveolar process. Posteriorly, the boundary between the palatine and alveolar processes is sharp. Anteriorly, the boundary is less well defined. The medial edge of the palatine process is for articulation with the opposite palatine process at the median palatine suture. Behind the central incisors, the medial edge shows evidence of the incisive fossa. Through this pass the nasopalatine nerves and branches of the greater palatine vessels. An incisive canal runs through the palatine process in the region of the incisive fossa. The medial edge is

thickened on its nasal surface to contribute to the nasal crest (a structure which articulates with the inferior border of the vomer). The crest is noticeably thickened anteriorly and is prolonged into the anterior nasal spine. Both the nasal and oral surfaces of the palatine process are concave. Unlike the nasal surface, the oral surface of the palatine process is rough and irregular, forming palatine grooves and spines. The posterior edge of the palatine process articulates with the horizontal plate of a palatine bone at the transverse palatine suture.

The alveolar process of the maxilla extends inferiorly from the body of the maxilla and supports the teeth within bony sockets. Each maxilla can contain a full quadrant of eight permanent teeth or five deciduous teeth. The form of the alveolus is related to the functional demands put upon the teeth. For example, when the teeth are extracted, the alveolus resorbs. Essentially, the alveolar process consists of two parallel plates of cortical bone, the buccal and palatal alveolar plates, between which lie the sockets of individual teeth. Between the sockets are inter-alveolar or interdental septa. The floor of the socket has been termed the fundus. Its rim is called the alveolar crest. The form and depth of each socket is defined by the form and length of the root it supports. The sockets thus show considerable variation. In multirooted teeth, the sockets are divided by interradicular septa. The apical regions of the sockets of anterior teeth are closely related to the nasal fossae, whereas those of posterior teeth are related to the maxillary sinus. In the midline, the alveolar processes of the maxillary bones meet at the intermaxillary suture. At the upper end of the suture lies a sharp bony projection termed the anterior nasal spine. Adjacent to the nasal spine, and forming the floor of the anterior nasal aperture, is a notch called the nasal notch.

The following muscles are attached to the maxilla:

- Buccinator

- Depressor septi

- Levator anguli oris

- Levator labii superioris

- Nasalis

- Orbicularis oculi

- Orbicularis oris

1.41 The contribution of the maxillary bone to the palate and the lateral wall of the nose

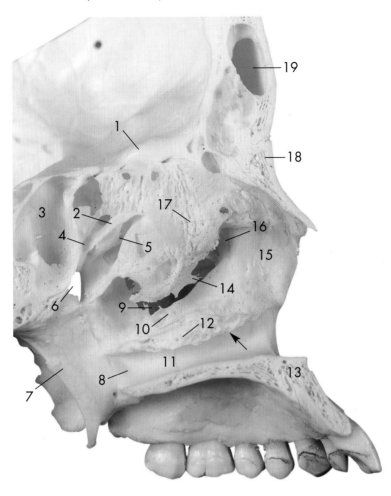

1 Cribriform plate of ethmoid
2 Superior concha
3 Sphenoidal sinus
4 Spheno-ethmoidal recess
5 Superior meatus
6 Sphenopalatine foramen
7 Medial pterygoid plate of sphenoid
8 Perpendicular plate of palatine bone
9 Opening of maxillary sinus
10 Middle meatus
11 Inferior meatus

12 Inferior concha
13 Hard palate
14 Uncinate process of ethmoid
15 Medial surface of maxilla
16 Lacrimal bone
17 Middle concha
18 Nasal bone
19 Frontal sinus

Arrow indicates position of opening of
nasolacrimal canal

The mandible (1.42–1.45)

The mandible consists of a horizontal, horseshoe-shaped body and two vertical rami. The body of the mandible supports the mandibular teeth within the alveolar process. The rami of the mandible articulate with the temporal bones at the temporomandibular joints.

The body of the mandible has important features on both the lateral and medial surfaces.

The lateral surface of the body of the mandible shows a ridge in the upper part of the midline which represents the site of the mandibular symphysis. Close to the inferior margin of the body lies a distinct prominence, the mental protuberance. On each side of the protuberance are the mental tubercles. The mental protuberance and tubercles together comprise the chin. Above the mental protuberance lies a shallow depression called the incisive fossa. Behind this fossa, a canine eminence overlies the root of the mandibular canine tooth. In the region of the premolar teeth is found the mental foramen. The mental branches of the inferior alveolar nerve and vessels pass onto the face through this foramen. During growth of the mandible, when the prominence of the chin develops, the opening of the mental foramen alters in direction from facing forwards to facing upwards and backwards. Rarely, there may be multiple mental foramina. The alveolus forms the superior margin of the body of the mandible. The junction of the alveolus and ramus is demarcated by a ridge, the external oblique line. This ridge is continuous with the anterior border of the ramus and passes downwards and forwards across the body of the mandible to terminate below the mental foramen.

The medial surface of the body of the mandible has two shallow depressions close to the midline on its inferior border. These are the digastric fossae, providing sites for the attachment of the anterior bellies of the digastric muscles. Above these fossae are the genial tubercles (mental spines). There are generally two inferior and two superior tubercles. They mark the sites of attachment of the geniohyoid and genioglossus muscles. Across the medial surface of the body of the mandible is a prominent ridge called the mylohyoid line (internal oblique line). To this is attached the mylohyoid muscle. The ridge arises between the genial tubercles and the digastric fossa and increases in prominence as it passes backwards and upwards to end on the anterior surface of the ramus. The surface of the mandible above and in front of the mylohyoid line presents a shallow depression in which lies the sublingual salivary gland. The depression is therefore termed the sublingual fossa. The shallow concavity below the mylohyoid line is the submandibular fossa in which lies the superficial portion of the submandibular salivary gland. At the posterior end of the mylohyoid line is attached the pterygomandibular raphe.

The alveolar process of the mandible continues upwards from the body. It consists of buccal and lingual alveolar plates joined by interdental and interradicular septa. Near the second and third molar teeth, the external oblique line is superimposed upon the buccal alveolar plate. The form and depth of the tooth sockets is related to the morphology of the roots of the mandibular teeth and to functional demands.

The ramus of the mandible meets the body of the mandible at an obtuse angle. The region where the inferior margin of the ramus meets the posterior margin is termed the angle of the mandible. This area provides attachment for the masseter and medial pterygoid muscles and for the stylomandibular ligament. Superiorly, are located the coronoid and condylar processes. These are separated by the mandibular notch. The lateral surface of the ramus is relatively featureless. It presents a surface for the attachment of the masseter muscle. In the centre of the medial surface of the ramus lies the mandibular foramen through which the inferior alveolar nerve and vessels pass into the mandibular canal. A bony process called the lingula extends from the anterosuperior surface of the foramen and gives attachment to the sphenomandibular ligament. A groove, the mylohyoid groove, runs down from the postero-inferior surface of the mandibular foramen. Below and behind the mylohyoid groove, the medial surface of the ramus is roughened around the angle for the attachment of the medial pterygoid muscle. Running down from the tip of the coronoid process is a ridge termed the temporal crest. This extends down to the bone just behind the third molar tooth. The triangular depression between the temporal crest and the anterior border of the ramus is called the retromolar fossa.

The coronoid process lies anterior to the condylar process. It is a triangular plate of bone which gives attachment to the temporalis muscle.

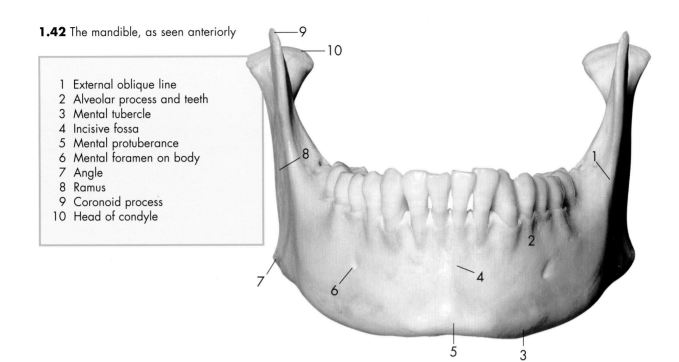

1.42 The mandible, as seen anteriorly

1 External oblique line
2 Alveolar process and teeth
3 Mental tubercle
4 Incisive fossa
5 Mental protuberance
6 Mental foramen on body
7 Angle
8 Ramus
9 Coronoid process
10 Head of condyle

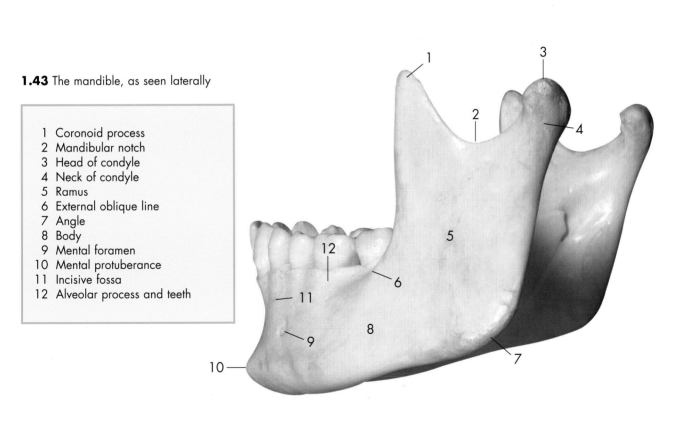

1.43 The mandible, as seen laterally

1 Coronoid process
2 Mandibular notch
3 Head of condyle
4 Neck of condyle
5 Ramus
6 External oblique line
7 Angle
8 Body
9 Mental foramen
10 Mental protuberance
11 Incisive fossa
12 Alveolar process and teeth

The condylar process lies considerably in terms of both shape and size. Its broad articular head joins the ramus through a thin bony projection termed the neck of the condyle. The anteroposterior dimension of the condylar head is approximately half the mediolateral dimension. The long axis of the condyle is not, however, at right angles to the ramus but diverges posteriorly from a strictly coronal plane such that the long axes of the two condyles, if extended medially, would meet to form an obtuse angle of approximately 150 degrees at the anterior border of the foramen magnum. The convex anterior and superior surfaces of the head of the condyle are the articular surfaces. The posterior surface of the head of the condyle is broad and flat. A small depression, the pterygoid fovea, is a site of attachment of the lateral pterygoid muscle. It is situated on the anterior part of the neck of the condyle.

The mandibular canal begins at the mandibular foramen and passes initially downwards and forwards in the ramus. It runs horizontally below the molar teeth in the body of the mandible. Near the premolar teeth, the canal bifurcates into incisive and mental canals. The narrow incisive canal continues forwards towards the midline beneath the incisor teeth. The mental canal runs upwards, outwards and backwards to open onto the face at the mental foramen.

Many muscles are attached to the mandible and comprise:

Muscles of mastication	Lateral pterygoid
	Masseter
	Medial pterygoid
	Temporalis
Muscles of facial expression	Buccinator
	Depressor anguli oris
	Depressor labii inferioris
	Mentalis
	Platysma
Suprahyoid muscles	Digastric
	Geniohyoid
	Mylohyoid
Muscles of tongue and pharynx	Genioglossus
	Superior constrictor

1.44 The internal surface of the mandible

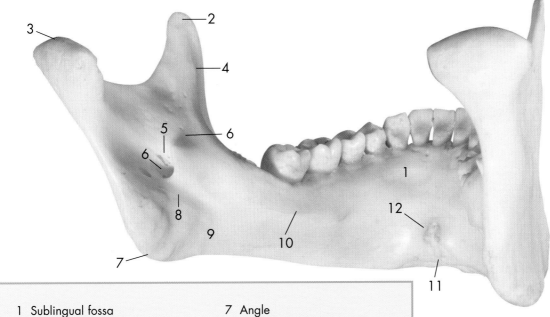

1 Sublingual fossa	7 Angle
2 Coronoid process	8 Mylohyoid groove
3 Head of condyle	9 Submandibular fossa
4 Temporal crest	10 Mylohoid (internal oblique) line
5 Lingula	11 Digastric fossa
6 Mandibular foramen	12 Mental spines (genial tubercles)

1.45 The mandibular dentition, as seen from above

1 Alveolar process and teeth on body
2 Mental foramen
3 External oblique line
4 Retro-molar fossa
5 Mental spines (genial tubercles)
6 Mental protuberance
7 Mental tubercle

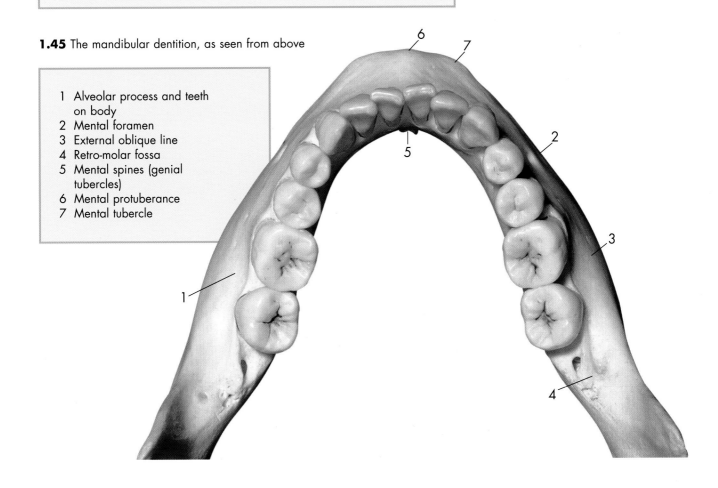

SKULL BONE ARTICULATIONS

The skull is usually considered either in terms of a fully articulated structure or in terms of the individual bones. A further appreciation of this most complex of osseous structures can be obtained by considering how the individual bones comprising a region articulate. This is of particular importance for understanding the osteology of the orbit, nose, cranial fossae and pterygopalatine fossa.

THE ORBITAL AND NASAL APERTURES

The orbital and nasal apertures of the facial skeleton are defined by the frontal, maxillary, nasal and zygomatic bones.

The orbital aperture (aditus of the orbit) is bounded above by the supra-orbital margin of the frontal bone, laterally by the zygomatic bone and the zygomatic process of the frontal bone, below by the zygomatic bone and the maxilla, and medially by the frontal bone and the anterior lacrimal crest of the frontal process of the maxilla.

The anterior nasal aperture (piriform aperture) is bounded mainly by the maxillary bones. The nasal bones form the superior margin of the aperture.

THE ORBIT (1.46, 1.47)

The orbital cavity is pyramidal in shape, with the apex pointing posteriorly. It has a roof, a floor, and medial and lateral walls. The bones which comprise the orbital cavity are the ethmoid, frontal, lacrimal, maxillary, palatine, sphenoid, and zygomatic bones.

The roof of the orbit is formed mainly by the orbital part of the frontal bone. The lesser wing of the sphenoid bone is situated posteriorly near the apex.

The floor of the orbit is composed of the orbital surfaces of the maxillary and the zygomatic bones, with the orbital process of the palatine bone near the apex.

The medial wall of the orbit begins at the anterior lacrimal crest of the frontal process of the maxilla. Behind this lies the lacrimal bone. Most of the medial wall behind the lacrimal bone is formed by the orbital plate of the ethmoid bone. The body of the sphenoid bone contributes to the medial wall posteriorly. Between the anterior lacrimal crest of the maxilla and the posterior lacrimal crest of the lacrimal bone is the fossa for the lacrimal sac.

The lateral wall of the orbit is formed by the orbital surface of the greater wing of the sphenoid bone and by the orbital surface of the zygomatic bone.

There are several prominent foramina and fissures within the orbit.

At the superior orbital margin are the supra-orbital notch (or foramen) and the frontal notch (or foramen). These transmit respectively the supra-orbital and the supratrochlear nerves and vessels.

In the floor of the orbit is found the infra-orbital groove and the infra-orbital canal for the infra-orbital nerve and vessels.

At the medial wall is situated the opening of the nasolacrimal canal, and the anterior and posterior ethmoidal foramina for the anterior and posterior ethmoidal nerves and vessels. The nasolacrimal canal is located antero-inferiorly, close to the orbital margin. The ethmoidal foramina lie at the junction with the roof of the orbital cavity.

At the lateral wall is the zygomatico-orbital foramen (occasionally foramina). Through this foramen pass the zygomatic branches of the maxillary division of the trigeminal nerve and accompanying vessels.

Near the apex of the orbital cavity are the optic canal, the superior orbital fissure and the inferior orbital fissure. The optic canal lies within the lesser wing of the sphenoid and transmits the optic nerve and ophthalmic artery. The superior orbital fissure lies between the greater and lesser wings of the sphenoid at the junction of the roof and lateral wall of the orbit. It transmits the oculomotor, trochlear, ophthalmic and abducent nerves, together with the ophthalmic veins. The inferior orbital fissure lies at the junction of the lateral wall and floor of the orbit. Through this fissure pass the infra-orbital and zygomatic branches of the maxillary division of the trigeminal nerve and accompanying vessels.

1.46 The osteology of the orbit

1 Orbital surface of greater
   wing of sphenoid
2 Orbital surface of
   zygomatic bone
3 Inferior orbital fissure
4 Infra-orbital groove
5 Infra-orbital foramen
6 Opening of nasolacrimal
   canal
7 Superior orbital fissure
8 Optic canal
9 Frontal notch
10 Supra-orbital notch

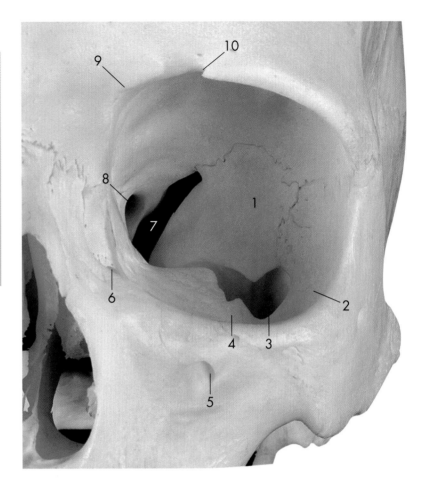

1.47 The medial wall of the orbit

1 Lesser wing of sphenoid
2 Zygomatic bone
3 Optic canal
4 Body of sphenoid
5 Orbital plate of ethmoid
6 Orbital surface of maxilla
7 Lacrimal bone
8 Posterior lacrimal crest
9 Fossa for lacrimal sac
10 Anterior lacrimal crest of
   maxilla
11 Anterior and posterior
   ethmoidal foramina
12 Orbital part of frontal bone
13 Zygomatic process of frontal
   bone

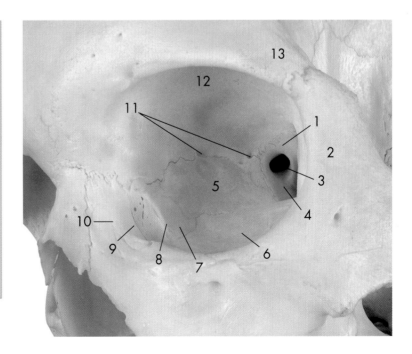

THE NASAL CAVITY (1.48, 1.49)

The nasal cavity is divided into two nasal fossae by a nasal septum. The external nose has a skeleton which is mainly cartilaginous (see page 192). Each nasal fossa has a roof, a floor, a lateral wall and a medial wall.

The medial wall is formed by the nasal septum (see page 194). It is composed of the septal cartilage anteriorly, the perpendicular plate of the ethmoid bone posterosuperiorly and the vomer postero-inferiorly. At the base of the nasal septum is the nasal crest formed by the maxillary and palatine bones.

The bones that comprise the remaining walls of the nasal fossa are the ethmoid, frontal, lacrimal, maxillary, nasal, palatine, sphenoid, and vomer bones and the bone of the inferior concha.

The roof of the nasal fossa is formed centrally by the cribriform plate of the ethmoid bone. Anteriorly lies the nasal bone and the nasal spine of the frontal bone. Posteriorly is located the body of the sphenoid overlapped by the ala of the vomer and the sphenoidal process of the palatine bone. The cribriform plate transmits olfactory nerves into the roof of the nasal cavity and also the anterior ethmoidal nerves and vessels.

The floor of the nasal fossa is formed by the palatine process of the maxilla anteriorly and the horizontal plate of the palatine bone posteriorly.

The lateral wall of the nasal fossa consists mainly of the medial surface of the maxilla, with the large maxillary hiatus being reduced in size by the overlapping of the lacrimal and ethmoid bones above, the palatine bone behind and the inferior concha below. From the lateral wall project the three nasal conchae. The superior and middle conchae are part of the labyrinth of the ethmoid bone. The inferior concha is a separate bone. The region above and behind the superior nasal concha is called the spheno-ethmoidal recess. The region between the superior and middle nasal conchae is the superior meatus. Between the middle and inferior conchae is located the middle meatus. Below the inferior nasal concha is the inferior meatus. The nasolacrimal canal on the lateral wall of the nasal fossa is formed by the lacrimal groove of the maxilla articulating with the descending process of the lacrimal bone and the lacrimal process of the inferior concha. The sphenopalatine foramen which links the nasal cavity with the pterygopalatine fossa lies high up in the posterior part of the lateral wall. It is formed by the notch between the orbital and sphenoidal processes of the perpendicular plate of the palatine bone articulating with the body of the sphenoid bone. This foramen transmits the nasopalatine and posterior superior nasal nerves and the sphenopalatine vessels.

The lateral wall of the nose is noted for being the site of drainage of the paranasal air sinuses. The sphenoidal sinus drains into the spheno-ethmoidal recess. The posterior ethmoidal air cells drain into the superior meatus. The frontal and maxillary air sinuses and the anterior and middle ethmoidal air cells drain into the middle meatus. The opening of the nasolacrimal canal lies in the inferior meatus.

1.48 The osteology of the lateral wall of the nose

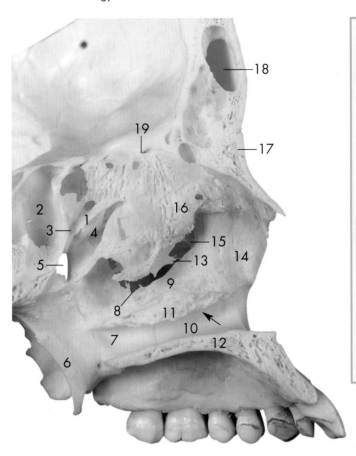

1 Superior concha
2 Sphenoidal sinus
3 Spheno-ethmoidal recess
4 Superior meatus
5 Sphenopalatine foramen
6 Medial pterygoid plate of sphenoid
7 Perpendicular plate of palatine bone
8 Opening of maxillary sinus
9 Middle meatus
10 Inferior meatus
11 Inferior concha
12 Hard palate
13 Uncinate process of ethmoid
14 Medial surface of maxilla
15 Hiatus semilinaris
16 Middle concha
17 Nasal bone
18 Frontal sinus
19 Cribriform plate of ethmoid

Arrow indicates position of opening of nasolacrimal canal

1.49 The osteology of the nasal septum

1 Cribriform plate of ethmoid
2 Frontal sinus
3 Nasal bone
4 Opening of incisive canal
5 Palatine process of maxilla
6 Horizontal process of palatine bone
7 Vomer
8 Perpendicular plate of ethmoid
9 Sphenoidal sinus
10 Body of sphenoid

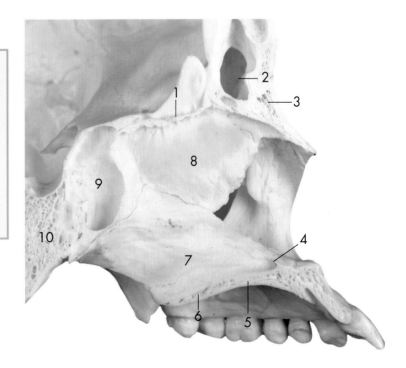

The posterior nasal apertures (choanae) link the nasal fossae with the nasopharynx. The bones which contribute to this region are the palatine, sphenoid and vomer bones. The posterior border of the vomer separates the two posterior nasal apertures. Each aperture is bounded below by the posterior border of the horizontal plate of the palatine bone, laterally by the medial pterygoid plate, and above by the body and vaginal process of the sphenoid bone and the ala of the vomer. A groove on the lower surface of the vaginal process of the sphenoid bone is converted into the palatovaginal canal by articulation with the upper surface of the sphenoidal process of the palatine bone. This canal transmits the pharyngeal branch of the pterygopalatine ganglion and the pharyngeal branch of the maxillary artery. The vomerovaginal canal lies between the upper surface of the vaginal process of the sphenoid bone and the ala of the vomer. The pharyngeal branch of the sphenopalatine artery passes through this occasional canal.

THE BASE OF THE SKULL (1.9)

The cranial base has already been described in detail (see pages 18–25).

Internally lies the anterior, middle and posterior cranial fossae.

The floor of the anterior cranial fossa is formed by the orbital parts of the frontal bone, the cribriform plate and crista galli of the ethmoid bone, and the lesser wings and jugum of the sphenoid bone.

The middle cranial fossa consists of a central part formed by the body of the sphenoid bone, and right and left lateral parts each formed by the greater wing of the sphenoid and the squamous and petrous parts of the temporal bone.

The posterior cranial fossa is formed by the basilar, lateral, and squamous parts of the occipital bone, by the petrous parts of the temporal bones, by the mastoid angles of the parietal bones, and by the dorsum sellae and posterior part of the body of the sphenoid bone.

The external surface of the base of the skull can be subdivided into three zones: the anterior, intermediate and posterior zones.

The anterior zone comprises the hard palate and is formed by the palatine processes of the maxillae and the horizontal plates of the palatine bones (1.50).

The intermediate and posterior zones are formed by the sphenoid bone anteriorly, the occipital bone posteriorly and the petrous parts of the temporal bones laterally.

The numerous foramina associated with the cranial base are described on pages 18–23.

1.50 The osteology of the hard palate

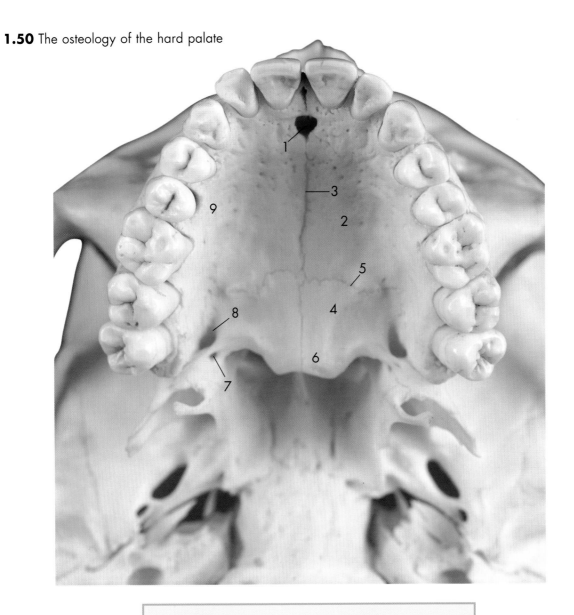

1 Incisive fossa
2 Palatine process of a maxillary bone
3 Median palatine suture
4 Horizontal plate of palatine bone
5 Transverse palatine suture
6 Posterior nasal spine
7 Lesser palatine foramen
8 Greater palatine foramen
9 Alveolus of a maxillary bone

THE PTERYGOPALATINE FOSSA (1.51, 1.52)

The pterygopalatine fossa lies between the infratemporal (posterior) surface of the maxilla and the pterygoid process of the sphenoid bone. It communicates with the infratemporal fossa through the pterygomaxillary fissure. The anterior wall of the fossa is the infratemporal surface of the maxilla. The posterior wall of the fossa is the pterygoid process. The medial wall is formed by the perpendicular plate of the palatine bone. The lateral wall shows the pterygomaxillary fissure. The pyramidal process of the palatine bone is situated inferiorly and articulates with the tuberosity of the maxilla. It fills the triangular gap between the lower ends of the medial and lateral pterygoid plates.

The pterygomaxillary fissure transmits the maxillary artery from the infratemporal fossa, the posterior superior alveolar branches of the maxillary division of the trigeminal nerve and the sphenopalatine veins. The fissure continues above with the posterior end of the inferior orbital fissure in the floor of the orbit. Passing through the inferior orbital fissure from the pterygopalatine fossa are the infra-orbital and zygomatic branches of the maxillary nerve, the orbital branches of the pterygopalatine ganglion and the infra-orbital blood vessels.

Entering the pterygopalatine fossa posteriorly are the foramen rotundum from the middle cranial fossa and the pterygoid canal from the region of the foramen lacerum at the base of the skull. The maxillary division of the trigeminal nerve passes through the foramen rotundum. The pterygoid canal transmits the nerve of the pterygoid canal (greater petrosal and deep petrosal nerves, see page 216) and an accompanying artery.

On the medial wall of the pterygopalatine fossa lies the sphenopalatine foramen. This foramen communicates with the nasal cavity. It transmits the nasopalatine and posterior superior nasal nerves (from the pterygopalatine ganglion) and the sphenopalatine vessels.

At the base of the pterygopalatine fossa, the greater and lesser palatine nerves (from the pterygopalatine ganglion), together with accompanying vessels, pass into the hard palate to emerge at the greater and lesser palatine foramina.

The full contents of the pterygopalatine fossa are described on page 210.

1.51 The pterygopalatine fossa

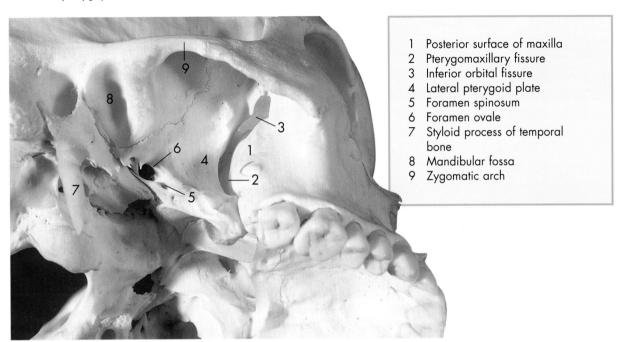

1	Posterior surface of maxilla
2	Pterygomaxillary fissure
3	Inferior orbital fissure
4	Lateral pterygoid plate
5	Foramen spinosum
6	Foramen ovale
7	Styloid process of temporal bone
8	Mandibular fossa
9	Zygomatic arch

1.52 The isolated sphenoid bone showing features related to the pterygopalatine fossa

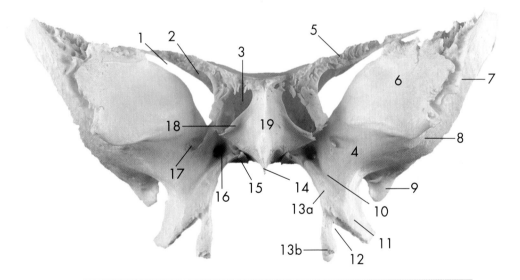

1	Superior orbital fissure	11	Lateral pterygoid plate
2	Optic canal	12	Pterygoid notch
3	Sphenoidal air sinus in body of sphenoid	13	Medial pterygoid plate (a) surmounted by pterygoid hamulus (b)
4	Maxillary surface of greater wing	14	Rostrum
5	Frontal margin of lesser wing	15	Vaginal process
6	Orbital surface of greater wing	16	Pterygoid canal
7	Temporal surface of greater wing	17	Foramen rotundum
8	Infratemporal crest of greater wing	18	Concha
9	Spine	19	Crest
10	Pterygoid process		

THE CERVICAL VERTEBRAE AND HYOID BONE

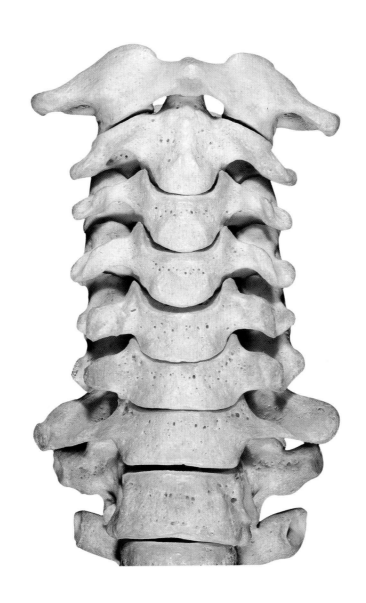

Chapter 2 THE CERVICAL VERTEBRAE AND HYOID BONE

The vertebral column forms that part of the skeleton known to the layman as the backbone or spine. Above, it supports the skull. Below, it gives attachment to the pelvic girdle which supports the lower limbs. To its thoracic component are attached the ribs. This part of the vertebral column is also associated with the pectoral girdles and the upper limbs. In addition to its obvious role in posture and locomotion, the vertebral column surrounds, and thus protects, the spinal cord.

The vertebral column is comprised of thirty-three bones, the vertebrae. There are seven cervical, twelve thoracic, five lumbar, five sacral and four coccygeal vertebrae. Whereas the cervical, thoracic and lumbar vertebrae are separate bones, the sacral and coccygeal vertebrae are fused. Between the bodies of individual vertebrae are the intervertebral discs.

The vertebral column exhibits four curvatures when viewed from the side. The cervical and lumbar curvatures are convex anteriorly. The thoracic and sacral curvatures are concave anteriorly. In the fetus, however, the vertebral column has a single curvature which is concave anteriorly. This is referred to as the primary curvature and is present throughout life in the thoracic and sacral regions. The development of the cervical curvature is associated with the ability of the baby to hold its head upright. The lumbar curvature develops later with standing and walking.

Of the seven cervical vertebrae, the lower five appear similar, although the seventh cervical vertebra has some distinctive features. The first cervical vertebra (atlas) and the second cervical vertebra (axis) show specialisations which are related to the articulation of the vertebral column with the skull (2.1).

2.1 Sagittal section of head showing cervical vertebrae

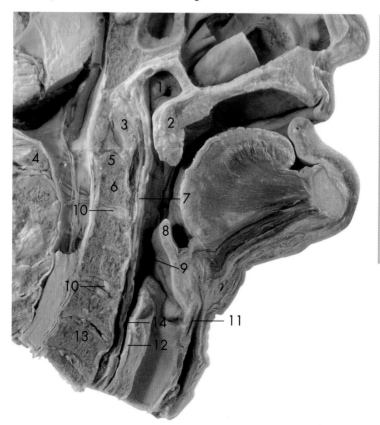

1 Eustachian tube
2 Soft palate
3 Anterior arch of atlas
4 Posterior arch of atlas
5 Dens of axis
6 Body of axis
7 Muscular wall of pharynx
8 Epiglottis
9 Inlet of larynx
10 Intervertebral disc
11 Thyroid cartilage
12 Lamina of cricoid cartilage
13 Body of sixth cervical vertebra
14 Retropharyngeal tissue space

2.2 The articulated cervical vertebrae, posterior aspect (cervical vertebrae numbered C1 to C7)

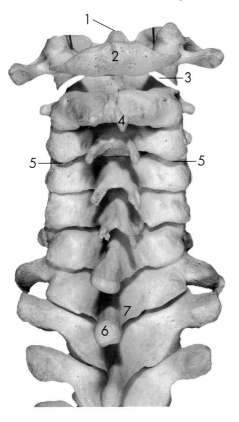

1	Dens of axis (C2)
2	Posterior arch of atlas (C1)
3	Lateral atlanto-axial joint
4	Bifid spine of axis (C2)
5	Zygopophysial joint
6	Spine of seventh cervical vertebra (non-bifid)
7	Lamina of seventh cervical vertebra

2.3 The articulated vertebrae, anterior aspect

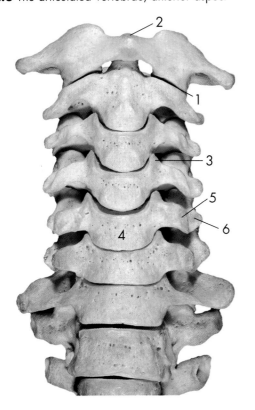

1	Lateral atlanto-axial joint
2	Tip of dens of axis (C2)
3	Lip or uncus of fourth cervical vertebra
4	Body of fifth cervical vertebra
5	Carotid tubercle of sixth cervical vertebra
6	Transverse process of sixth cervical vertebra

TYPICAL CERVICAL VERTEBRA (2.2–2.6)

The typical cervical vertebra (representing the third to the sixth cervical vertebrae) is comprised of two main components, a body anteriorly and a vertebral arch posteriorly. These components surround the vertebral foramen which houses the spinal cord.

The body is small compared with the body of a vertebra in other regions. It is nearly cylindrical, but is flattened anteroposteriorly. The anterior surface is convex, with depressions on either side for the attachments of the longus colli muscles. The posterior surface is flattened and forms the anterior wall of the vertebral foramen. This surface may exhibit one or more foramina related to basivertebral veins. The superior and inferior surfaces of the body are concave. The peripheries of these surfaces are smooth but centrally they are roughened. This difference relates to a difference in embryological origin (from the annular epiphysis peripherally and from the centrum centrally). The lower border of the vertebra anteriorly overlaps the upper border of the vertebra below. A lip or uncus is present at each side of the upper surface posteriorly.

The vertebral arch can be subdivided into several components. The arch is attached to the posterolateral aspects of the body by the pedicles which are directed backwards and outwards. The superior and inferior borders of the pedicles are notched. When adjacent vertebrae are articulated, the notches form intervertebral foramina for the passage of spinal nerves. Continuous with the pedicles are the laminae. These are thin, narrow plates of bone which are directed backwards and medially to fuse in the midline. Associated with the vertebral arch are seven processes: four articular processes, two transverse processes and a spine.

There are two superior and two inferior articular processes.

They project from the junctions between the pedicles and laminae. The articular facets of the superior processes face backwards and upwards, whereas the facets of the inferior processes face downwards and forwards.

The transverse processes are small. They project laterally and are situated just anterior to the articular processes. The most characteristic feature of the transverse process of a cervical vertebra is the presence of the foramen transversarium. This foramen is circular and transmits the vertebral vessels. The foramen subdivides the transverse process into three parts: anterior and posterior roots joined laterally by a costotransverse bar. The free extremities of the anterior and posterior roots project as the anterior and posterior tubercles. The anterior tubercle is particularly prominent for the sixth cervical vertebra. It is termed the carotid tubercle since the adjacent internal carotid artery can be compressed against it. Within the groove between the anterior and posterior tubercles lies the ventral rami of a cervical spinal nerve. The anterior tubercle and the costotransverse bar comprise the costal element of the vertebra. Occasionally, this may be sufficiently well-developed to produce a small cervical rib.

The spine is short and projects backwards in the midline where the two laminae meet. It is bifid and each projection terminates as a tubercle. The spines and laminae of the fifth and sixth cervical vertebrae are directed downwards as well as backwards.

The vertebral foramen cervically is triangular in outline and larger than in other regions of the vertebral column. When vertebrae are articulated to form the vertebral column, the serial vertebral foramina constitute the vertebral canal.

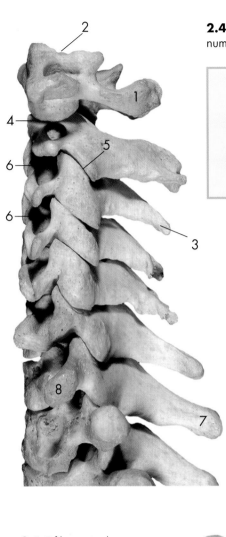

2.4 The articulated cervical vertebrae, lateral aspect (cervical vertebrae numbered C1 to C7)

1 Posterior arch of atlas (C1)	6 Intervertebral foramen
2 Tip of dens of axis (C2)	7 Spine of seventh cervical
3 Spine of third cervical	vertebra
vertebra	8 Transverse process of
4 Lateral atlanto-axial joint	seventh cervical vertebra
5 Zygopophysial joint	

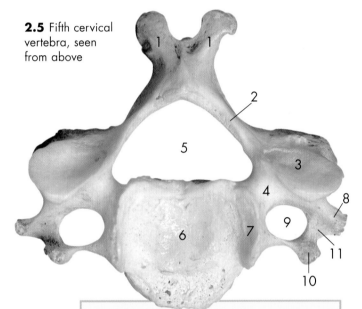

2.5 Fifth cervical vertebra, seen from above

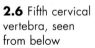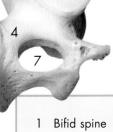

2.6 Fifth cervical vertebra, seen from below

1 Bifid spine
2 Lamina
3 Superior articular process
4 Pedicle
5 Triangular outline of vertebral foramen
6 Body
7 Lip or uncus of body
8 Posterior tubercle of transverse process
9 Foramen transversarium
10 Anterior tubercle of transverse process
11 Groove for spinal nerve

1 Bifid spine	5 Vertebral foramen
2 Lamina	6 Body
3 Inferior articular process	7 Foramen transversarium
4 Pedicle	in transverse process

SEVENTH CERVICAL VERTEBRA (2.7, 2.8)

This vertebra has the largest spine of any cervical vertebra. The spine is directed downwards and, as it is readily palpated, the vertebra has been termed the vertebra prominens. The spine is not bifid, but is thickened and terminates in a single tubercle. The transverse processes are larger than those of the other cervical vertebrae. The foramen transversarium is not circular but is oval. The main vertebral vessels do not pass through this foramen. Instead, it usually transmits an accessory vertebral vein. The posterior tubercle of the transverse process is particularly prominent and gives attachment to the suprapleural membrane. If there is a cervical rib, it is almost always associated with the seventh cervical vertebra.

FIRST CERVICAL VERTEBRA (2.9, 2.10)

The first cervical vertebra can also be termed the atlas. It is the vertebra which articulates with the skull. Unlike the other vertebrae, it does not have a body, this being incorporated into the second cervical vertebra as the dens. There is also no spine. The atlas takes the form of a thin ring of bone with anterior and posterior arches. Between the arches are situated the lateral masses. These show the articular facets and the transverse processes.

The anterior arch of the atlas is only slightly curved. There is an anterior tubercle at the midpoint of its anterior surface. On its posterior surface is an oval facet for articulation with the dens.

The posterior arch of the atlas has a pronounced curvature. There is a posterior tubercle at the midpoint of its posterior surface. The superior surface of the posterior arch shows grooves just behind the lateral masses. These grooves are related to the vertebral arteries as they wind around the lateral masses before entering the cranial cavity through the foramen magnum. The dorsal rami of the first cervical nerves also lie in these grooves.

Each lateral mass has articular facets on both the superior and inferior surfaces. The superior articular facet is oval and concave. It faces upwards and inwards to articulate with an occipital condyle. The inferior articular facet is flat. It faces downwards and inwards and articulates with the facet of a superior articular process of the second cervical vertebra. The posterior surface of the lateral mass is grooved above the level of the posterior arch by the vertebral artery as it passes backwards and inwards from the foramen transversarium. A small tubercle may be present on the inner surface of the lateral mass. This is the site of attachment of the transverse ligament of the atlas.

The transverse processes of the atlas are large and they project further laterally than all but the seventh cervical vertebra. Each process ends in a single, prominent tubercle. This tubercle is homologous with the posterior tubercle of the other cervical vertebrae. The foramen transversarium is slightly oval.

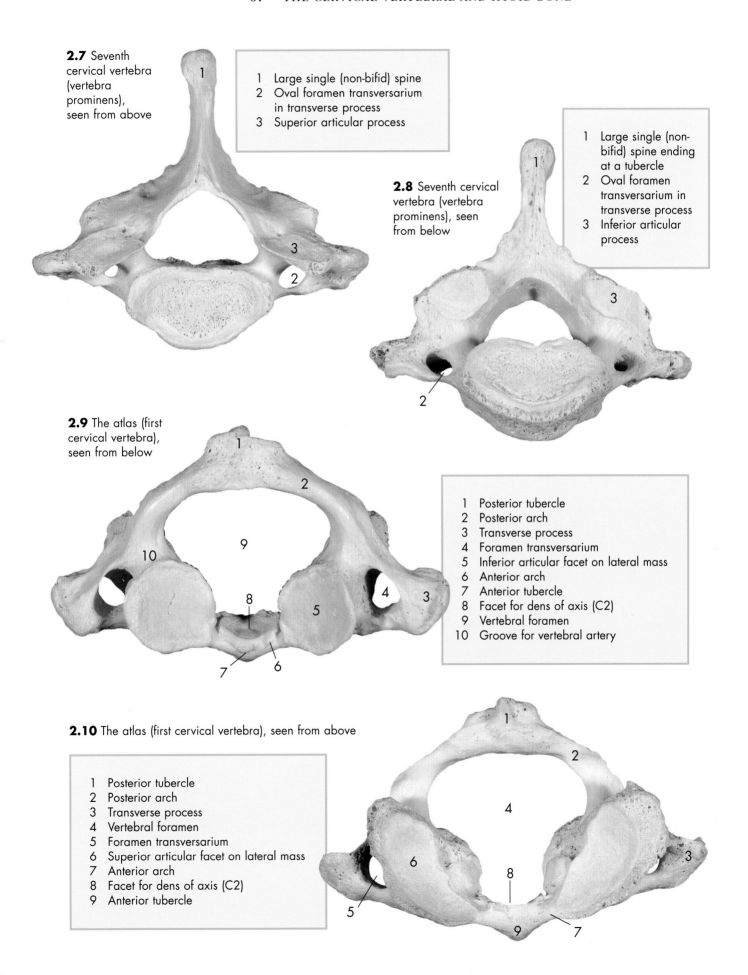

2.7 Seventh cervical vertebra (vertebra prominens), seen from above

1 Large single (non-bifid) spine
2 Oval foramen transversarium in transverse process
3 Superior articular process

2.8 Seventh cervical vertebra (vertebra prominens), seen from below

1 Large single (non-bifid) spine ending at a tubercle
2 Oval foramen transversarium in transverse process
3 Inferior articular process

2.9 The atlas (first cervical vertebra), seen from below

1 Posterior tubercle
2 Posterior arch
3 Transverse process
4 Foramen transversarium
5 Inferior articular facet on lateral mass
6 Anterior arch
7 Anterior tubercle
8 Facet for dens of axis (C2)
9 Vertebral foramen
10 Groove for vertebral artery

2.10 The atlas (first cervical vertebra), seen from above

1 Posterior tubercle
2 Posterior arch
3 Transverse process
4 Vertebral foramen
5 Foramen transversarium
6 Superior articular facet on lateral mass
7 Anterior arch
8 Facet for dens of axis (C2)
9 Anterior tubercle

SECOND CERVICAL VERTEBRA (2.11, 2.12)

The second cervical vertebra is also called the axis. It can be distinguished from the other cervical vertebrae by the presence of a tooth-like process called the dens (odontoid process). The dens projects upwards in the midline from the anterior surface of the body. It articulates with the facet on the posterior surface of the anterior arch of the atlas. Rotation of the head occurs at this joint.

The body of the axis resembles the bodies of the other cervical vertebrae. The anterior overlap of the inferior border, and the depressions associated with the longus colli muscles, are especially prominent. The dens originates from the middle of the upper surface of the body of the axis. The tip of the dens is termed the apex and is the site of attachment of the apical ligament. The anterior surface of the dens bears a convex facet which articulates with the facet on the anterior arch of the atlas. The lateral surfaces slope downwards and outwards and give attachment to alar ligaments. The posterior surface of the dens, near its connection with the body, is grooved by the transverse ligament of the atlas.

The pedicles and laminae of the axis are thicker than those of the other cervical vertebrae. There are no superior vertebral notches on the pedicles. The laminae meet posteriorly in a relatively broad, bifid spine. Unlike the lower cervical vertebrae, the articular processes of the axis do not lie in the same plane. The superior articular processes are located anterior to the inferior processes. The superior articular facets are larger than those of the lower cervical vertebrae and they point in a different direction, facing upwards and slightly outwards. In addition, they are situated anterior and medial to the foramina transversaria. Because of the absence of superior vertebral notches, the superior articular processes extend over the lateral surfaces of the body of the axis towards the base of the dens. The inferior articular processes are similar to those of the lower cervical vertebrae.

The transverse processes of the axis are small. Each ends laterally in a single tubercle which is homologous with the posterior tubercle on a lower cervical vertebra. Because the vertebral vessels pass outwards as well as upwards to reach the foramen transversarium of the atlas, the foramen transversarium in the axis is directed upwards and outwards.

The following muscles are attached to the cervical vertebrae (from above downwards):

- Rectus capitis anterior
- Rectus capitis lateralis
- Rectus capitis posterior minor
- Superior
- Oblique scalenus medius
- Splenius cervicis
- Levator scapulae
- Intertransverse rectus capitis
- Posterior major semispinalis cervicis
- Spinalis cervicis
- Semispinalis thoracis
- Multifidis interspinalis
- Scalenus anterior
- Scalenus posterior
- Longus capitis
- Longus colli
- Longissimus cervicis and capitis iliocostalis cervicis
- Trapezius
- Rhomboideus minor
- Serratus posterior
- Superior scalenus
- Minimus levatores costarum

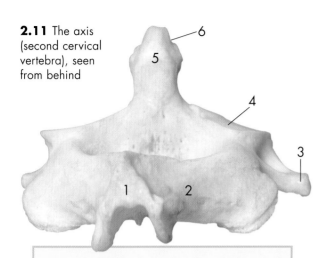

2.11 The axis (second cervical vertebra), seen from behind

1   Spine (bifid)
2   Lamina
3   Transverse process
4   Superior articular process
5   Posterior articular surface of dens
6   Impression for alar ligament

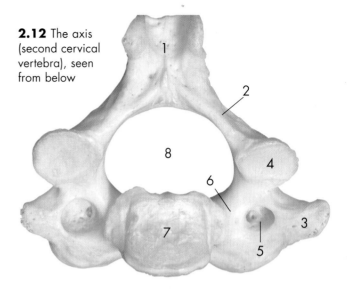

2.12 The axis (second cervical vertebra), seen from below

1   Bifid spine
2   Lamina
3   Transverse process
4   Inferior articular process
5   Foramen transversarium
6   Pedicle
7   Body
8   Vertebral foramen

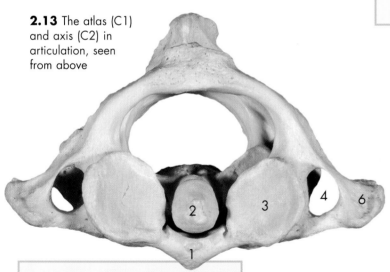

2.13 The atlas (C1) and axis (C2) in articulation, seen from above

1   Anterior tubercle and arch of atlas
2   Dens of axis
3   Superior articular facet on lateral mass of atlas
4   Foramen transversarium of atlas
5   Posterior arch of atlas
6   Transverse process

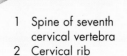

2.14 Lateral view of seventh cervical vertebra possessing a cervical rib

1   Spine of seventh cervical vertebra
2   Cervical rib
3   True first rib

JOINTS OF THE CERVICAL VERTEBRAE

JOINTS BETWEEN THE VERTEBRAL BODIES (2.15, 2.17–2.19)

With the exception of the atlas which lacks a body, the bodies of the cervical vertebrae are joined by secondary cartilaginous joints (symphyses). The intervening fibrocartilaginous discs are termed the intervertebral discs. These discs increase the stability and strength of the vertebral column and act as shock absorbers. They are thicker anteriorly, conforming to the curvature of the cervical part of the spine. Each disc has a central gelatinous mass termed the nucleus pulposus and a peripheral fibrous ring called the annulus fibrosus. The annulus fibrosus is attached to the smooth peripheral region of the vertebral body. The nucleus pulposus joins with the roughened central region lined by hyaline cartilage.

The joints are strengthened by anterior and posterior longitudinal ligaments. These run in the midline along the anterior and posterior surfaces of the bodies of the vertebrae. They are attached to the intervertebral discs. The anterior longitudinal ligament is stronger and is attached above to the anterior tubercle of the atlas and to the basilar part of the occipital bone. The posterior longitudinal ligament runs inside the vertebral canal and is attached above to the body of the axis.

JOINTS BETWEEN THE VERTEBRAL ARCHES (2.16, 2.18, 2.19)

The articular facets of adjacent vertebrae are united by synovial joints. Concerning the ligaments associated with the vertebral arches, passing between adjacent laminae is the ligamentum flavum. This is composed primarily of elastic fibres. Whereas the tips of the spinous processes in other parts of the vertebral column are joined by interspinous and supraspinous ligaments, these are poorly developed in the cervical region and the ligamentum nuchae is present. This is a triangular fibro-elastic septum which lies between the postvertebral muscles in the midline. Its posterior border extends from the external occipital protuberance to the spine of the seventh cervical vertebra. Its anterior border is attached to the spines of the cervical vertebrae and to the posterior tubercle of the atlas. Its superior border is attached to the external occipital crest.

2.15 The cervical vertebral column *in situ,* seen in a sagittal section

1 Anterior margin of foramen magnum
2 Cervical spinal cord
3 Anterior arch of atlas
4 Dens of axis
5 Body of axis
6 Intervertebral disc
7 Anterior longitudinal ligament
8 Posterior longitudinal ligament

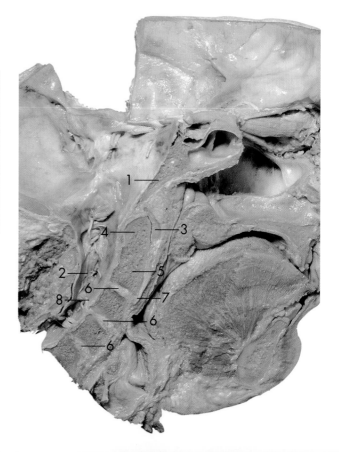

2.16 The cervical vertebral column, posterior aspect (cervical vertebrae numbered)

1 Ligamentum flavum
2 Supraspinous ligament

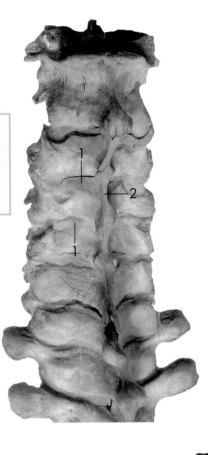

2.17 The cervical vertebral column, anterior aspect (cervical vertebrae numbered)

1 Anterior longitudinal ligament

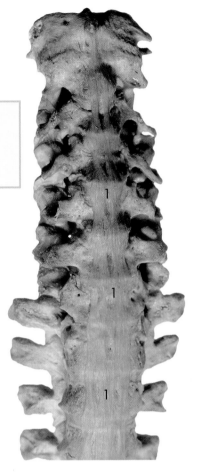

2.18 The cervical vertebral column, lateral aspect (cervical vertebrae numbered)

1 Interspinous ligament
2 Supraspinous ligament
3 Anterior longitudinal ligament

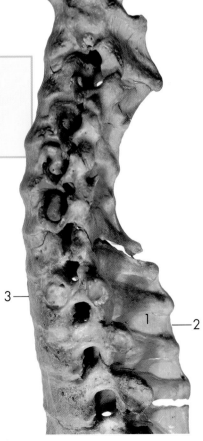

ATLANTO-AXIAL JOINTS (2.13, 2.19–2.21)

These joints differ from the joints between the other cervical vertebrae because of the absence of a body for the atlas and the presence of the dens on the axis. There is no intervertebral disc. In front, the body of the axis is joined to the anterior tubercle of the atlas by the anterior longitudinal ligament. The inferior articular facets of the atlas articulate with the superior articular facets of the axis at the lateral atlanto-axial joints.

Another synovial joint is present in the midline between the articular facet on the anterior surface of the dens of the axis and the articular facet on the posterior surface of the anterior arch of the atlas. This joint is the median atlanto-axial joint. The dens is held in position by the transverse ligament of the atlas. This ligament is attached on either side of the dens to the small tubercles on the lateral masses of the atlas. The posterior articular surface of the dens forms a synovial joint with the cartilage-covered, anterior surface of the transverse ligament. Sometimes this joint is continuous with the joint cavity of one of the lateral atlanto-axial joints. Vertical extensions from the transverse ligament pass upwards and downwards in the midline. The upward extension is called the superior longitudinal band and is attached to the inner surface of the anterior margin of the foramen magnum. The downward extension is the inferior longitudinal band. This is attached to the posterior surface of the body of the axis. Because of the cross-shaped appearance of the transverse ligament and its vertical extensions, it is referred to as the cruciform ligament. Viewed posteriorly, the cruciform ligament is covered by an upward continuation of the posterior longitudinal ligament which is termed the membrana tectoria. This membrane is attached to the inner surface of the anterior margin of the foramen magnum.

The dens is further stabilised by three ligaments which run to the occipital bone. These are the apical ligament and the two alar ligaments. As the name indicates, the apical ligament arises from the apex of the dens. It passes vertically upwards to be attached to the anterior margin of the foramen magnum (in front of the superior longitudinal band of the cruciform ligament). Each alar ligament arises from the side of the upper part of the dens. It passes upwards and outwards to be inserted onto the medial surface of the occipital condyle.

ATLANTO-OCCIPITAL JOINTS (2.19)

The superior articular facets on the lateral masses of the atlas articulate with the occipital condyles at the atlanto-occipital joints. The upper border of the anterior arch of the atlas is connected to the anterior margin of the foramen magnum by the anterior atlanto-occipital membrane. An upward extension from the anterior longitudinal ligament of the vertebral column runs in front of the membrane to the basilar part of the occipital bone. A posterior atlanto-occipital membrane passes between the upper border of the posterior arch of the atlas and the posterior border of the foramen magnum. Between the lateral margins of the membrane and the lateral masses of the atlas pass the vertebral arteries and the first cervical nerves.

2.19 Median sagittal section through the base of the skull and the upper cervical vertebrae to illustrate some of the vertebral joints and ligaments

1 Ligamentum flavum
2 Ligamentum nuchae
3 Posterior atlanto-occipital membrane
4 Opening for vertebral artery
5 Membrana tectoria
6 Apical ligament of dens
7 Anterior atlanto-occipital membrane
8 Superior longitudinal band of cruciform ligament
9 Anterior arch of atlas
10 Synovial joints of dens
11 Transverse ligament of atlas
12 Inferior longitudinal band of cruciform ligament
13 Anulus fibrosus – intervertebral disc
14 Nucleus pulposus – intervertebral disc
15 Hyaline cartilage
16 Anterior longitudinal ligament
17 Posterior longitudinal ligament

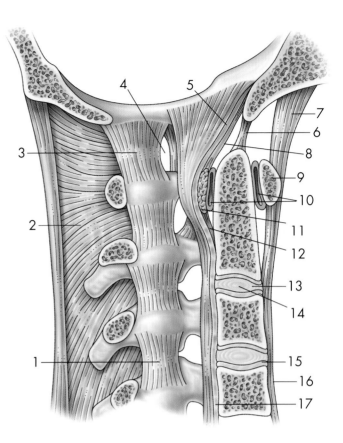

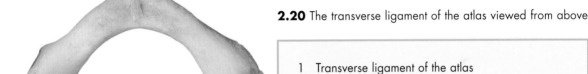

2.20 The transverse ligament of the atlas viewed from above

1 Transverse ligament of the atlas
2 Anterior arch of atlas

21.1 The atlanto-axial joint viewed posteriorly

1 Inferior longitudinal band of cruciform ligament
2 Transverse ligament of atlas
3 Superior longitudinal band of cruciform ligament
4 Alar ligament
5 Posterior longitudinal ligament
6 Transverse process of atlas

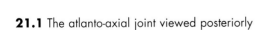

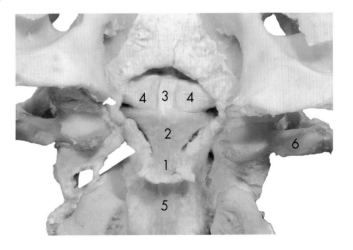

VASCULATURE OF THE CERVICAL VERTEBRAL COLUMN (2.22–2.24)

The cervical vertebrae derive their arterial supply from the vertebral arteries, with spinal branches passing through the intervertebral foramina to enter the vertebral canal (2.22, 2.23).

The veins associated with the cervical vertebrae are situated in two rich plexuses, one external and one internal. The plexuses freely intercommunicate both locally and with other parts of the vertebral column to form a series of venous rings at the level of each vertebra and particularly around the foramen magnum. The external vertebral venous plexus is located on both the anterior surface of the bodies (anterior external vertebral plexus) and on the posterior surfaces of the vertebral arches (posterior external vertebral plexus). The internal vertebral venous plexus lies between the meninges surrounding the spinal cord and the wall of the vertebral canal. It forms a complete ring around the vertebral canal and can be subdivided into a pair of anterior and a pair of posterior plexuses. Passing out from foramina on the posterior surfaces of the bodies of the vertebrae are basivertebral veins. These drain into the anterior part of the internal vertebral venous plexus. The basivertebral veins are also connected to the anterior external plexus by veins passing through the vertebral bodies. Intervertebral veins passing through the intervertebral foramina link the vertebral plexuses to veins in other regions. The vertebral veins are valveless. Leaving the foramen transversarium of the sixth cervical vertebra, it runs anterolateral to the vertebral artery and subclavian vein to drain usually into the brachiocephalic vein. An accessory vertebral vein usually runs through the foramen transversarium of the seventh cervical vertebra, also draining into the brachiocephalic vein.

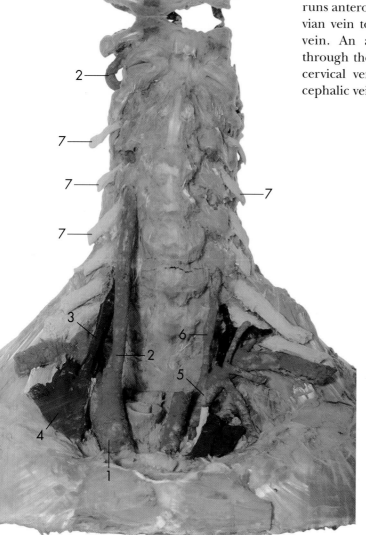

2.22 Root of the neck and anterior surface of the vertebral column showing the vertebral vessels and the cervical spinal nerves

1	Right subclavian artery
2	Right vertebral artery
3	Right vertebral vein
4	Right subclavian vein
5	Left subclavian artery
6	Left vertebral artery
7	Cervical spinal nerves

2.23 Cervical part of vertebral column viewed posterior to show course of upper part of vertebral artery

1 Transverse process of atlas
2 Vertebral artery lying in groove on posterior arch of atlas
3 Posterior arch of atlas
4 Spinal cord
5 Dens of atlas
6 Posterior (dorsal) ramus of second cervical spinal nerve

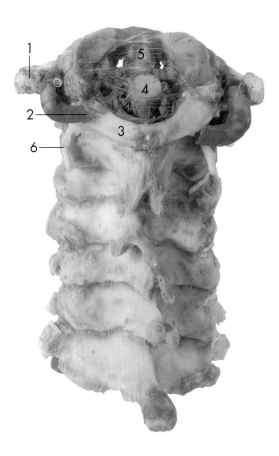

2.24 The veins associated with the cervical vertebrae

1 Anterior and posterior internal vertebral venous plexuses
2 Posterior external vertebral venous plexus
3 Intervertebral vein
4 Anterior external vertebral venous plexus
5 Basivertebral vein

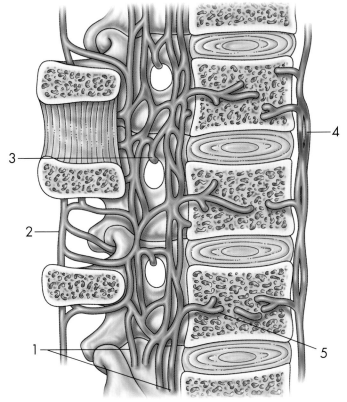

THE HYOID BONE (2.25)

The hyoid bone is situated in the upper part of the front of the neck, just posterior to and a little below the inferior border of the chin. It lies at the level of the third cervical vertebra. The bone is horseshoe-shaped and consists of a central body spanning the midline, with greater and lesser horns on each side.

The body of the hyoid bone is quadrilateral. It is curved such that its anterior surface appears convex viewed from the front. A vertical median ridge is frequently present on the anterior surface. Transverse ridges may also be found. The posterior surface is smooth and concave.

The greater horns of the hyoid bone project backwards from the lateral margins of the body. At their posterior tips, they end in tubercles.

The lesser horns of the hyoid bone are very small. They project upwards at the junctions between the body and the greater horns. The union of the lesser horns with the rest of the hyoid bone may be osseous. In most instances, however, they are connected by fibrous tissue (occasionally by synovial joints).

The hyoid bone is maintained in its position by means of the considerable number of muscles, ligaments and membranes attached to it. The muscles attached to the hyoid bone are:

- Genioglossus

- Geniohyoid

- Hyoglossus (and chondroglossus)

- Middle constrictor of pharynx

- Mylohyoid

- Omohyoid

- Sternohyoid

- Stylohyoid

- Thyrohyoid

The hyoid bone is suspended from the styloid processes of the temporal bones by the stylohyoid ligaments. These ligaments are attached to the lesser horns. The thyrohyoid membrane passes from the superior border of the thyroid cartilage of the larynx to the upper and posterior surface of the hyoid bone. A bursa intervenes between the membrane and the bone. There is also a hyo-epiglottic ligament which connects with the anterior surface of the epiglottis.

2.25 Lateral oblique view of the hyoid bone

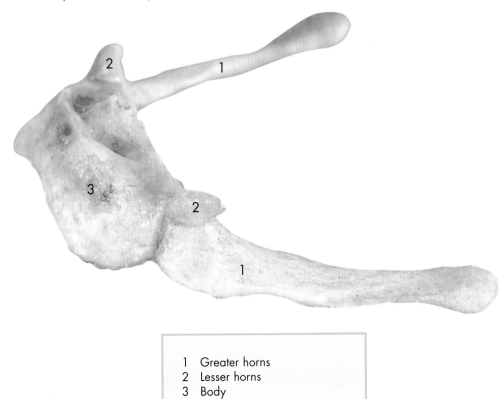

1   Greater horns
2   Lesser horns
3   Body

chapter 3
THE FACE

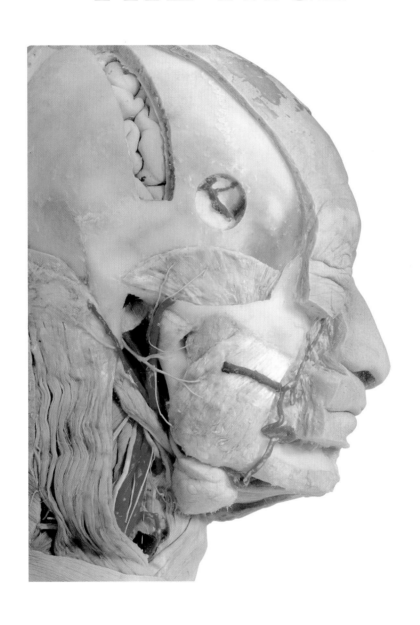

Chapter 3 THE FACE

The face lies anterior to the auricles and extends from the hair margin to the chin. Its main functions are related to the presence of many of the organs of special sense and to two prominent openings, the oral and nasal apertures, which mark the entrances to the digestive and respiratory tracts. The face also plays an important role in communication, being concerned with both speech and facial expression. Furthermore, each individual is recognised by the idiosyncratic variations in the shape of the face.

SURFACE MARKINGS OF THE FACE (3.1–3.3)

The shape of the face relies not only upon the form of the facial skeleton but also upon the disposition of the soft tissues. The skin creases depend upon the arrangement of the underlying facial muscles and within the cheek there may be a prominent mass of fat (the buccal pad of fat).

The essential surface anatomy of the face is familiar. For descriptive convenience, the face is usually subdivided into: the forehead, the temporal region, the orbital region, the external nose, the cheek, the oral region and chin.

The forehead extends from the hair margin to the eyebrows and is a region common to both the face and the scalp. It is relatively featureless. On each side, about half-way up, the forehead sometimes appears bossed (corresponding to the frontal tuberosities of the frontal bone). There are a variable number of long, transverse creases in the skin which become particularly prominent when expressing surprise or fright. Between the eyebrows lies a small elevation termed the glabella. Vertical wrinkles are produced here when frowning.

The temporal region is situated on the lateral aspect of the face, in front of the external ear and above the zygomatic arch of the cheek. It is demarcated superiorly by the temporal crest. This crest indicates the upper limit of the temporalis muscle. The muscle becomes obvious when the teeth are clenched. The skin of the temple closest to the ear is particularly hirsute and is sometimes referred to as the 'beard part of the temple'. The region in front of this may consequently be called the 'non-beard part of the temple'. The superficial temporal vessels are often visible here, especially in the elderly.

The orbital region is bounded by the bony rim of the orbit which can be readily palpated around its entire extent. A supra-orbital notch may be located on the upper or supra-orbital margin, marking the site of exit of the supra-orbital nerve and vessels onto the forehead. A frontal notch may also be found towards the bridge of the nose. This is associated with the supratrochlear nerve and vessels. Above the supra-orbital margin is the eyebrow.

Protecting the front of the eye are the eyelids (superior and inferior palpebrae), the upper eyelid being larger and more mobile. The interval between the eyelids is termed the palpebral fissure. Extending from the margins of the eyelids are the eyelashes (cilia). The eyelashes are arranged in two or three rows. Near the attachment of the eyelashes lie the openings of a series of glands. The lower eyelid may be everted to reveal its inner surface which is normally red and vascular. The upper eyelid cannot be everted readily, sufficiently to reveal the superior fornix. Tarsal glands may be visualised as yellowish streaks on the inner surfaces of both eyelids. The lateral and medial angles of the eyelids are referred to as the lateral (or outer) and medial (or inner) canthi. The lateral canthus is relatively featureless.

3.1 Surface markings on the face

1	Glabella
2	Zygomatic arch
3	Supra-orbital notch
4	Frontal notch
5	Upper eyelid
6	Lower eyelid
7	Medical canthus
8	Root of nose
9	Dorsum of nose
10	Apex of nose

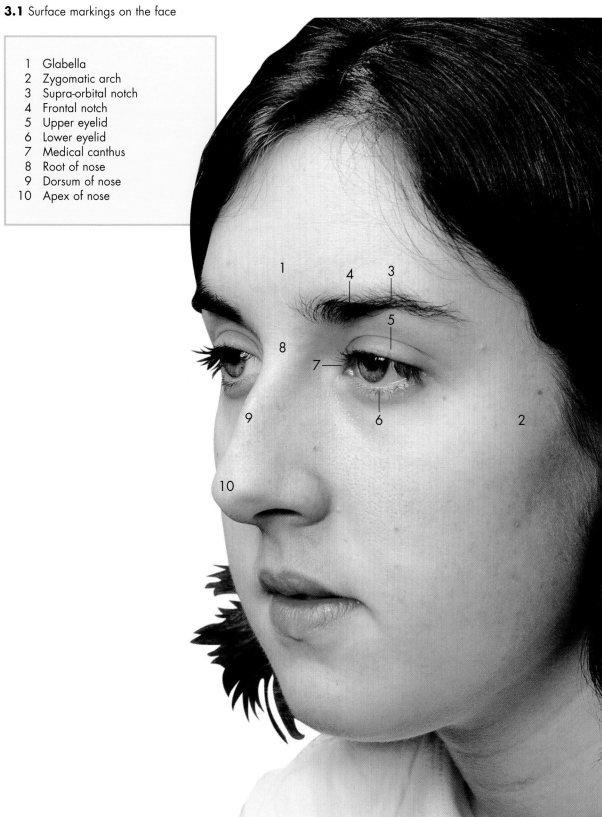

The medial canthus shows a number of features. The medial canthus is separated from the eyeball by a small triangular space, the lacrimal lake (lacus lacrimalis). Here also lies a small, reddish body containing sebaceous and sweat glands, the lacrimal caruncle. Lateral to the caruncle is the plica semilunaris, a fold of conjunctiva believed by some to be a vestige of the nictitating membrane of other animals. The medial end of each lid margin has no eyelashes. In this region lies a small elevation (the lacrimal papilla) on which is found a fine opening termed the punctum lacrimale. The punctum opens into the lacrimal canaliculus through which tears from the lacrimal lake pass into the lacrimal sac. The anterior surface of the eyeball shows many features. The peripheral part is the relatively avascular sclera, forming the 'white of the eye'. The sclera is seen through the thin, mucous membrane layer (bulbar conjunctiva) which contains a fine vascular network. The sclera becomes transparent over the central portion of the eye as the cornea. The boundary between the sclera and cornea is called the sclerocorneal junction or limbus. The dark, circular, central opening is the pupil. Surrounding the pupil is the iris. The iris acts as a diaphragm which controls the size of the pupil. Its colour depends on the amount and distribution of pigment.

The external nose is essentially pyramidal in shape. Superiorly, it is confluent with the forehead at the root of the nose where it is supported by the nasal bones at the bridge. This part of the nose is immobile. Inferiorly, the tip of the nose is termed the apex. The ridge connecting the root and apex is referred to as the dorsum of the nose. The apex and the dorsum are supported by cartilage and are mobile. The nostrils (anterior or external nares) are separated by a septum which joins the apex of the nose to the philtrum of the upper lip. The nostrils lead into the nasal vestibule. Here, the skin is characterised by having coarse hairs. The flared, lateral margins of the nose are known as the alae. The nasolabial grooves of the upper lip continue around the alae to form alar grooves.

The cheek is an extensive area of the face below the temporal region. It can be subdivided into two. There is an upper and anterior region overlying the bone of the zygomatic arch and body of the maxilla, and a lower and posterior region overlying the buccinator muscle, the ramus of the mandible and the parotid gland. The masseter muscle, parotid duct and condyle of the mandible may be visualised and/or palpated.

The oral region presents the red zone of the lip (the vermilion) which is a characteristic of man. The sharp junction of the red zone and the skin is termed the vermilion border. In the upper lip, the red zone protrudes in the midline to form the tubercle. The lower lip shows a slight depression in the midline corresponding to the tubercle. In passing from the midline to the corners of the mouth, the lips widen and then narrow. Laterally, the upper lip is separated from the cheeks by nasolabial grooves. With age, similar grooves appear at the corners of the mouth delineating the lower lip from the cheeks (labiomarginal sulci). A labiomental groove separates the lower lip from the chin. In the midline, running from the upper lip to the septum of the nose is the philtrum. The corners of the lips (labial commissures) are usually located at the level of the maxillary canine and mandibular first premolar teeth. The lips exhibit sexual dimorphism; as a general rule the skin of the male is thicker, firmer, more hirsute, but is less mobile.

The chin is also a facial feature characteristic of man. It forms a distinct protuberance in the midline of the lower jaw. Passing laterally from the chin, the inferior border of the mandible is readily discernible. Where the anterior border of the masseter meets the lower border of the mandible, the facial vessels are to be found. The junction of the posterior and inferior borders of the mandible is termed the angle of the mandible.

3.2 Surface features of the right eye

1	Medial canthus
2	Lacrimal caruncle
3	Plica semilnaris
4	Lacrimal papilla
5	Sclera
6	Sclerocorneal junction (limbus)
7	Pupil
8	Iris

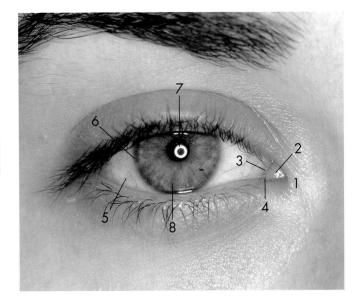

3.3 Surface features of the mouth and nose

1	Dorsum of nose
2	Apex of nose
3	Nostril
4	Ala of nose
5	Nasolabial groove
6	Vermillion zone
7	Tubercle of upper lip
8	Labiomarginal sulcus
9	Labiomental groove
10	Philtrum
11	Chin

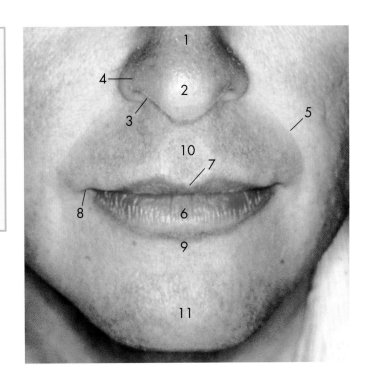

SUPERFICIAL STRUCTURES OF THE FACE

On reflecting the skin of the face, the following main structures are revealed:

- Muscles of facial expression

- Facial nerve

- Cutaneous branches of the trigeminal nerve and the great auricular nerve

- Facial and superficial temporal vessels

- Parotid gland and duct

- Buccal pad of fat

- Facial lymph nodes

MUSCLES OF FACIAL EXPRESSION

The face differs from most regions of the body in not having a deep membranous fascia beneath the skin. Instead, many small slips of muscle are attached to the facial skeleton and insert into the skin. These muscles cause movement of the facial skin to reflect emotions. The muscles are grouped mainly around the orifices of the face. Indeed, it can be argued that their primary function is to act as sphincters and dilators of the facial orifices and that the function of facial expression has developed secondarily.

The muscles of facial expression vary considerably between individuals in terms of size, shape and strength. In many instances, the names given to the muscles describe their actions. Muscles of facial expression not only lie in the face, but also in the scalp (occipitofrontalis, see page 150) and in the neck (platysma, see page 322).

THE ORBITAL GROUP (3.4)

The chief muscle is orbicularis oculi; its fibres run circumferentially around the orbit and within the eyelids. In addition, there is the corrugator supercilii muscle.

The orbicularis oculi muscle

Attachments: This muscle is composed of three parts, the orbital, palpebral and lacrimal.

The orbital part is the largest and extends onto the face some distance beyond the orbital rim. It arises from three sites: from the nasal part of the frontal bone, from the frontal process of the maxilla and, between these two sites, from the medial palpebral ligament. The fibres then pass around the orbit in concentric loops.

The palpebral part is the central part and is confined to the eyelids. It arises mainly from the medial palpebral ligament and runs across the eyelids (in front of the tarsal plates) to insert into the lateral palpebral raphe.

The lacrimal part is a muscular slip which arises from the lacrimal bone. It passes behind the lacrimal sac where some fibres insert into the lacrimal fascia. Other fibres insert into the tarsi of the eyelids near the lacrimal canaliculi and into the lateral palpebral raphe.

Innervation: The muscle is supplied by temporal and zygomatic branches of the facial nerve.

Vasculature: The arterial supply is derived from branches of the superficial temporal, facial, maxillary (infra-orbital branch) and ophthalmic arteries.

Actions: The orbicularis oculi muscle may be regarded as a sphincter of the eyelids. The orbital part is involved in forced closure (i.e. 'screwing up' the eye). The palpebral part of orbicularis oculi is involved in closing the eyelids without effort (i.e. involuntary closure during blinking). By pulling on the lacrimal fascia, the lacrimal part of the muscle is said to dilate the lacrimal sac and so aid the flow of tears into the sac.

Some fibres from the upper part of the orbicularis oculi muscle are inserted into the eyebrow and have been termed the **depressor supercilii muscle**. As the name suggests, this muscle depresses the eyebrow.

3.4a Lateral view of face showing orbicularis oculi muscle and adjacent musculature

1 Frontal belly of occipitofrontalis muscle
2 Procerus muscle
3 Orbicularis oculi muscle – orbital part
4 Orbicularis oculi muscle – palpebral part
5 Levator labii superioris alaeque nasi muscle
6 Nasalis muscle
7 Zygomaticus minor muscle
8 Zygomaticus major muscle

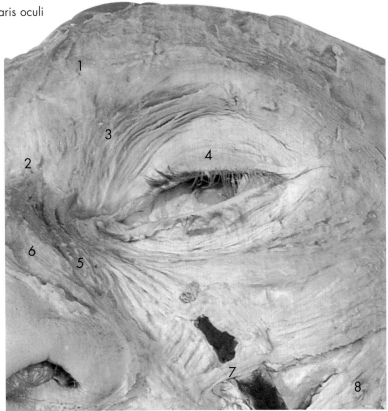

3.4b Frontal view of face showing orbicularis oculi muscle and adjacent musculature

1 Procerus muscle
2 Orbicularis oris muscle – orbital part
3 Orbicularis oris muscle – palpebral part
4 Levator labii superioris alaeque nasi muscle
5 Levator palpebrae superioris muscle
6 Facial artery
7 Zygomaticus major muscle

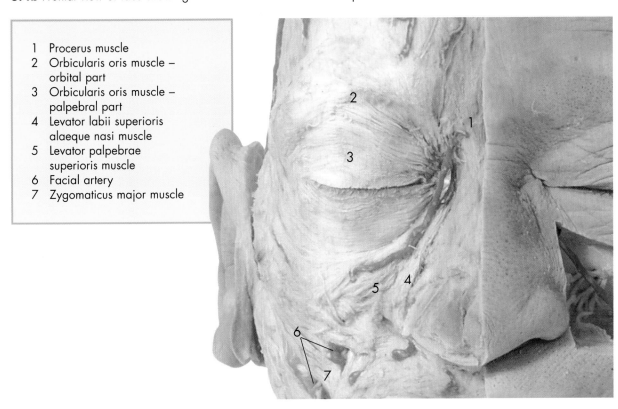

The corrugator supercilii muscle

Attachments: This muscle originates from the medial end of the supra-orbital ridge on the frontal bone, deep to the orbicularis oculi muscle. It passes upwards and outwards through orbicularis oculi to insert into the skin of the middle of the eyebrow.

Innervation: This is derived from the temporal and (upper) zygomatic branches of the facial nerve.

Vasculature: Branches from the superficial temporal artery are the muscle's chief source of blood supply.

Actions: The corrugator supercilii is the principal muscle in the expression of suffering. It produces vertical ridges above the bridge of the nose when frowning by drawing the eyebrows downwards and inwards.

THE NASAL GROUP (3.4–3.6)

Four muscles can be included within this group: procerus, compressor naris, dilator naris, and depressor septi. The compressor naris and the dilator naris muscles are often considered to be components of the nasalis muscle. The levator labii superioris alaeque nasi muscle can also be included in this group, although it is usually considered with the oral group of muscles.

The procerus muscle

Attachments: It arises from the nasal bone and the lateral nasal cartilage. Its fibres pass upwards to insert into the skin overlying the bridge of the nose.

Innervation: The procerus muscle is supplied by the temporal and (lower) zygomatic branches of the facial nerve. However, it has been reported that it is innervated only by the buccal branch of the facial nerve.

Vasculature: Its arteries are derived mainly from the facial artery (angular branch).

Actions: It produces transverse wrinkles over the bridge of the nose. Consequently, some consider procerus to be a member of the orbital group of facial muscles.

3.5 Some of the nasal group of muscles

1   Procerus
2   Levator labii superioris alaeque nasi
3   Compressor naris
4   Depressor septi

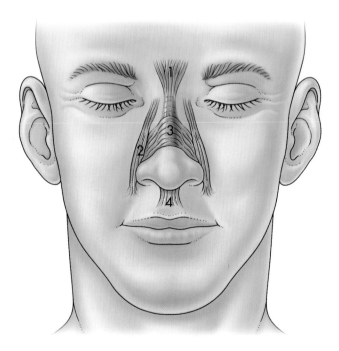

The compressor naris muscle (transverse part of nasalis)

Attachments: This muscle arises from the maxilla in the region overlying the root of the canine tooth. Its fibres pass over the dorsum of the nose to join the muscle from the opposite side.

Innervation: It is supplied by the buccal branch of the facial nerve, although there may also be a contribution from the zygomatic branch.

Vasculature: The arterial supply is derived from branches of the facial and maxillary (infra-orbital branch) arteries.

Actions: As indicated by the name, it compresses the nasal aperture.

The dilator naris muscle (alar part of nasalis)

Attachments: This muscle originates from the maxilla in the region of the lateral incisor. It inserts into the greater nasal cartilage.

Innervation and Vasculature: As for compressor naris.

Actions: It draws the ala of the nose downwards and laterally to dilate the nostril.

The depressor septi muscle

Attachments: This muscle arises from the incisor region of the maxilla and passes upwards from beneath the orbicularis oris muscle to insert into the cartilaginous nasal septum.

Innervation: This is provided by the buccal branch (sometimes the zygomatic branch) of the facial nerve.

Vasculature: The facial artery (superior labial branch) supplies the depressor septi muscle.

Actions: It pulls the nasal septum downwards and constricts the nostril.

THE AURICULAR GROUP

This group is composed of the anterior, superior and posterior auricular muscles. The muscles are often rudimentary and show considerable variation. The most constant is the superior auricular muscle.

The anterior, superior and posterior auricular muscles

Attachments: The anterior auricular muscle arises from the epicranial aponeurosis. It passes downwards and backwards to insert into the helix of the auricle. The superior auricular muscle also arises from the epicranial aponeurosis. It passes downwards to be inserted into the upper part of the cranial surface of the auricle. The posterior auricular muscle arises from the base of the mastoid process of the temporal bone. It passes upwards to be inserted into the convexity of the concha.

Innervation: These muscles are not usually under voluntary control. The anterior and superior auricular muscles are supplied by the temporal branches of the facial nerve, the posterior auricular muscle by the posterior auricular branch.

Vasculature: The arteries are derived from the posterior auricular and superficial temporal arteries.

Actions: The auricular muscles usually show little activity. However, they may cause elevation and forward and backward movements of the ear.

THE CIRCUM-ORAL GROUP (3.6, 3.7)

The muscles which comprise this group show a complex arrangement. They may be subdivided into the orbicularis oris muscle itself and the muscles which radiate around it.

The orbicularis oris muscle

This muscle is the sphincter of the orifice of the mouth. Its fibres are said to encircle the orifice, lying within the upper and lower lips. However, it is possible that many fibres are derived from the other facial muscles which pass into the lips, so that relatively few fibres are truly intrinsic. The muscle may appear stratified, in which case the deep layer contains the buccinator muscle and the superficial layer comprises the other muscles merging into the lips. The arrangement of the intrinsic fibres is complex. There are oblique fibres which pass through the full thickness of the lips to connect the skin and mucous membrane. Other intrinsic fibres pass outwards from the alveolar bone in the incisor region to the angle of the mouth. It is believed that the philtrum of the upper lip is produced by the interlacing and crossing over of the intrinsic fibres of the orbicularis oris muscle in the midline.

Innervation: The muscle is innervated by the buccal and marginal mandibular branches of the facial nerve.

Vasculature: The main blood supply comes from the facial artery (superior and inferior labial branches), from the maxillary artery (mental and infra-orbital branches), and from the superficial temporal artery.

Actions: The orbicularis oris muscle is capable of various movements, including closure, protrusion and pursing of the lips.

The muscles of the lips which are arranged around orbicularis oris can be subdivided into superficial and deep muscles. The superficial muscles of the upper lip are the levator labii superioris and the zygomaticus major and minor muscles. The levator anguli oris muscle is the deep muscle of the upper lip. The superficial muscle of the lower lip is the depressor anguli oris muscle. The depressor labii inferioris and the mentalis muscles are the deep muscles of the lower lip. At the corners of the mouth lie the buccinator and risorius muscles.

The levator labii superioris muscle

Attachments: It arises from the maxilla at the inferior margin of the orbit, above the infra-orbital foramen. Here, the muscle is deep to the orbicularis oculi muscle. Some of its fibres pass downwards to be inserted into the skin overlying the lateral side of the upper lip. Other fibres merge with those of orbicularis oris. A small slip of muscle arises from the frontal process of the maxilla, close to the side of the nose. This is usually termed the levator labii superioris alaeque nasi (also referred to as the angular head of the levator labii superioris). This inserts into the skin and the greater nasal cartilage of the nose and into the skin and musculature of the upper lip.

Innervation: The zygomatic and buccal branches of the facial nerve innervate this muscle.

Vasculature: The muscle is supplied by branches from the facial and maxillary (infra-orbital branch) arteries.

Actions: The primary function of the levator labii superioris muscle is to elevate the upper lip. The levator labii superioris alaeque nasi muscle also dilates the nostril.

The zygomaticus major muscle

Attachments: This muscle takes origin from the lateral surface of the zygomatic bone, just in front of the zygomaticotemporal suture. It passes obliquely downwards to the corner of the mouth where it mingles with the orbicularis oris muscle.

Innervation: The muscle is supplied by the zygomatic and buccal branches of the facial nerve.

Vasculature: The arterial supply is derived from the facial artery (superior labial branch).

Actions: The muscle pulls the corner of the mouth upwards and outwards, as in laughing.

3.6 Lateral-oblique view of the face showing the circum-oral muscles of facial expression

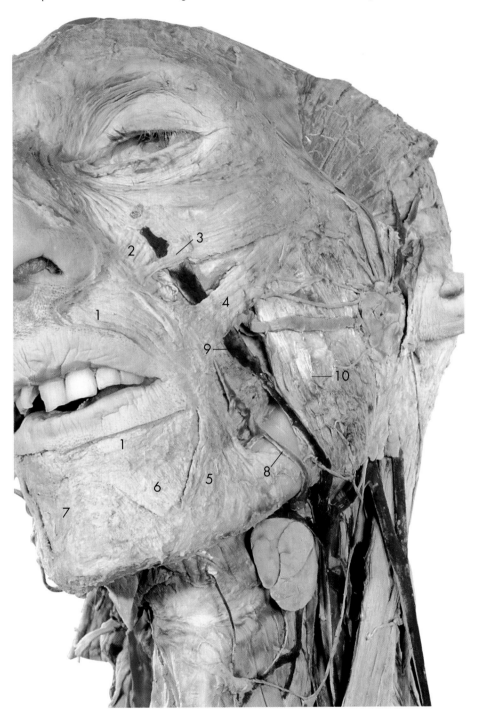

1	Orbicularis oris muscle	6	Depressor labii inferioris muscle
2	Levator labii superioris muscle	7	Mentalis muscle
3	Zygomaticus minor muscle	8	Facial artery
4	Zygomaticus major muscle	9	Facial vein
5	Depressor anguli oris muscle	10	Masseter muscle

The zygomaticus minor muscle
Attachments: From its attachment on the zygomatic bone (in front of the origin of zygomaticus major), zygomaticus minor runs downwards and forwards to insert into the lateral part of the upper lip.

Innervation: It receives its nerve supply from the zygomatic and buccal branches of the facial nerve.

Vasculature: Its blood supply is derived from the facial artery (superior labial branch).

Actions: The muscle elevates the upper lip. Acting with other facial muscles, it produces the expression of disdain. The nasolabial furrow is associated with this muscle.

The levator anguli oris muscle
Attachments: It arises from the canine fossa of the maxilla (immediately below the infra-orbital foramen) and passes downwards towards the corner of the mouth. Some fibres continue around the corner of the mouth to mingle with orbicularis oris in the lower lip.

Innervation: This is derived from the zygomatic and buccal branches of the facial nerve.

Vasculature: The blood supply arises from the facial (superior labial branch) and maxillary (infra-orbital branch) arteries.

Actions: The levator anguli oris muscle elevates the corner of the mouth.

The depressor anguli oris muscle
Attachments: It arises from an extensive area around the external oblique line of the mandible. Its fibres pass upwards to the corner of the mouth. It is partly inserted here and partly into the orbicularis oris in the upper lip.

Innervation: The muscle is innervated by the buccal and mandibular branches of the facial nerve.

Vasculature: The facial (inferior labial branch) and maxillary (mental branch) arteries supply the muscle.

Actions: The muscle depresses the corner of the mouth. It is said to be associated with the expression of grief.

The depressor labii inferioris muscle
Attachments: This muscle arises from the mandible just in front of the mental foramen (here it is covered by the anterior fibres of depressor anguli oris). The fibres pass upwards and medially to converge with the orbicularis oris muscle in the lower lip.

Innervation: It is supplied by the marginal mandibular branch of the facial nerve.

Vasculature: The blood supply is derived from the facial (inferior labial branch) and maxillary (mental branch) arteries.

Actions: It depresses the lower lip and draws it laterally. The muscle is associated with the expression of irony.

The mentalis muscle
Attachments: The muscle originates from the incisive fossa of the mandible. Its fibres descend to insert into the skin of the chin.

Innervation: This is provided by the marginal mandibular branch of the facial nerve.

Vasculature: It receives blood from the facial (inferior labial branch) and maxillary (mental branch) arteries.

Actions: The mentalis muscle raises and protrudes the lower lip (as during the expression of doubt or disdain).

3.7 Lateral view of face showing circum-oral muscles of facial expression

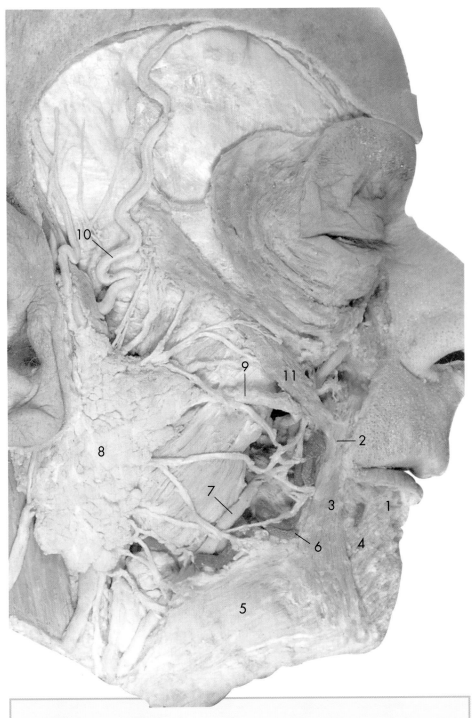

1	Orbicularis oris muscle	6	Facial artery
2	Levator anguli oris muscle	7	Facial vein
3	Depressor anguli oris muscle	8	Parotid gland
4	Depressor labii inferioris muscle	9	Parotid duct
5	Platysma muscle	10	Superficial temporal artery
		11	Zygomaticus major muscle

The risorius muscle

Attachments: This muscle is usually poorly developed. Unlike the other facial muscles, it does not arise from bone but originates from the connective tissue overlying the parotid gland. The muscle runs horizontally across the face to insert into skin at the corner of the mouth. In some cases, risorius is indistinguishable from the facial portion of the platysma muscle.

Innervation: The muscle is supplied by the buccal and zygomatic branches of the facial nerve.

Vasculature: This is derived from the facial artery (superior labial branch).

Actions: Risorius pulls the corner of the mouth laterally as in grinning.

The buccinator muscle (3.8, 3.25)

This forms the musculature of the cheek. Although classified with the muscles of facial expression, the buccinator muscle functions principally during mastication. An important relationship is with the parotid duct which pierces the muscle opposite the maxillary third molar and then runs forwards to open into the oral cavity opposite the maxillary second molar.

Attachments: The buccinator muscle has two main origins. Firstly, it arises from the anterior margin of the pterygomandibular raphe (the superior constrictor muscle of the pharynx arising from the posterior margin). Secondly, it is attached to the alveolar margins of the maxilla and mandible in the region of the molar teeth. A few fibres also arise from a tendinous band bridging the interval between the pterygoid hamulus and the maxillary tuberosity. Initially lying deep to the ramus of the mandible, the muscle emerges into the cheek by crossing the retromolar fossa of the mandible (behind the third molar). The fibres eventually run into the orbicularis oris muscle (where they form the deep layer of this muscle). The upper and lower fibres of the buccinator muscle pass into the substance of the corresponding lip, whereas the more centrally positioned fibres (arising mainly from the pterygomandibular raphe) decussate at the corner of the mouth to pass into the opposite lip.

Innervation: This is derived from the buccal branch of the facial nerve.

Vasculature: The arterial supply is from branches of the facial artery and from the maxillary (buccal branch) artery.

Actions: The main function of the buccinator muscle is to aid in mastication by maintaining the bolus of food between the molar teeth. In addition, it is involved in sucking and in expelling air forcibly (e.g. in whistling or playing a wind instrument).

It may be appreciated from the descriptions of the circum-oral musculature that several muscles converge and interlace at the corners of the mouth. This is said to produce a nodular region termed the modiolus which is palpable. The modiolus may be fixed by the action of some of the muscles to provide a base for the action of other muscles.

3.8 Lateral view of infratemporal fossa showing buccinator muscle

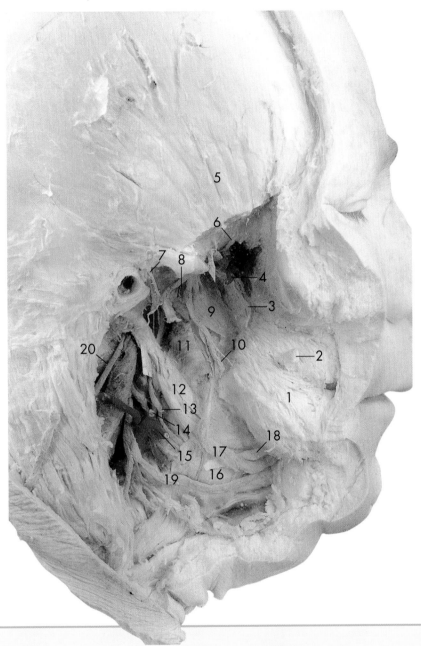

1	Buccinator muscle	12	Styloglossus muscle
2	Parotid duct (cut end)	13	Glossopharyngeal nerve
3	Buccal branch of mandibular nerve	14	Facial artery
4	Maxillary artery (cut end)	15	Lingual artery lying on middle constrictor muscle
5	Temporalis muscle		
6	Temporal branch of mandibular nerve	16	Hyoglossus muscle
7	Auriculotemporal nerve	17	Lingual nerve
8	Middle meningeal artery	18	Submandibular duct
9	Tensor palati muscle	19	Hypoglossal nerve
10	Inferior alveolar nerve	20	Spinal accessory nerve
11	Superior constrictor muscle		

THE NERVES OF THE FACE

Both motor and sensory nerves are found on the face. The motor nerves are derived from the facial nerve (cranial nerve VII). The sensory innervation is primarily from the three divisions of the trigeminal nerve with a small contribution from the cervical plexus via the great auricular nerve.

THE FACIAL NERVE (3.7, 3.9, 3.12, 3.14)

After emerging from the base of the skull at the stylo-mastoid foramen, the facial nerve gains access to the face by passing through the substance of the parotid gland.

Branches in the face include:

- Posterior auricular nerve

- Nerve to digastric and stylohyoid muscles

- Temporal branches

- Zygomatic branches

- Buccal branches

- Marginal mandibular nerve

- Cervical branch

The *posterior auricular nerve* arises close to the stylo-mastoid foramen. It supplies the occipital belly of the occipitofrontalis and some of the ear muscles (see pages 107 and 150).

The *nerves to the posterior belly of the digastric and the stylohyoid muscles* also arise close to the stylomastoid foramen.

Just before entering the parotid gland, the facial nerve divides into temporo-facial and cervico-facial trunks, the former being the larger. Within the substance of the parotid gland, the trunks show a variable pattern of branching to form a parotid plexus. From this plexus five distinct sets of branches from the antero-medial surface of the gland usually emerge.

The *temporal branches* (usually three or four) leave the superior surface of the gland and cross the zygomatic arch to reach the forehead. They cross the superficial temporal vessels and auriculotemporal nerve and supply the auricular muscles, the frontal belly of the occipitofrontalis muscle in the scalp and part of the orbicularis oculi muscle.

The *zygomatic branches* may be up to three in number. The upper branch passes above the orbit to supply the frontal belly of the occipitofrontalis muscle and the orbicularis oculi. The lower branch passes below the orbit to supply the lower part of orbicularis oculi and to contribute to the innervation of muscles in the upper lip and nose.

The *buccal branch* (sometimes two in number) passes across the face usually below the parotid duct. It supplies the buccinator muscle and contributes to the innervation of the muscles of the upper lip and nose. Where two branches are present, one lies above the parotid duct.

The (*marginal*) *mandibular branches* (usually two but sometimes one or three) emerges from the lower border of the parotid gland and runs near the inferior border of the mandible. Initially, it may pass into the neck below the angle of the mandible, but at the anterior border of the masseter muscle it crosses back onto the face in all but 5% of cases. Its function is to supply the muscles of the lower lip.

The *cervical branch* passes (two branches in 20% of cases) downwards from the lower border of the parotid gland to supply the platysma muscle in the neck, roughly at the level of the hyoid bone.

It is not known to what extent sensory fibres are present in the facial nerve after it exits the stylomastoid foramen. In some animals, 15% of the sensory fibres of the nerve may emerge at the stylomastoid foramen. Many of these are thought to be distributed to the concha of the auricle and sometimes to an area behind the ear. Others claim that some sensory fibres travel with the motor fibres to the face. Indeed, some believe the facial nerve may be involved in the appreciation of deep pain in the face as well as proprioceptive functions for the facial musculature.

The course and distribution of the facial nerve is complicated by the presence of communicating branches with other nerves. On the face, these nerves are branches from the trigeminal nerve and the cervical plexus. Though the significance of these communications is not fully known, it is thought that they may represent proprioceptive contributions from the trigeminal nerve to the facial muscles.

3.9 Lateral view of face showing dissection of facial nerve

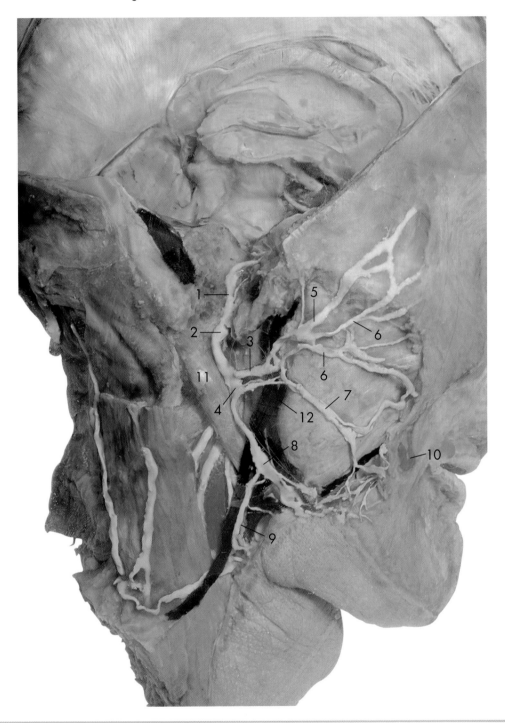

1	Intracranial part of facial nerve	7	Buccal branch of facial nerve
2	Facial nerve exiting skull at stylomastoid foramen	8	Mandibular branch of facial nerve
3	Temporofacial trunk of facial nerve	9	Cervical branch of facial nerve
4	Cervicofacial trunk of facial nerve	10	Facial artery
5	Temporal branch of facial nerve	11	Posterior belly of digastric muscle
6	Zygomatic branches of facial nerve	12	Retromandibular vein and external carotid artery

THE CUTANEOUS INNERVATION OF THE FACE (3.10, 3.14, 4.3)

Three large areas of the face can be mapped out to indicate the peripheral nerve fields associated with the three divisions of the trigeminal nerve. The fields are not horizontal but curve upwards. It is claimed that the reason for this is that the skin moves upwards with growth of the brain. Embryologically, each division of the trigeminal nerve is associated with a developing facial process which gives rise in the adult to a particular area of the face. The ophthalmic nerve is associated with the frontonasal process, the maxillary nerve with the maxillary process and the mandibular nerve with the mandibular process.

The ophthalmic nerve

This nerve has three branches (frontal, nasociliary and lacrimal) which are distributed to the face. The area supplied is extensive, including the forehead, the upper eyelid and much of the external surface of the nose. Five nerves are concerned with the cutaneous innervation.

The *supra-orbital nerve* is the largest ophthalmic branch on the face. It is one of the two terminal branches of the frontal nerve. It emerges from the orbit through the supra-orbital notch (or foramen) and supplies much of the forehead and most of the upper eyelid.

The *supratrochlear nerve* supplies a small area of skin over the medial part of the forehead and over the medial part of the upper eyelid. It is also a terminal branch of the frontal nerve and emerges from the orbit medial to the supra-orbital nerve. Its name indicates that it runs above the trochlea associated with the superior oblique muscle of the eye.

The *infratrochlear nerve* is one of the two terminal branches of the nasociliary nerve (the other being the anterior ethmoidal nerve). It supplies skin over the bridge of the nose and at the medial corner of the upper eyelid. As its name suggests, it leaves the orbit below the trochlea associated with the superior oblique muscle.

The *external nasal nerve* is the terminal part of the anterior ethmoidal nerve. It supplies the skin of the nose below the nasal bones (excluding the ala portion around the external nares).

The *lacrimal nerve* is the smallest branch of the ophthalmic nerve. It emerges from the upper lateral margin of the orbit to supply the lateral part of the upper eyelid.

The maxillary nerve

The maxillary nerve supplies the skin of the lower eyelid, the prominence of the cheek, the ala part of the nose, part of the temple, and the upper lip. It has three cutaneous branches.

The *infra-orbital nerve*, the largest cutaneous branch of the maxillary nerve, emerges onto the face through the infra-orbital foramen. As well as supplying skin overlying the maxilla, it gives off palpebral branches to the lower eyelid, nasal branches to the ala of the nose and labial branches to the upper lip.

The *zygomaticofacial nerve* is one of the two branches of the zygomatic nerve. It emerges from the orbit onto the face at the zygomaticofacial foramen. It supplies skin overlying the prominence of the cheek.

The *zygomaticotemporal nerve* is the remaining branch of the zygomatic nerve. It enters the temporal fossa via the zygomaticotemporal foramen on the deep surface of the zygomatic bone. It supplies skin over the anterior part of the temple (non-beard part of temple).

3.10a The cutaneous innervation of the face

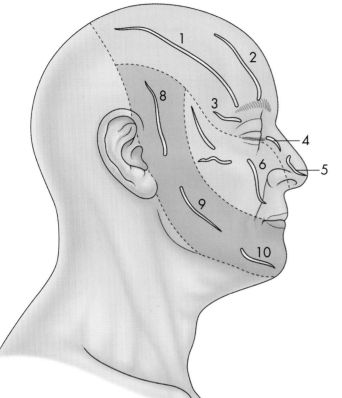

1	Supra-orbital nerve – V_1
2	Supratrochlear nerve – V_1
3	Lacrimal nerve – V_1
4	Infratrochlear nerve – V_1
5	External nasal nerve – V_1
6	Infra-orbital nerve – V_2
7	Zygomaticofacial and zygomaticotemporal nerves – V_2
8	Auriculotemporal – V_3
9	Buccal nerve – V_3
10	Mental nerve – V_3

3.10b Frontal view of face showing the cutaneous innervation

1	Supra-orbital nerve and artery
2	Supratrochlear nerve and artery
3	External nasal nerve
4	Branch of lacrimal nerve
5	Infra-orbital nerve
6	Mental nerve

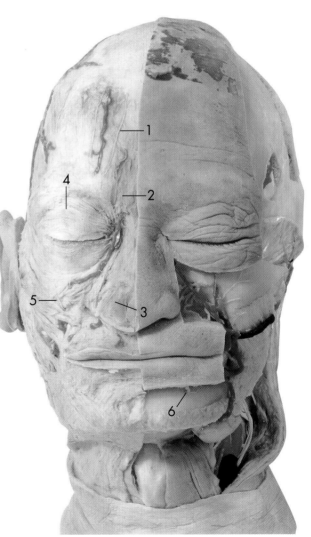

The mandibular nerve

The area supplied by the mandibular nerve includes the skin overlying the mandible, the lower lip, the fleshy part of the cheek, part of the auricle, and part of the temple. It has three cutaneous branches.

The *mental nerve* is a branch of the inferior alveolar nerve. It emerges onto the face through the mental foramen of the mandible. It supplies the skin of the lower lip and the skin overlying the mandible (except around the angle of the mandible).

The *buccal branch of the mandibular nerve* is sometimes referred to as the long buccal nerve to distinguish it from the buccal branch of the facial nerve. It emerges onto the face from behind the ramus of the mandible to supply the skin overlying the fleshy part of the cheek.

The *auriculotemporal nerve* appears on the face behind the temporomandibular joint, and ascends over the zygomatic arch. It supplies the tragus, concha, external auditory meatus and tympanic membrane of the ear, and the posterior part of the temple (beard part of the temple).

The great auricular nerve

One part of the face which does not receive its cutaneous innervation from the trigeminal nerve is the angle of the mandible. The skin in this region is supplied by the great auricular nerve (see page 320). This nerve is derived from the cervical plexus (anterior primary rami of the second and third cervical nerves). Appearing at the posterior border of the sterno-cleidomastoid muscle, it passes forwards and upwards across the muscle to reach the angle of the mandible.

THE ARTERIES OF THE FACE

The main arterial supply to the face comes from the facial and superficial temporal arteries. These are both branches of the external carotid artery. Blood also reaches the face from some of the branches of the maxillary and ophthalmic arteries. The various branches are joined by numerous anastomoses.

THE FACIAL ARTERY (3.11–3.14)

After its origin from the external carotid artery in the neck, the facial artery passes upwards and forwards towards the inferior border of the mandible. This cervical course is described further on page 344.

The facial artery first makes its appearance on the external surface of the mandible at the anterior border of the masseter muscle. At this point, it pierces the deep fascia to pass onto the face. It then continues upwards and medially, following a tortuous course towards the bridge of the nose. It lies deep to the zygomatic and risorius muscles, but superficial to the buccinator and the levator anguli oris muscles. It passes either superficial or deep to levator labii superioris. Thus, it is generally only visible on the cheek between the zygomaticus and risorius muscles. Alongside the nose, it is closely related to the levator labii superioris alaeque nasi muscle. Here, it is termed the angular artery. Throughout its course on the face, it usually lies anterior to the facial vein.

The chief branches of the facial artery on the face are the inferior labial, superior labial and angular arteries. The inferior and superior labial arteries have a tortuous course in the lower and upper lip respectively. If the margin of each lip is compressed between the thumb and index fingers, the pulsations of the labial arteries may be felt. These arteries are situated deep to the orbicularis oris muscle, lying just beneath the labial mucosa. The superior labial artery has a branch supplying the nasal septum. The angular artery gives off small branches to the nose but, where there is a large branch, it has been termed the lateral nasal artery. In addition, the submental artery (which arises in the neck) runs along the lower border of the mandible to supply the chin and lower lip.

3.11 Lateral view of face showing the course of the facial artery

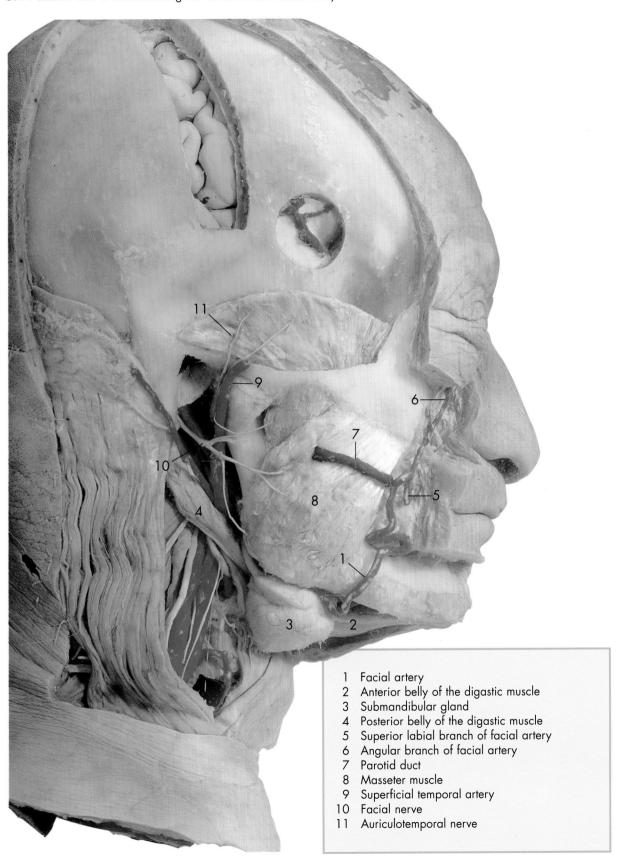

1 Facial artery
2 Anterior belly of the digastic muscle
3 Submandibular gland
4 Posterior belly of the digastic muscle
5 Superior labial branch of facial artery
6 Angular branch of facial artery
7 Parotid duct
8 Masseter muscle
9 Superficial temporal artery
10 Facial nerve
11 Auriculotemporal nerve

THE SUPERFICIAL TEMPORAL ARTERY (3.11–3.14)

This is one of the terminal branches of the external carotid artery within the parotid gland. Emerging from the superior surface of the gland, the artery passes upwards towards the scalp, crossing the zygomatic process of the temporal bone. It then divides into anterior and posterior branches (these may also be termed frontal and parietal branches, indicating their region of supply on the scalp). Glandular branches are given off to the parotid gland.

A transverse facial artery arises from the superficial temporal artery within the parotid gland. It crosses the masseter muscle above the parotid duct. The transverse facial artery gives branches to both the gland and the duct, to the masseter muscle, and to adjacent skin. The superficial temporal artery also gives off a middle temporal artery which pierces the temporal fascia to supply the temporalis muscle, auricular branches to supply the external lower part of the ear, and a zygomatico-orbital branch to the orbicularis oris muscle.

FACIAL BRANCHES FROM THE MAXILLARY ARTERY (3.13, 3.14)

The maxillary artery is a terminal branch of the external carotid artery. It provides three branches to the face.

The mental artery arises from the first part of the maxillary artery as a terminal branch of the inferior alveolar artery. It emerges onto the face from the mandibular canal at the mental foramen. The mental artery supplies muscles and skin in the chin region and anastomoses with the inferior labial and submental arteries.

The buccal artery is a branch of the second part of the maxillary artery. It emerges onto the face from the infratemporal fossa and crosses the buccinator muscle to supply the cheek. The buccal artery anastomoses with the infra-orbital artery and with branches of the facial artery.

The infra-orbital artery arises from the third part of the maxillary artery. It runs through the infra-orbital foramen and onto the face, supplying the lower eyelid, the lateral aspect of the nose and the upper lip. The infra-orbital artery has extensive anastomoses with the transverse facial, ophthalmic and buccal arteries and with branches of the facial artery.

FACIAL BRANCHES FROM THE OPHTHALMIC ARTERY (3.13, 4.3)

The ophthalmic artery is a branch of the internal carotid artery. Five branches arise from the ophthalmic artery within the orbit to supply the face.

The supra-orbital artery leaves the orbit through the supra-orbital notch (or foramen). It supplies much of the upper eyelid, forehead and scalp. It anastomoses with the supratrochlear and superficial temporal arteries.

The supratrochlear artery emerges from the orbit onto the face at the frontal notch. It supplies the medial parts of the upper eyelid, forehead and scalp.

The lacrimal artery appears on the face at the upper lateral corner of the orbit to supply the lateral part of the eyelids. Within the orbit, the lacrimal artery gives off a zygomatic artery which subdivides into zygomaticofacial and zygomaticotemporal arteries. The zygomaticofacial artery then passes through the lateral wall of the orbit to emerge onto the face at the zygomaticofacial foramen, supplying the region overlying the prominence of the cheek. The zygomaticotemporal artery also passes through the lateral wall of the orbit, via the zygomaticotemporal foramen, to supply the skin over the non-beard part of the temple. The lacrimal artery anastomoses with the deep temporal branch of the maxillary artery and the transverse facial branch of the superficial temporal artery.

The dorsal nasal artery accompanies the infratrochlear nerve. It exits the orbit at the upper medial corner. The artery supplies a region of skin around the bridge of the nose, anastomosing with the angular branch of the facial artery.

The external nasal artery is the terminal branch of the anterior ethmoidal artery from the ophthalmic artery. It supplies skin on the external nose, emerging at the junction of the nasal bone and the lateral nasal cartilage.

3.12 Lateral view of face showing superficial temporal and facial arteries

1   Superficial temporal artery
2   Parotid gland
3   Parotid duct
4   Facial artery
5   Accessory parotid gland

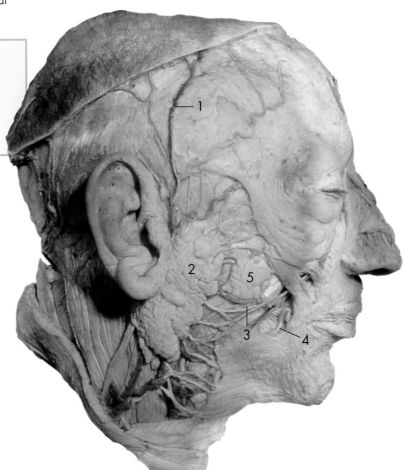

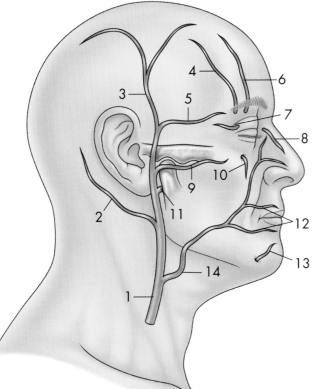

3.13 The arteries of the face

1   External carotid artery
2   Posterior auricular artery
3   Superficial temporal artery
4   Supra-orbital artery
5   Zygomatico-orbital artery
6   Supratrochlear artery
7   Lacrimal artery
8   External nasal artery
9   Transverse facial artery
10 Infra-orbital artery
11 Maxillary artery
12 Superior and inferior labial arteries
13 Mental artery
14 Facial artery

THE VEINS OF THE FACE

The veins show a similar distribution to the arteries of the face, although there is greater variability. The chief vein is the facial vein.

THE FACIAL VEIN (3.7, 3.14, 3.16)

This begins as the angular vein at the medial corner of the eye, the angular vein being formed by the confluence of the supra-orbital and supratrochlear veins. The facial vein soon divides into a part which communicates with the superior ophthalmic vein in the orbit and a part which remains superficial and which passes downwards close behind the facial artery. The facial vein passes over the inferior border of the mandible near the anterior attachment of the masseter muscle. In the submandibular region, it receives the anterior branch of the retromandibular vein (forming what was once called the common facial vein) and, crossing the submandibular gland and the facial artery, drains into the internal jugular vein. The tributaries of the facial vein include nasal, deep facial, and the superior and inferior labial veins. The deep facial vein connects the facial vein with the pterygoid venous plexus in the infratemporal fossa (3.42).

The *superior ophthalmic and infra-orbital veins* are also important when considering the connections of the facial vein. The superior ophthalmic vein links the angular vein with the cavernous sinus and can receive veins from the scalp, forehead, and upper eyelid (3.42). As the facial vein has no valves, pressure or blockage may result in blood flowing into the cavernous sinus. The infra-orbital vein links the facial vein with the pterygoid venous plexus in the infratemporal fossa. It can receive veins from the lower eyelid, lateral part of the nose, and upper lip.

THE SUPERFICIAL TEMPORAL VEIN (3.14, 3.16)

This vein is formed above the zygomatic arch by the union of anterior and posterior tributaries. The superficial temporal vein then enters the substance of the parotid gland. Here, it unites with the maxillary vein to form the retromandibular vein (see page 124). It receives the transverse facial vein and veins from the parotid gland and ear.

Buccal and mental veins drain veins from the cheek and the chin into the pterygoid venous plexus.

THE LYMPHATICS OF THE FACE

Both the distribution of the lymph nodes and the arrangement of the lymphatic vessels in the face show considerable variation.

3.14 Lateral view of face showing
superficial temporal and facial veins

1   Superificial temporal vein
    and artery
2   Branches of facial nerve
3   Supra-orbital nerve
4   Supratrochlea nerve
5   Transverse facial artery
6   Great auricular nerve on
    sternocleidomastoid muscle
7   External jugular vein
8   Submandibular gland
9   Internal jugular vein
10 Facial vein
11 Facial artery
12 Buccinator muscle
13 Inferior labial artery
14 Superiro labial artery
15 Mental nerve and artery
16 Lesser occipital nerve
17 Greater occipital nerve
18 Occipital artery

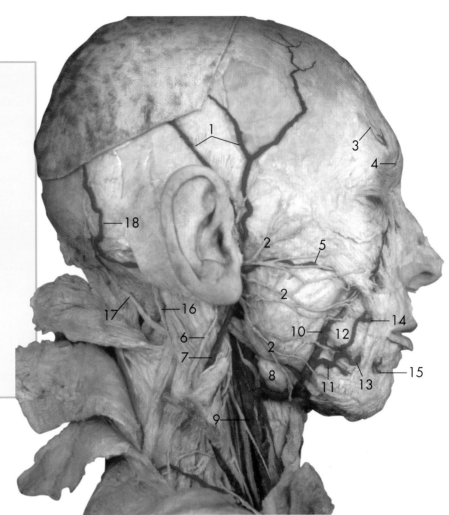

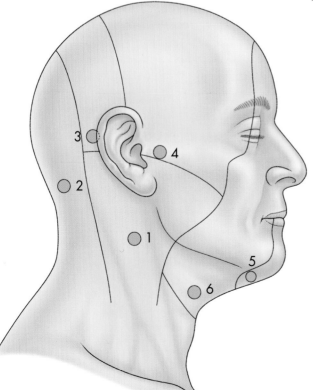

3.15 The lymphatics of the face

1   Superficial cervical nodes
2   Occipital nodes
3   Retro-auricular nodes
4   Parotid nodes
5   Submental nodes
6   Submandibular nodes

THE PAROTID GLAND
(3.7, 3.14, 3.16, 3.17)

This is the largest of the major paired salivary glands. It occupies the region between the ramus of the mandible and the mastoid process, extending upwards to the external acoustic meatus. The gland is surrounded by an unyielding capsule, the parotid capsule, derived from the investing layer of deep cervical fascia.

Within the gland lies the facial nerve, the external carotid artery and its terminal branches, and the retromandibular vein (and its formative vessels). Lymph nodes are present both within, and on the surface of the gland. The parotid gland is a serous gland (though a small mucous component is present in the neonate) and the secretions travel in the main parotid duct to discharge into the oral cavity close to the crown of the upper second molar tooth.

In addition to the main gland, a small portion of glandular tissue may be situated above the parotid duct. This part is called the accessory parotid gland (3.12).

The parotid gland is essentially pyramidal in shape. The base (superior surface) is closely moulded around the external acoustic meatus and is termed the glenoid lobe. The superficial temporal vessels and the auriculotemporal nerve appear at the superior surface and pass upwards to be distributed to the temple. The apex (inferior surface) of the gland extends beyond the angle of the mandible to overlap the digastric triangle. The lateral surface (superficial surface) has an irregular, lobulated appearance. It is covered only by skin, superficial fascia, and part of the platysma muscle. The great auricular nerve from the cervical plexus crosses this part of the gland to be distributed to the surrounding skin and the parotid fascia. The medial surface (deep surface) rests on the 'parotid bed'. It can be divided into two parts. The anterior part is applied to the masseter muscle, the posterior border of the ramus, the medial pterygoid muscle, and the condyle of the mandible. The posterior part rests on the sternocleidomastoid muscle, the mastoid process, and the styloid group of muscles. At the junction between anteromedial and posteromedial surfaces a flange of glandular tissue may extend beyond the posterior border of the mandible to reach the wall of the pharynx.

STRUCTURES WITHIN THE PAROTID GLAND

The deepest of the three main structures within the gland is the external carotid artery. The artery enters the posteromedial surface of the gland from the neck. Here, it divides into the maxillary and superficial temporal arteries. The maxillary artery emerges from the anteromedial surface of the gland and passes forwards between the neck of the mandible and the sphenomandibular ligament to enter the infratemporal fossa (see page 144). The superficial temporal artery passes upwards to leave the gland at its superior surface. Within the substance of the gland, it gives off the transverse facial artery. This emerges at the anterior border of the parotid gland and runs above the parotid duct. The posterior auricular artery may also arise within the parotid gland.

The veins within the parotid gland are superficial to the arteries. The superficial temporal and maxillary veins join within the upper part of the gland to form the retromandibular vein. The retromandibular vein near the apex of the gland usually divides into anterior and posterior branches. Outside the gland, the anterior branch joins the facial vein; the posterior branch unites with the posterior auricular vein to form the external jugular vein.

The facial nerve is the most superficial of the structures within the parotid gland. Emerging from the stylomastoid foramen, the nerve enters the parotid gland in the upper part of its posteromedial surface (after about 1.3 cm). It crosses the styloid process, the retromandibular vein, and the external carotid artery before dividing into a plexus in the region of the temporomandibular joint. Five main branches (which may be single or multiple) arise from the plexus and emerge from the anterior and inferior margin of the parotid gland. These are temporal, zygomatic, buccal, mandibular and cervical branches (see page 114). Some anatomists subdivide the parotid gland into superficial and deep parts with reference to the facial nerve.

The auriculotemporal nerve is a branch of the mandibular nerve which is a division of the trigeminal nerve. It appears within the superior surface of the parotid gland having passed from behind the temporomandibular joint from the infratemporal fossa (see page 140). The auriculotemporal nerve then ascends over the posterior part of the zygomatic process of the temporal bone behind the superficial temporal vessels.

3.16 Lateral view of face to show form and relations of the parotid gland

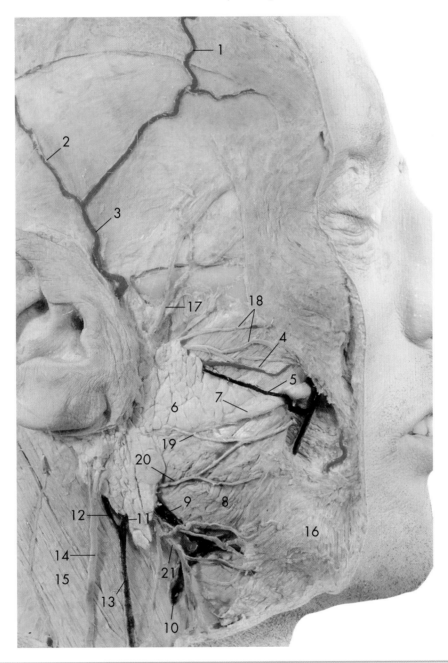

1	Frontal branch of superficial temporal artery	11	Posterior division of retromandibular vein
2	Parietal branch of superficial temporal artery	12	Posterior auricular vein
3	Superficial temporal artery	13	External jugular vein
4	Transverse facial branch of superficial temporal artery	14	Great auricular nerve
5	Transverse facial vein	15	Sternocleidomastoid muscle
6	Parotid gland	16	Platysma muscle
7	Parotid duct	17	Temporal branch of facial nerve
8	Masseter muscle	18	Zygomatic branch of facial nerve
9	Anterior division of retromandibular vein	19	Buccal branch of facial nerve
10	Common facial vein	20	Mandibular branch of facial nerve
		21	Cervical branch of facial nerve

The parotid capsule

The parotid gland is surrounded by a fibrous capsule which is a continuation of the investing layer of deep cervical fascia. This fascia is traditionally described as splitting to enclose the gland within a superficial and a deep layer. The superficial layer is attached above to the zygomatic process of the temporal bone, the cartilaginous part of the external acoustic meatus, and the mastoid process. The deep layer is attached to the mandible, and to the tympanic plate and the styloid and mastoid processes of the temporal bone. However, recent studies suggest that the superficial layer of parotid fascia is not derived from the investing layer of deep cervical fascia, but should be considered as superficial fascia. Between the styloid process and the angle of the mandible, the fascia is thickened to form the stylomandibular ligament. This separates the parotid and submandibular glands. A mandibulostylo-hyoid ligament (angular tract) passes between the angle of the mandible and the stylohyoid ligament.

The parotid duct (3.7, 3.11, 3.12, 3.16)

This duct appears at the anterior border of the parotid gland. It passes horizontally across the masseter muscle, approximately at a level midway between the angle of the mouth and the zygomatic arch. Here, the duct lies below the transverse facial artery and receives one or more ducts from the accessory parotid gland. The parotid duct bends sharply around the anterior border of the masseter to pierce the buccal pad of fat and the buccinator muscle at the level of the upper third molar tooth. A further bend in the duct is found as it passes forwards beneath the oral mucosa before opening into the vestibule. The duct usually opens into the oral cavity opposite the crown of the upper second molar tooth. Adjacent to the opening is a small elevation of the mucosa (the parotid papilla).

The innervation and vasculature of the parotid gland

The innervation is related to the otic parasympathetic ganglion (3.18, 3.40).

The parasympathetic secretomotor supply is from the inferior salivatory nucleus of the brain stem. Passing with the glossopharyngeal nerve, the fibres run in the tympanic branch which contributes to the tympanic plexus on the promontory of the middle ear (see page 306). From this plexus arises the lesser petrosal nerve. This exits the middle ear, runs in a groove on the petrous portion of the temporal bone, and then passes through the foramen ovale (or the petrosal/in-nominate foramen) to the otic ganglion. Synapsing at the ganglion, postganglionic fibres leave to join the nearby auriculotemporal nerve which distributes the fibres to the parotid gland. There is some evidence that secretomotor fibres from the chorda tympani branch of the facial nerve may also supply the parotid gland.

The sympathetic supply to the parotid gland is derived initially from the superior cervical sympathetic ganglion. From this ganglion, the innervation reaches the gland via the plexus around the middle meningeal artery, the otic ganglion (without synapsing) and eventually the auriculotemporal nerve. It seems likely that an alternative source of sympathetic fibres is derived directly from the sympathetic plexuses accompanying the vessels supplying the parotid gland.

Sensory fibres to the connective tissue within the parotid gland are derived directly from the auriculotemporal nerve. In passing back to the parent mandibular nerve, they run through the otic ganglion (without synapsing) via a connecting branch.

The parotid fascia is innervated by the great auricular nerve from the cervical plexus of the neck.

The parotid gland receives its blood supply from branches of the external carotid artery which lie within the gland. Blood drains into the veins found locally. Lymphatics pass into the parotid (pre-auricular) lymph nodes.

3.17 Lateral view of face showing contents and deep relations of the parotid gland

1	Facial nerve at stylomastoid faramen
2	Temporofacial branch of facial nerve
3	Cervicofacial branch of facial nerve
4	Temporal branch of facial nerve
5	Zygomatic branch of facial nerve
6	Buccal branch of facial nerve
7	Mandibular branch of facial nerve
8	Cervical branch of facial nerve
9	Posterior belly of digastic muscle
10	Retromandibular vein and external carotid artery
11	Spinal accessory nerve
12	Sternocleidomastoid muscle
13	Lesser occipital nerve

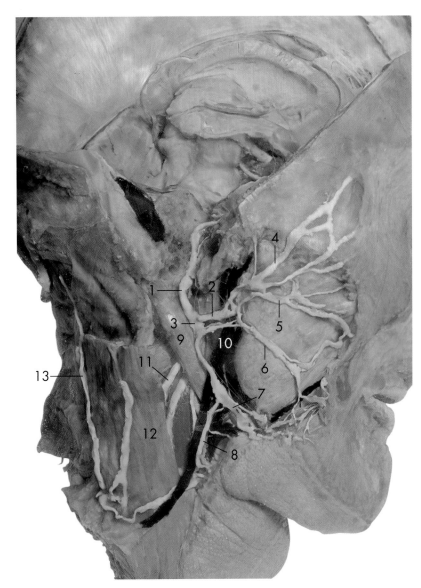

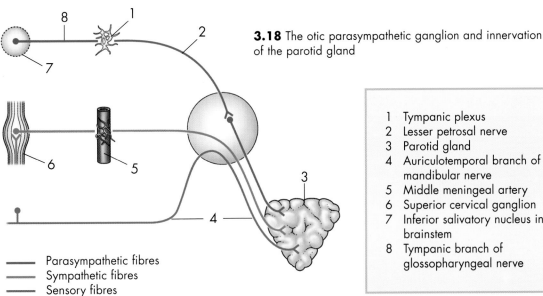

3.18 The otic parasympathetic ganglion and innervation of the parotid gland

1	Tympanic plexus
2	Lesser petrosal nerve
3	Parotid gland
4	Auriculotemporal branch of mandibular nerve
5	Middle meningeal artery
6	Superior cervical ganglion
7	Inferior salivatory nucleus in brainstem
8	Tympanic branch of glossopharyngeal nerve

—— Parasympathetic fibres
—— Sympathetic fibres
—— Sensory fibres

DEEP DISSECTION OF THE FACE

Removal of the parotid gland and the superficial structures in the face reveals the ramus of the mandible and structures associated with it. Thus, a description of the deep dissection of the face includes consideration of the muscles of mastication, the temporomandibular joint and the infratemporal fossa deep to the ramus.

THE MUSCLES OF MASTICATION

Although many muscles in the head and neck are involved in mastication, the term 'muscles of mastication' is usually reserved for the four pairs of muscles — the masseter, temporalis, and lateral and medial pterygoid muscles — which are primarily responsible for moving the mandible during the comminution and processing of food prior to swallowing.

The masseter and temporalis muscles lie relatively superficial in the face. The pterygoid muscles are situated deep to the ramus of the mandible and are thus considered later with the infratemporal fossa.

All four muscles of mastication develop from the mesenchyme of the first branchial arch. They therefore derive their innervation from the mandibular branch of the trigeminal nerve.

The masseter muscle (3.19)

Attachments: The muscle consists of three overlapping layers. A superficial part arises from the zygomatic process of the maxilla and from the anterior two-thirds of the lower border of the zygomatic arch. A middle part originates from the deep surface of the anterior two-thirds of the zygomatic arch and from the lower border of the posterior one-third of the arch. A deep part arises from the deep surface of the zygomatic arch. The three layers merge as the fibres pass downwards and backwards to insert into the lateral surface of the angle, ramus and coronoid process of the mandible.

Innervation: The muscle is innervated by the masseteric nerve from the anterior division of the mandibular nerve.

Vasculature: The arterial supply is derived from the superficial temporal (transverse facial branch), the maxillary artery (masseteric branch) and the facial arteries.

Actions: The masseter muscle elevates the mandible.

The temporalis muscle (3.20)

Attachments: The muscle arises from the floor of the temporal fossa and from the overlying temporal fascia. The attachment of the muscle is limited above by the inferior temporal line. The fibres converge towards their insertion onto the apex, the anterior and posterior borders, and the medial surface of the coronoid process. Indeed, the insertion extends down the anterior border of the ramus almost as far as the third molar tooth. The posterior fibres pass horizontally forwards, the anterior fibres pass vertically down onto the coronoid process. In order to reach the coronoid process, the temporalis muscle runs beneath the zygomatic arch. Many of the fibres (but not all) have a tendinous insertion.

Innervation: The muscle receives its nerve supply from the anterior division of the mandibular nerve.

Vasculature: This is derived from the superficial temporal (middle temporal branch) and maxillary (deep temporal branches) arteries.

Actions: The anterior (vertical) fibres of the temporalis muscle elevate the mandible, the posterior (horizontal) fibres retract it.

The *temporal fascia* is a strong membrane which covers the temporal fossa and the temporalis muscle. It is attached above to the superior temporal line on the cranium. Near the zygomatic arch it splits into two layers. The superficial layer is attached onto the superior margin of the zygomatic arch. The deep layer merges with connective tissue beneath the masseter muscle. As mentioned above, the temporal fascia contributes to the origin of the temporalis muscle, producing a bipennate form to the muscle. Pennate muscles are found where considerable power is required within a limited space.

3.19 Lateral view of face showing masseter and temporalis muscle

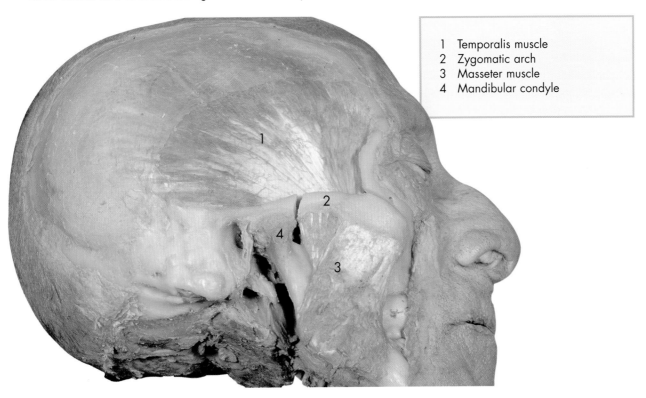

1	Temporalis muscle
2	Zygomatic arch
3	Masseter muscle
4	Mandibular condyle

3.20 Lateral view of face with zygomatic arch and masseter reflected to show attachment of temporalis muscle

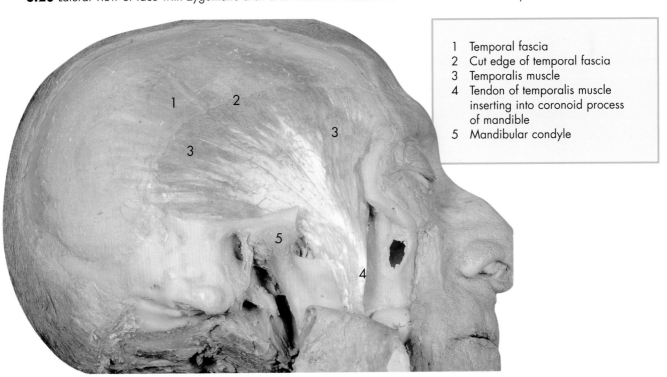

1	Temporal fascia
2	Cut edge of temporal fascia
3	Temporalis muscle
4	Tendon of temporalis muscle inserting into coronoid process of mandible
5	Mandibular condyle

THE TEMPOROMANDIBULAR JOINT (3.21–3.28)

The temporomandibular joint is a synovial joint. It is formed by the condyle of the mandible articulating in the mandibular fossa (glenoid fossa) of the temporal bone. Unlike most other synovial joints, the joint cavity is divided into two by an intra-articular disc. Although basically a hinge joint, the temporomandibular joint also allows for some gliding movements. Movement of the condylar head occurs within the mandibular fossa and down a bony prominence termed the articular tubercle which is located immediately anterior to the mandibular fossa.

The articular surfaces of the temporomandibular joint are lined by fibrous tissue. This reflects the development of the joint. Unlike all other synovial joints whose articular surfaces develop endochondrally and are therefore lined by hyaline cartilage, the temporomandibular joint develops in membrane.

The mandibular fossa (3.21, 3.22)

The mandibular fossa is an oval depression in the temporal bone lying immediately anterior to the external acoustic meatus. It is bounded anteriorly by the articular tubercle, laterally by the zygomatic process, and posteriorly by the tympanic plate. The petrotympanic fissure separates the mandibular fossa from the petrous part of the temporal bone. Occasionally, a ridge of bone (the postglenoid process) forms a prominence at the posterior boundary of the fossa.

The shape of the mandibular fossa does not exactly conform to the shape of the mandibular condyle, the articular disc moulding together the joint surfaces. The bone of the central part of the fossa is thin. This indicates that masticatory loads are not dissipated through the mandibular fossa but through the teeth and thence the facial bones and base of the cranium.

3.21 Lateral view of the skull showing the bones forming the temporomandibular joint

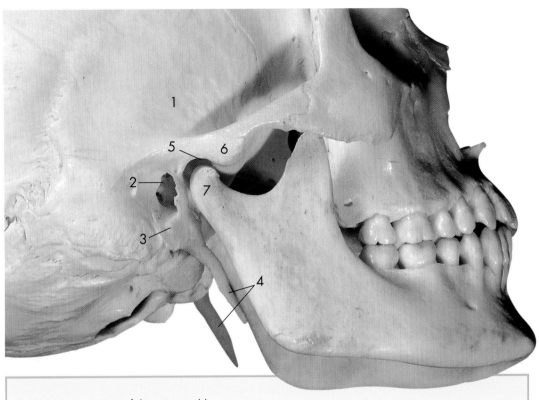

1 Squamous part of the temporal bone	
2 External auditory meatus	5 Mandibular fossa of temporal bone
3 Tympanic part of temporal bone	6 Articular eminence of temporal bone
4 Styloid process of temporal bone	7 Condyle of mandible

1 Zygomatic process of temporal bone
2 Articular eminence
3 Mandibular fossa
4 Tympanic part of temporal bone
5 Petrotympanic fissure

3.22 Base of skull showing the mandibular fossa

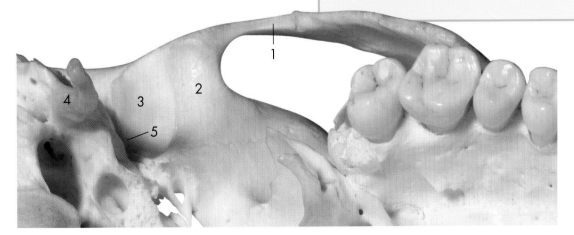

The mandibular condyle (3.23, 3.24)

The mandibular condyle varies considerably both in size and shape. The anteroposterior dimension of the condyle is approximately half the mediolateral dimension. The long axis of the condyle is not however at right angles to the ramus, but diverges posteriorly from a strictly coronal plane; if the long axes of the two condyles were extended, they would meet at an obtuse angle (approximately 150 degrees) at the anterior border of the foramen magnum.

The articular surfaces of the condyle are the anterior and superior surfaces. These surfaces are convex. The posterior surface of the condyle is broad and flat.

The condyle is composed of a core of cancellous bone covered by a thin layer of compact bone. During the period of growth, however, a layer of hyaline cartilage lies immediately beneath the fibrous articulating surface of the condyle.

The articular head of the condyle joins the ramus through a thin bony projection termed the neck of the condyle. A small depression (the pterygoid fovea) marks part of the attachment of the lateral pterygoid muscle. This fovea is situated on the anterior surface of the neck, below the articular surface.

The articular disc (3.25, 3.26, 3.32)

The articular disc is fibrous and is moulded to the bony joint surfaces. When viewed in sagittal section, the upper surface of the disc is concavo-convex from before backwards and the lower surface is concave. The disc is of variable thickness, being thinnest centrally. Its margins merge with the joint capsule. Anteriorly, it is attached to the lateral pterygoid muscle and fibrous bands connect it to the anterior margin of the articular tubercle above and to the anterior margin of the condyle below. Posteriorly, the disc becomes bilaminar, the upper part attaching to the anterior margin of the squamotympanic fissure, the lower part attaching to the posterior margin of the condyle; the elasticity of the upper part may aid in retracting the disc.

The capsule and ligaments of the temporomandibular joint (3.28)

The joint capsule is attached to the neck of the condyle and to the margins of the mandibular fossa. The capsule is thin although posteriorly it forms a thick, vascular, but loosely arranged connective tissue (the retrodiscal pad).

Synovial membrane lines the joint capsule, but not the intra-articular disc.

The joint capsule is strengthened by the lateral ligament (temporomandibular ligament). From the articular tubercle the ligament passes downwards and backwards to attach onto the lateral surface and posterior border of the neck of the condyle.

The accessory ligaments of the temporomandibular joint are the stylomandibular ligament, the spheno-mandibular ligament, and the pterygomandibular raphe. However, none have any significant influence upon mandibular movements. The stylomandibular ligament is a reinforced lamina of the deep cervical fascia as it passes medial to the parotid salivary gland. It extends from the tip of the styloid process and from the stylohyoid ligament to the angle of the mandible. The sphenomandibular ligament is a remnant of the perichondrium of cartilage of the embryonic first branchial arch. It runs from the spine of the sphenoid bone to the lingula near the mandibular foramen. The pterygomandibular raphe passes from the ptery-goid hamulus to the posterior end of the mylohyoid line in the retromolar region of the mandible. A retinacular ligament, passing from the articular eminence into fascia overlying the masseter muscle at the angle of the mandible has been described.

The innervation and vasculature of the temporomandibular joint

The innervation of the joint is provided mainly from the auriculotemporal branch of the mandibular division of the trigeminal nerve. Additional fibres are supplied by the masseteric branch of the mandibular nerve.

The vascular supply is derived from the superficial temporal artery and the maxillary artery (deep auricular branch).

3.23 Lateral view of ramus of mandible showing mandibular condyle

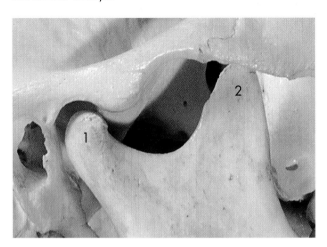

3.24 Frontal view of condyle showing the pterygoid fovea

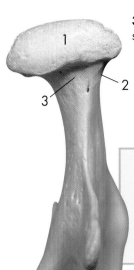

1 Head of mandibular condyle
2 Neck of mandibular condyle
3 Pterygoid fovea

1 Mandibular condyle
2 Coronoid process

3.25 Lateral view of deep face showing the articular disc of the temporomandibular joint

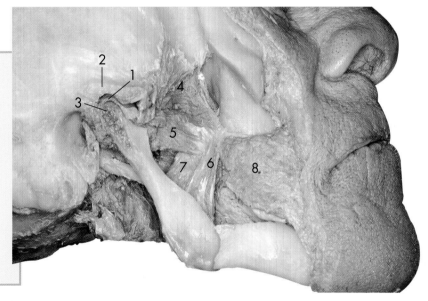

1 Articular disc of temporomandibular joint
2 Mandibular fossa
3 Mandibular condyle
4 Upper head of lateral pterygoid muscle
5 Lower head of lateral pterygoid muscle
6 Superficial head of medial pterygoid muscle
7 Deep head of medial pterygoid muscle
8 Buccinator muscle

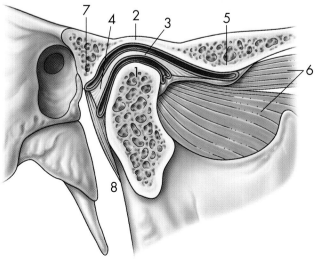

3.26 The articular disc and attachments of the lateral pterygoid muscle

1 Articular surface of condyle
2 Mandibular fossa
3 Thin central part of articular disc
4 Thick peripheral part of articular disc
5 Articular eminence
6 Two heads of lateral pterygoid muscle
7 Position of squamolymphanic fissure
8 Posterior margin of condyle

Movements of the mandible at the temporomandibular joint

Mandibular movements may be classified either as bilaterally symmetrical or bilaterally asymmetrical. Because the mandible is a single bone, movement through one temporomandibular joint cannot occur without a similar co-ordinating or dissimilar reactive movement in the other joint. Depression, elevation, protrusion and retrusion of the mandible are bilaterally symmetrical movements as they require similar co-ordinated movements through both temporomandibular joints. Lateral excursions (side-to-side movements) are bilaterally asymmetrical as there are dissimilar activities at the joints.

It is said that the joint space above the articular disc is associated with anterior gliding movements, whereas the joint space below the disc is associated with hinge movements. Retrusion of the mandible takes the condyle from a position on the articular tubercle back into the mandibular fossa. Little backward movement is possible from within the fossa.

Movements of the mandible are produced principally by the four muscles of mastication, although depression is aided by the activity of other muscles.

Depression of the mandible is produced mainly by the lateral pterygoid muscles, aided by the suprahyoid musculature. With slow and conscious activity, there are initially hinge movements (in the lower joint spaces) followed by sliding of the condylar processes and the articular discs forwards and downwards along the articular tubercles (involving the upper joint spaces).

Elevation of the mandible is produced by the masseter and the medial pterygoid muscles and by the anterior fibres of the temporalis muscles. The condylar processes and the articular discs are pulled upwards and backwards along the articular tubercles into the mandibular fossae. This is accompanied by hinge movements. Hinging may precede retrusion in slow, conscious closure.

Protrusion of the mandible is produced by the activity of the lateral and medial pterygoid muscles on both sides. The lateral pterygoids draw the condyles and the articular discs forwards along the slopes of the articular tubercles while the medial pterygoids maintain the teeth in contact.

Retrusion of the mandible is produced by the posterior (horizontal) fibres of the temporalis muscles which draw the condyles and the articular discs backwards and upwards along the articular tubercles, the masseter muscles maintaining the teeth in contact.

Lateral movement of the mandible is produced by the activity of the medial and lateral pterygoid muscles on one side only. Thus, for the jaw to move to the left, the right pterygoid muscles cause protrusion of the condyle down the articular tubercle on the right side with the condyle on the left remaining within its mandibular fossa (although showing some rotation around a laterally shifting axis).

3.28a Lateral view of temporomandibular joint showing joint capsule and temporomandibular ligament

1	Temporomandibular ligament

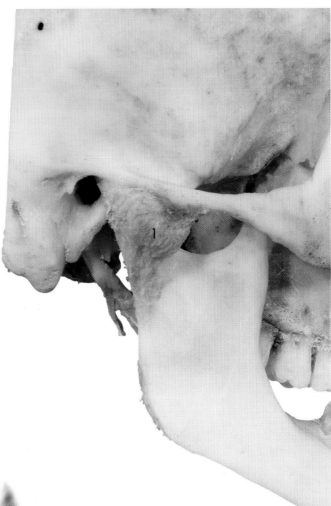

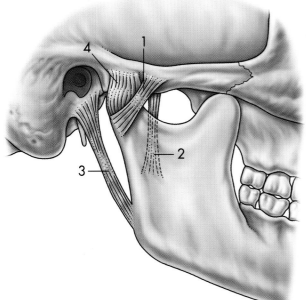

3.28b The temporomandibular joint and ligaments

1	Temporomandibular ligament
2	Sphenomandibular ligament
3	Stylomandibular ligament
4	Capsule

THE INFRATEMPORAL FOSSA

The infratemporal fossa is the space located deep to the ramus of the mandible (3.29).

The fossa is bounded anteriorly by the posterior surface of the maxilla and posteriorly by the styloid apparatus, carotid sheath and deep part of the parotid gland. Medially lies the lateral pterygoid plate and the superior constrictor muscle of the pharynx. Laterally lies the ramus of the mandible. The roof is formed by the infratemporal surface of the greater wing of the sphenoid. The infratemporal fossa has no anatomical floor, being continuous with tissue spaces in the neck.

The infratemporal fossa communicates with the temporal fossa deep to the zygomatic arch. It also communicates with the pterygopalatine fossa through the pterygomaxillary fissure. At the base of the cranium, the foramen ovale and foramen spinosum enter the fossa through the sphenoid bone. The foramen lacerum and the petrotympanic, squamotympanic and petrosquamous fissures are also found close to the infratemporal fossa. On the medial surface of the ramus of the mandible is the mandibular foramen.

Major structures which occupy the infratemporal fossa are:

* Lateral and medial pterygoid muscles

* Mandibular division of the trigeminal nerve

* Chorda tympani branch of the facial nerve

* Otic parasympathetic ganglion

* Maxillary artery and branches

* Pterygoid venous plexus

The key to understanding the relationships of structures within the infratemporal fossa is the lateral pterygoid muscle. This lies in the roof of the fossa, running anteroposteriorly in a horizontal plane from the region of the pterygoid plates to the mandibular condyle. It consists of two heads, an upper head and a lower head. Deep to the muscle arise the branches of the mandibular nerve and the main origin of the medial pterygoid muscle. Superficially lies the maxillary artery. The buccal branch of the mandibular nerve passes between the two heads of the lateral pterygoid muscle. Emerging below the inferior border of the muscle are the medial pterygoid muscle and the lingual and inferior alveolar nerves. At the upper border emerge the deep temporal nerves and vessels. Concentrated around and within the lateral pterygoid muscle lies a venous network, the pterygoid venous plexus.

The lateral pterygoid muscle (3.25, 3.30–3.32, 3.34)
Attachments: The bulk of the muscle is formed by its lower head. This arises from the lateral surface of the lateral pterygoid plate of the sphenoid bone. The smaller upper head takes origin from the infratemporal surface of the greater wing of the sphenoid in the roof of the fossa. The two heads converge near the point of insertion. The fibres of the upper head insert primarily into the capsule and medial aspect of the articular disc of the temporomandibular joint. The fibres from the lower head insert into the pterygoid fovea on the mandibular condyle.

Innervation: The nerves to the lateral pterygoid (one for each head) arise from the anterior trunk of the mandibular nerve, deep to the muscle.

Vasculature: The arterial supply is derived from the maxillary artery (pterygoid branches) as it crosses the lateral pterygoid muscle.

Actions: The main action of the muscle is to assist in opening the jaws by pulling forwards the mandibular condyle and the articular disc of the temporomandibular joint. In addition, the muscle is involved in protrusion and in lateral movements of the mandible.

3.29 Lateral view of skull showing osteology of infratemporal fossa

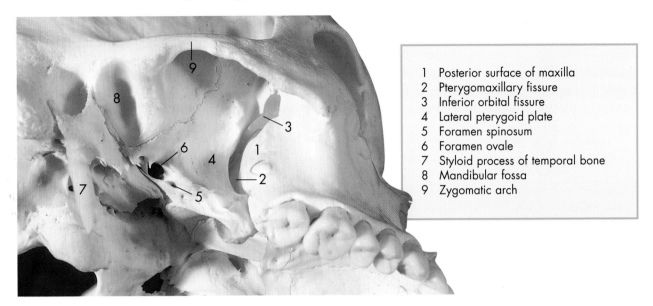

1	Posterior surface of maxilla
2	Pterygomaxillary fissure
3	Inferior orbital fissure
4	Lateral pterygoid plate
5	Foramen spinosum
6	Foramen ovale
7	Styloid process of temporal bone
8	Mandibular fossa
9	Zygomatic arch

3.30 Lateral view of deep face showing the contents of the infratemporal fossa, including the pterygoid muscles

1	Capsule of temporo-mandibular joint
2	Upper head of lateral pterygoid muscle
3	Lower head of lateral pterygoid muscle
4	Maxillary artery
5	Buccal nerve
6	Superficial head of medial pterygoid muscle
7	Lingual nerve
8	Inferior alveolar nerve
9	Buccinator muscle
10	Facial vein
11	Facial artery
12	Posterior belly of digastric muscle
13	External carotid artery
14	Facial nerve
15	Deep head of medial pterygoid muscle

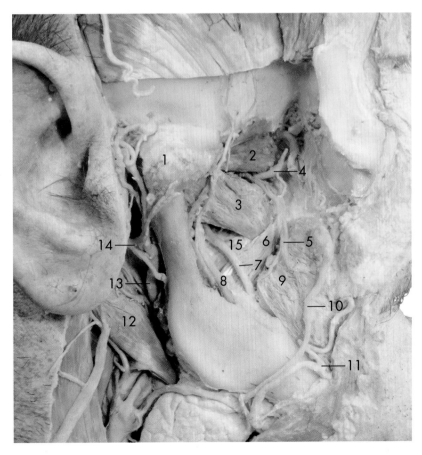

The medial pterygoid muscle (3.25, 3.30–3.32, 3.34)

Attachments: This muscle is the deepest of the four muscles of mastication. It consists of two heads. The bulk of the muscle arises as a deep head from the medial surface of the lateral pterygoid plate. Thus, the lateral pterygoid plate of the sphenoid bone gives rise to both pterygoid muscles. A common mistake is the belief that the medial pterygoid muscle arises from the medial pterygoid plate. However, the medial pterygoid plate gives origin only to a small portion of the superior constrictor muscle of the pharynx. The smaller superficial head of the medial pterygoid muscle originates from the maxillary tuberosity and the neighbouring part of the palatine bone (pyramidal process). From these sites, the fibres pass downwards and backwards to insert into the roughened surface of the angle of the mandible on its medial aspect.

Innervation: The nerve to the medial pterygoid muscle arises from the mandibular nerve (deep to the lateral pterygoid muscle), before the latter nerve divides into anterior and posterior trunks.

Vasculature: Like the lateral pterygoid muscle, the medial pterygoid derives its arterial supply from the maxillary artery.

Actions: The medial pterygoid muscle is an elevator of the mandible. Additionally, it assists in lateral and protrusive movements.

The mandibular nerve (3.30, 3.31, 3.33–3.36)

This is the largest division of the trigeminal nerve and is the only one to contain motor as well as sensory fibres. Developmentally, it is the nerve of the first branchial arch and is thus responsible for supplying structures derived from it. Its sensory fibres supply the mandibular teeth and their supporting structures, the mucosa of the anterior two-thirds of the tongue and the floor of the mouth, the skin of the lower part of the face (including the lower lip) and parts of the temporal region and auricle. Its motor fibres supply the four 'muscles of mastication' and the mylohyoid, anterior belly of digastric, tensor veli palatini and tensor tympani muscles.

The mandibular nerve is formed in the infratemporal fossa by the union of the sensory and motor roots immediately after they leave the skull at the foramen ovale. At this point, the nerve lies on the tensor veli palatini muscle and is covered by the lateral pterygoid muscle. After a short course, the nerve divides into a small anterior trunk and a larger posterior trunk. Prior to this division, the main trunk gives off two branches — the meningeal branch and the nerve to medial pterygoid. The anterior trunk of the mandibular nerve is mainly motor, the posterior trunk mainly sensory.

Branches of the mandibular nerve include:

- Meningeal branch (nervus spinosus)

- Nerve to medial pterygoid

- Anterior trunk:
    Masseteric nerve
    Deep temporal nerves
    Nerve to lateral pterygoid
    Buccal nerve

- Posterior trunk:
    Auriculotemporal nerve
    Lingual nerve
    Inferior alveolar nerve

3.31 Medial view of infratemporal fossa showing the medial pterygoid muscle and the mandibular nerve

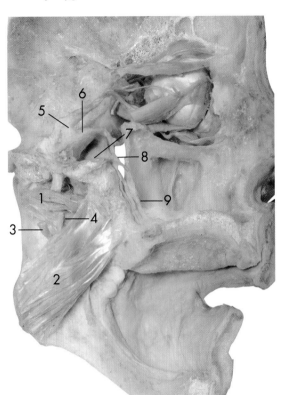

3.32 Infratemporal fossa of left side viewed posteriorly showing pterygoid muscles

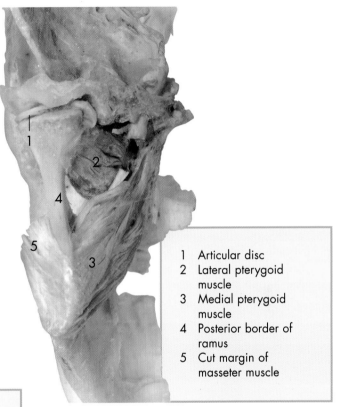

1	Lateral pterygoid muscle
2	Medial pterygoid muscle
3	Inferior alveolar nerve
4	Lingual nerve
5	Trigeminal ganglion
6	Maxillary nerve
7	Nerve of pterygoid canal
8	Pterygopalatine ganglion
9	Greater palatine nerve

1	Articular disc
2	Lateral pterygoid muscle
3	Medial pterygoid muscle
4	Posterior border of ramus
5	Cut margin of masseter muscle

3.33 The mandibular nerve.

1	Incisive branch
2	Mental nerve
3	Submandibular ganglion on hyoglossus muscle
4	Buccal branch
5	Lateral pterygoid nerve
6	Deep temporal nerve
7	Medial pterygoid nerve
8	Meningeal nerve
9	Auriculotemporal nerve
10	Chorda tympani nerve
11	Lingual nerve
12	Mylohyoid nerve
13	Inferior alveolar nerve
14	Molar branch

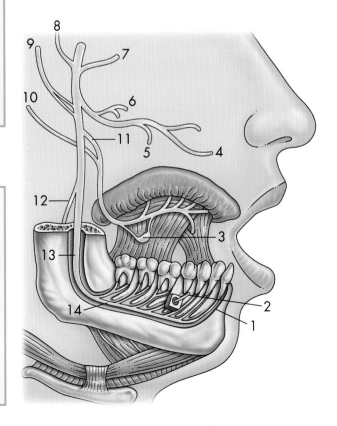

The *meningeal branch of the mandibular nerve* (nervus spinosus) arises from the main trunk of the mandibular nerve. It is a 'recurrent nerve' as it runs back into the middle cranial fossa through the foramen spinosum. It supplies the dura mater lining the middle cranial fossa and the mucosa of the mastoid antrum and mastoid air cells.

The *nerve to the medial pterygoid muscle* enters the deep surface of the muscle and also gives slender branches which pass uninterrupted through the otic ganglion to supply the tensor tympani and tensor veli palatini muscles.

The *masseteric nerve* is usually the first branch of the anterior trunk of the mandibular nerve. It passes above the upper border of the lateral pterygoid muscle and crosses the mandibular notch (between the condylar and coronoid processes) to be distributed into the masseter muscle. It also gives an articular branch to the temporomandibular joint.

The *anterior and posterior deep temporal nerves* also pass above the lateral pterygoid muscle. They subsequently enter the deep surface of the temporalis muscle.

The *nerve to the lateral pterygoid muscle* may arise separately or may run with the buccal nerve before entering the deep surface of the lateral pterygoid muscle.

The *buccal branch of the mandibular nerve* is the only sensory branch of the anterior trunk of the mandibular nerve. On emerging between the heads of the lateral pterygoid muscle, it passes downwards and forwards across the lower head to contact the medial surface of the temporalis muscle as it inserts onto the coronoid process of the mandible. It then clears the ramus of the mandible to lie on the lateral surface of the buccinator muscle in the cheek. At this point, it is close to the retromolar fossa of the mandible. It now gives branches to the skin of the cheek before piercing buccinator to supply its lining mucosa, the buccal sulcus, and the buccal gingiva

related to the mandibular molar and premolar teeth. It may also carry secretomotor fibres to minor salivary glands in the buccal mucosa, these being post-ganglionic fibres from the otic ganglion.

The *auriculotemporal nerve* is the first branch of the posterior trunk of the mandibular nerve. It is essentially sensory but it also distributes autonomic fibres to the parotid gland derived from the otic ganglion. It arises as two roots which encircle the middle meningeal artery and unite behind the artery. The nerve then runs backwards under the lateral ptery-goid muscle to lie beneath the mandibular condyle (between the condyle and the sphenomandibular ligament). On entering the parotid region, it turns to emerge superficially between the temporoman-dibular joint and the external acoustic meatus. From the upper surface of the parotid gland, the auriculo-temporal nerve ascends on the side of the head with the superficial temporal vessels, passing over the posterior part of the zygomatic arch. It gives several branches along its course:

- Ganglionic branches which communicate with the otic ganglion.

- Articular branches which enter the posterior part of the temporomandibular joint; these carry proprioceptive information important in mastication.

- Parotid branches which convey parasympathetic secretomotor fibres and sympathetic fibres to the parotid gland; these fibres are related to the otic ganglion. Sensory fibres from the auriculotemporal nerve supply the gland (with the exception of the capsule which is innervated by the great auricular nerve).

- Auricular branches (usually two) which supply the tragus and crus of the helix of the auricle, part of the external acoustic meatus, and the outer (lateral) surface of the tympanic membrane.

- Superficial temporal branches which are cutaneous nerves supplying part of the skin of the temple.

3.34 Lateral view of the infratemporal fossa showing the distribution of the mandibular nerve and the maxillary artery

1 Maxillary artery
2 Deep temporal arteries
3 Buccal nerve
4 Lower head of lateral pterygoid muscle
5 Lingual nerve
6 Inferior alveolar nerve
7 Medial pterygoid muscle
8 Buccinator muscle
9 Facial artery
10 Facial vein
11 Anterior branch of retromandibular vein
12 Posterior superior alveolar artery

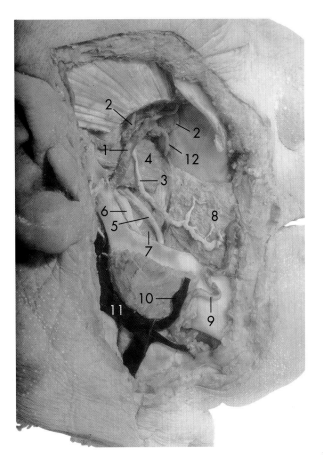

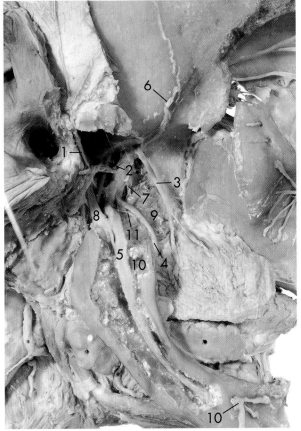

3.35 Lateral view of the infratemporal fossa showing branches of the mandibular nerve

1 Auriculotemporal nerve (two roots surrounding middle meningeal artery)
2 Middle meningeal artery
3 Buccal nerve
4 Lingual nerve
5 Inferior alveolar nerve with mylohyoid branch
6 Deep temporal nerve
7 Nerve to medial pterygoid muscle
8 Sphenomandibular ligament
9 Medial pterygoid muscle
10 Mental nerve
11 Chorda tympani nerve

The *lingual nerve* is the second branch of the posterior trunk of the mandibular nerve. It is essentially a sensory nerve but, following union with the chorda tympani branch of the facial nerve, it also contains parasympathetic fibres. Initially, the nerve lies on the tensor veli palatini muscle deep to the lateral pterygoid muscle. Here, the chorda tympani nerve (which has entered the infratemporal fossa via the petrotympanic fissure) joins the posterior surface of the lingual nerve. Emerging from the inferior border of the lateral pterygoid muscle, the lingual nerve curves downwards and forwards in the space between the ramus of the mandible and the medial pterygoid muscle (pterygomandibular space). At this level, it lies anterior to, and slightly deeper than, the inferior alveolar nerve. This completes the course of the nerve in the infratemporal fossa. It then passes towards the floor of the mouth (see page 178).

The *chorda tympani branch of the facial nerve* is distributed through the lingual nerve and has two types of fibres. Sensory fibres are associated with taste to the anterior two-thirds of the tongue. Parasympathetic fibres are preganglionic to the submandibular ganglion. Postganglionic fibres are secretomotor to the submandibular and sublingual glands.

The *inferior alveolar nerve* is the third branch of the posterior trunk of the mandibular nerve. Although it is essentially a sensory nerve, it also carries motor fibres which are given off as the mylohyoid nerve. Indeed, the mylohyoid nerve contains all the motor fibres of the posterior trunk of the mandibular nerve. The inferior alveolar nerve descends deep to the lateral pterygoid muscle, posterior to the lingual nerve. Here, it is crossed by the maxillary artery. On emerging at the inferior border of the muscle, it passes between the sphenomandibular ligament and the ramus of the mandible to enter the mandibular foramen.

The mylohyoid nerve is given off just before the mandibular foramen. It pierces the sphenomandibular ligament and runs in a groove (the mylohyoid groove) which lies immediately below the mandibular foramen. The mylohyoid nerve supplies the mylohyoid muscle and the anterior belly of the digastric.

The main distribution of the inferior alveolar nerve is to the mandibular teeth and their supporting structures, there being molar and incisive branches. The mental nerve is a cutaneous branch which supplies the skin of the chin and the lower lip. It arises within the mandible in the premolar region but soon exits onto the face via the mental foramen. For details of the course and distribution of the inferior alveolar nerve within the mandible see page 174.

The otic ganglion (3.37, 3.40, 5.30)

This parasympathetic ganglion lies immediately below the foramen ovale on the medial surface of the main trunk of the mandibular nerve. It is concerned primarily with supplying the parotid gland. Like other parasympathetic ganglia in the head, three types of fibres are associated with it: parasympathetic, sympathetic and sensory fibres. However, only the parasympathetic fibres synapse in the ganglion. The preganglionic parasympathetic fibres originate from the inferior salivatory nucleus in the brain stem. The fibres pass out in the glossopharyngeal nerve, appearing as the lesser (superficial) petrosal nerve from the tympanic plexus in the middle ear cavity (see page 306). The lesser petrosal nerve reaches the otic ganglion by a complex course. Passing through the petrous part of the temporal bone, the lesser petrosal nerve comes to lie in the floor of the middle cranial fossa. Here, it is lateral to the greater (superficial) petrosal branch of the facial nerve. The lesser petrosal nerve usually enters the infratemporal fossa through the foramen ovale to join the otic ganglion. The sympathetic root of the otic ganglion is derived from postganglionic fibres from the superior cervical ganglion. They are said to reach the otic ganglion from the plexus on the middle meningeal artery. The sensory root is derived from the auriculo-temporal nerve. The postganglionic parasympathetic fibres (with sympathetic and sensory components) reach the parotid gland by way of the auriculotemporal nerve. Parasympathetic fibres may also innervate the minor salivary glands in the cheek, passing with the buccal branch of the mandibular nerve.

The innervation of tensor veli palatini and tensor tympani is derived from the nerve to medial pterygoid by a branch which passes through the otic ganglion.

3.36 Medial view of the infratemporal fossa showing branches of the mandibular nerve

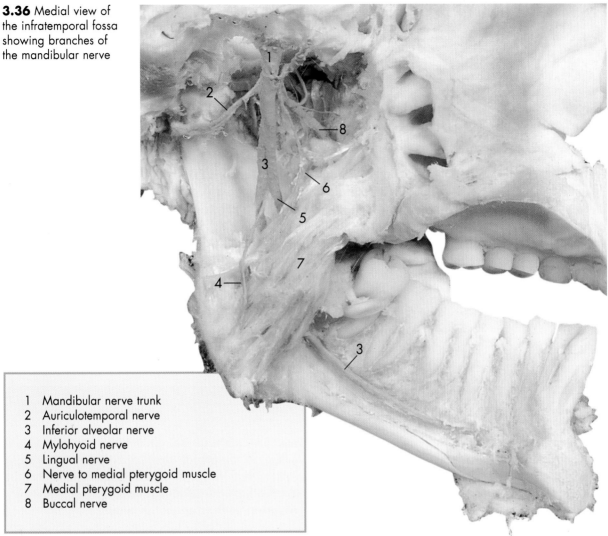

1 Mandibular nerve trunk
2 Auriculotemporal nerve
3 Inferior alveolar nerve
4 Mylohyoid nerve
5 Lingual nerve
6 Nerve to medial pterygoid muscle
7 Medial pterygoid muscle
8 Buccal nerve

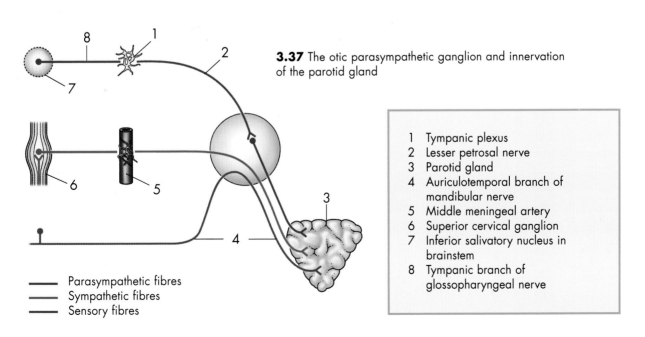

3.37 The otic parasympathetic ganglion and innervation of the parotid gland

1 Tympanic plexus
2 Lesser petrosal nerve
3 Parotid gland
4 Auriculotemporal branch of mandibular nerve
5 Middle meningeal artery
6 Superior cervical ganglion
7 Inferior salivatory nucleus in brainstem
8 Tympanic branch of glossopharyngeal nerve

—— Parasympathetic fibres
—— Sympathetic fibres
—— Sensory fibres

The maxillary artery (3.38–3.41)

The maxillary artery is a terminal branch of the external carotid artery. It arises within the parotid gland at the level of the neck of the condyle of the mandible. It enters the infratemporal fossa between the deep surface of the condyle and the spheno-mandibular ligament. At this point, it lies below the auriculotemporal nerve and above the maxillary vein. In the infratemporal fossa, it is closely related to the lateral pterygoid muscle. Initially, it lies near the inferior border of the muscle where it crosses the inferior alveolar nerve. Its subsequent course is variable, although it usually passes superficial to the lower head of the lateral pterygoid before entering the pterygopalatine fossa through the pterygomaxillary fissure.

The maxillary artery has many branches. It is convenient to subdivide the artery into three parts, before the lateral pterygoid muscle (first or mandibular part), on the lateral pterygoid muscle (second or pterygoid part) and in the pterygopalatine fossa (third or pterygopalatine part).

The first part of the maxillary artery has five branches and all enter bone. The first branch is the deep auricular artery, supplying the skin of the external acoustic meatus and part of the tympanic membrane. A small branch contributes to the arterial supply of the temporomandibular joint. The second branch, the anterior tympanic artery, passes through the petrotympanic fissure to supply part of the lining of the middle ear. This is the companion artery to the chorda tympani nerve. The middle meningeal artery is the main source of blood to the meninges and to the bones of the vault of the skull. It ascends between the two roots of the auriculotemporal nerve and leaves the infratemporal fossa through the foramen spinosum. Its course within the cranium is described further on page 280. An accessory meningeal artery runs through the foramen ovale into the middle cranial fossa to supply the trigeminal ganglion and the dura lining the floor of the middle cranial fossa. The inferior alveolar artery accompanies the inferior alveolar nerve and has a similar distribution. Immediately before the artery enters the mandible (at the mandibular foramen), it gives off a mylohyoid branch. In the mandibular canal, it gives off branches supplying the cheek teeth before terminating in mental and incisive branches. The mental artery passes through the mental foramen onto the face to supply the lower lip, the chin and the labial mucosa related to the anterior teeth. The incisive branch continues along the incisive canal to supply the anterior teeth.

The second part of the maxillary artery also has five branches, but they differ from those of the first part in not entering bone. Muscular branches include deep temporal arteries (anterior and posterior), pterygoid arteries and masseteric arteries. The masseteric arteries also supply the temporomandibular joint. A buccal artery accompanies the buccal nerve to supply structures in the cheek. A small lingual branch may be given off to accompany the lingual nerve and supply structures in the floor of the mouth.

Branches of the third part of the maxillary artery are described with the pterygopalatine fossa (see page 218).

3.38 The maxillary artery in the infratemporal fossa

1 First (mandibular) part of maxillary artery
2 Second (pterygoid) part of maxillary artery, in this dissection passing superficial to lower head of lateral pterygoid
3 Third (pterygopalatine) part of maxillary artery
4 Superficial temporal artery
5 Facial nerve
6 Inferior alveolar artery (cut end)
7 External carotid artery
8 Posterior auricular artery
9 Posterior belly of digastic muscle
10 Stylohyoid muscle
11 Sublingual gland
12 Lingual nerve
13 Submandibular ganglion
14 Hypoglossal nerve

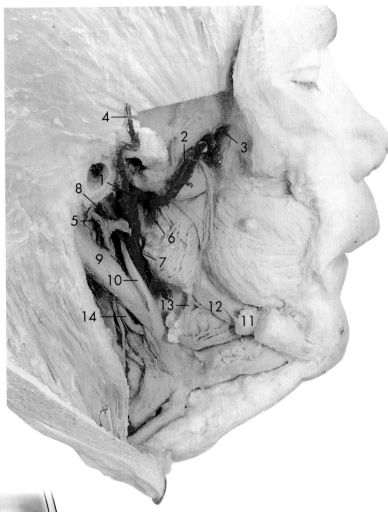

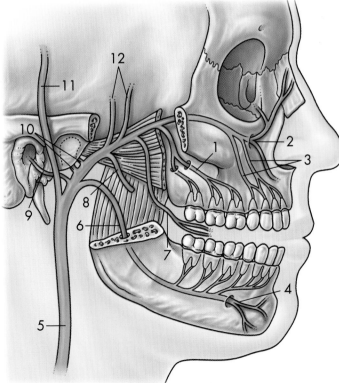

3.39 The maxillary artery

1 Posterior superior alveolar artery
2 Infra-orbital artery
3 Anterior and middle superior alveolar arteries
4 Mental artery
5 External carotid artery
6 Inferior alveolar artery
7 Buccal artery
8 Lingual branch
9 Deep auricular artery
10 Meningeal arteries
11 Superficial temporal artery
12 Deep temporal arteries

3.40 Maxillary artery viewed medially

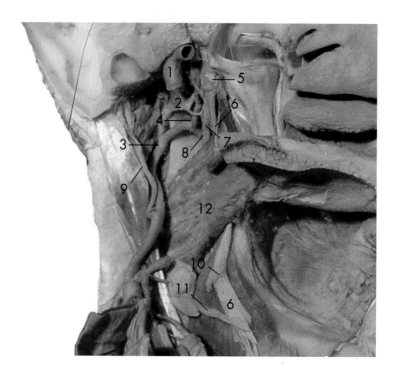

1	Internal carotid artery
2	Auriculotemporal nerve
3	Maxillary artery
4	Middle meningeal artery
5	Otic ganglion
6	Lingual nerve
7	Chorda tympani nerve
8	Inferior alveolar nerve
9	Occipital artery
10	Submandibular ganglion
11	Submandibular duct
12	Medial pterygoid muscle

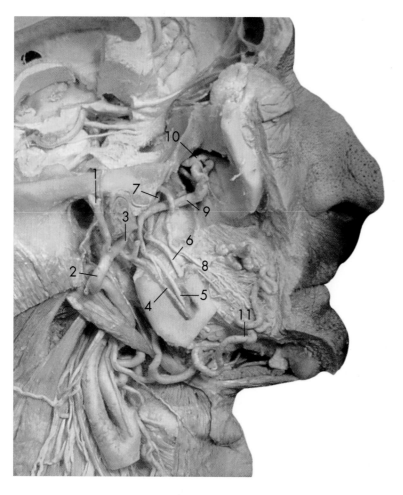

3.41 Maxillary artery in the infratemporal following removal of the pterygoid muscles

1	Superficial temporal artery
2	External carotid artery
3	First (mandibular) part of maxillary artery
4	Inferior alveolar artery
5	Inferior alveolar nerve (with mylohyoid nerve)
6	Lingual nerve
7	Middle meningeal artery
8	Buccal branch of mandibular nerve
9	Second (pterygoid) part of maxillary artery
10	Third (pterygopalatine) part of maxillary artery
11	Facial artery

The pterygoid venous plexus (3.42)

This is situated around and within the lateral pterygoid muscle and it surrounds the maxillary artery. Its tributaries correspond to the various branches of the maxillary artery. Although it is difficult to demonstrate in the cadaver, it is very prominent in life.

The plexus communicates with the cavernous sinus, the facial vein, the inferior ophthalmic vein and the pharyngeal plexus. The connections with the cavernous sinus are via emissary veins passing through the foramen ovale, foramen lacerum and, where present, the emissary sphenoidal foramen. The communication with the facial vein is via the deep facial vein which accompanies the buccal nerve. The inferior ophthalmic vein communicates with the pterygoid plexus through a branch passing through the inferior orbital fissure.

The pterygoid venous plexus drains posteriorly into the maxillary vein. The maxillary vein runs with the first part of the maxillary artery, passing deep to the neck of the condyle of the mandible to enter the parotid gland. Here, it joins the superficial temporal vein to form the retromandibular vein.

Other features of the infratemporal fossa

In addition to the major contents described above, the infratemporal fossa also contains the spheno-mandibular ligament, the tensor veli palatini muscle, the insertion of the temporalis muscle onto the coronoid process of the mandible, the maxillary nerve as it passes from the pterygopalatine fossa into the inferior orbital fissure, the posterior superior alveolar nerve(s), and a loop of the facial artery (together with its ascending palatine and tonsillar branches). These structures are considered in detail elsewhere.

3.42 The veins of the neck and face showing the connections of the pterygoid venous plexus

1	Deep facial vein
2	Pterygoid plexus
3	Facial vein
4	Lingual vein
5	Pharyngeal vein
6	Superior thyroid vein
7	Anterior jugular vein
8	Middle thyroid vein
9	Inferior thyroid vein
10	Brachiocephalic vein
11	Subclavian vein
12	Suprascapular vein
13	Transverse cervical vein
14	Vertebral vein
15	External jugular vein
16	Posterior external jugular artery
17	Posterior auricular vein
18	Internal jugular vein
19	Sigmoid sinus
20	Superficial temporal vein
21	Cavernous sinus

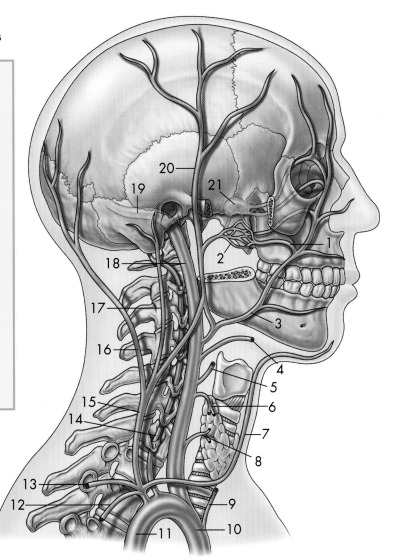

chapter 4
THE SCALP

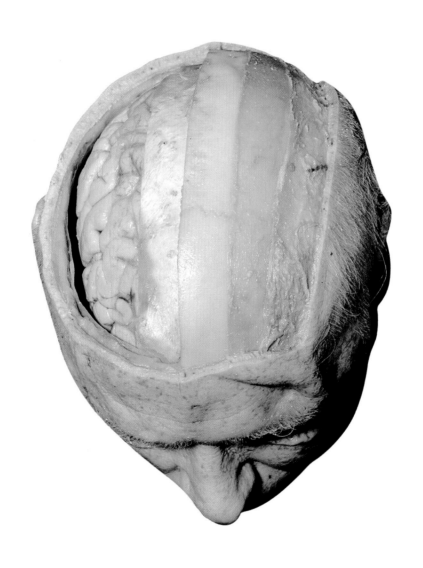

Chapter 4 THE SCALP

The skin, connective tissue and muscles covering the calvaria collectively comprise the scalp. The scalp extends from the eyebrows and forehead to the superior nuchal line in the occipital region. Laterally, the scalp extends down to the zygomatic arches. Thus, the forehead and the temple are areas common to both the scalp and the face.

THE LAYERS OF THE SCALP (4.1)

The scalp consists of five layers. Listed from the surface inwards, these are:

- Skin, which is thick and contains the hair

- Dense connective tissue which is richly vascularised

- The epicranial aponeurosis with the occipitofrontalis muscle

- Loose connective tissue, forming a potential subaponeurotic space

- Pericranium, the periosteum on the outer surface of the cranial vault

The three outer layers are closely adherent and can be readily separated from the underlying tissues. Consequently, they have been termed by some the scalp proper.

THE EPICRANIAL APONEUROSIS (4.1, 4.2)

The epicranial aponeurosis may also be termed the galea aponeurotica. It is a continuous musculomembranous sheet which extends from the external occipital protuberance and the supreme nuchal lines to the eyebrows. The aponeurosis is continuous laterally with the temporal fascia overlying the temporalis muscle. Although mainly membranous, it also contains the occipitofrontalis muscles.

The occipitofrontalis muscle (4.2)

Attachments: Each occipital belly arises from the lateral two-thirds of the supreme nuchal line of the occipital bone and from the mastoid process of the temporal bone. It extends forwards to become continuous with the epicranial aponeurosis. The two occipital bellies are separated in the midline by the aponeurosis as it attaches onto the external occipital protuberance. Each frontal belly arises from the anterior margin of the epicranial aponeurosis and passes forwards to merge with the orbital part of the orbicularis oculi muscle and with the muscle and connective tissue over the bridge of the nose.

Innervation: The occipitofrontalis muscle is innervated by the facial nerve, the occipital belly by the posterior auricular branch and the frontal belly by the temporal and zygomatic branches.

Vasculature: The muscle is supplied by branches from the superficial temporal, ophthalmic, posterior auricular, and occipital arteries.

Actions: The main function of the occipitofrontalis muscle is to elevate the eyebrows to express surprise or horror, or to produce transverse furrows of the forehead.

The *temporoparietalis muscle* is the name given to occasional muscle fibres present at the side of the scalp between the frontal belly of occipitofrontalis and the auricular muscles.

THE SUBAPONEUROTIC SPACE

This potential tissue space is limited by the attachments of the epicranial aponeurosis and the occipitofrontalis muscles. Posteriorly, therefore, it is limited by the supreme nuchal lines and laterally by the zygomatic arches. Anteriorly, however, the subaponeurotic space is continuous with the eyelids and the bridge of the nose.

4.1 The layers of the scalp

1	Skin
2	Epicranial aponeurosis
3	Frontal belly of occipito-frontalis muscle
4	Superficial temporal vessels
5	Supra-orbital nerve and vessels
6	Pericranium and loose connective tissue
7	Calvaria
8	Meninges (dura)
9	Layer of arachnoid meninges
10	Cerebral hemisphere of the brain

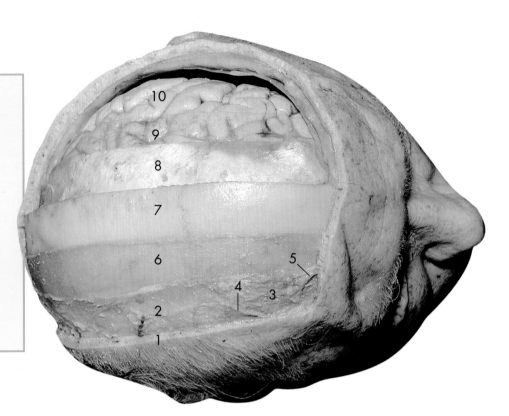

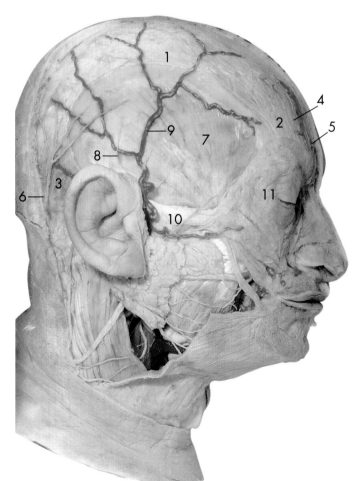

4.2 The scalp, as seen from the lateral aspect

1	Epicranial aponeurosis
2	Frontal belly of occipito-frontalis muscle
3	Occipital belly of occipito-frontalis muscle
4	Supra-orbital nerve
5	Supratrochlear nerve
6	Greater occipital nerve
7	Temporalis muscle
8	Auriculotemporal nerve
9	Superficial temporal artery
10	Zygomatic arch
11	Orbicularis oculi muscle

THE CUTANEOUS INNERVATION OF THE SCALP (4.2, 4.3)

Anteriorly and medially, the innervation is derived from the supratrochlear and supra-orbital branches of the ophthalmic nerve. Posteriorly, the skin is supplied by the dorsal ramus of the second cervical nerve (greater occipital nerve) and the third cervical nerves (third occipital nerve). Laterally, the zygomaticotemporal branch of the maxillary nerve, the auriculotemporal branch of the mandibular nerve, and the lesser occipital nerve from the cervical plexus, all contribute to the sensory innervation.

THE VASCULATURE OF THE SCALP (4.2–4.4)

The *arteries* are derived from branches of the external and internal carotid arteries. Both the arteries and the nerves enter the scalp from below (an important clinical consideration). The branches from the external carotid artery are the superficial temporal and posterior auricular arteries which supply the scalp laterally, and the occipital artery which supplies the posterior aspect. The scalp anteriorly is supplied by branches from the internal carotid, namely the supratrochlear and supra-orbital branches of the ophthalmic artery. All of the arteries in the scalp freely anastomose.

The *veins* have a similar distribution to the arteries, each artery in the scalp being usually accompanied by a pair of veins (venae comitantes). In addition, the veins of the scalp may communicate with the venous sinuses inside the skull via emissary veins which pass through the mastoid and parietal foramina.

The *lymphatic drainage of the scalp* involves submandibular, parotid, retro-auricular, occipital and superficial cervical nodes.

4.3 The innervation and arterial supply of the scalp

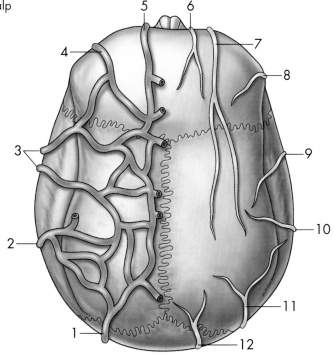

1	Occipital artery
2	Posterior auricular artery
3	Superficial temporal artery
4	Supra-orbital artery
5	Supratrochlear artery
6	Supratrochlear nerve
7	Supra-orbital nerve
8	Zygomaticotemporal nerve
9	Auriculotemporal nerve
10	Lesser occipital nerve
11	Greater occipital nerve
12	Third occipital nerve

4.4 Arterial supply to the face and scalp

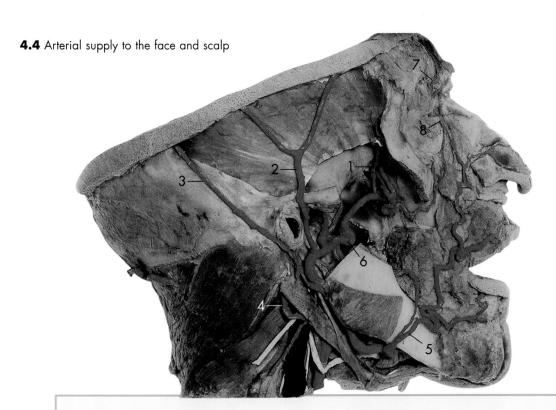

1	Deep temporal artery	5	Facial artery
2	Superficial temporal artery	6	Maxillary artery
3	Posterior auricular artery	7	Supra-orbital artery
4	Occipital artery	8	Infra-orbital artery

chapter 5
THE MOUTH
AND PALATE

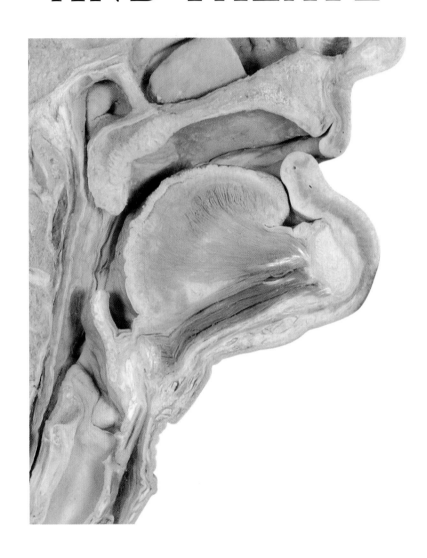

Chapter 5 THE MOUTH AND PALATE

THE MOUTH AND PALATE

The *mouth* or *oral cavity* extends from the lips and cheeks externally to the anterior pillars of the fauces internally, where it continues into the oropharynx. The mouth can be subdivided into the vestibule external to the teeth and the oral cavity proper internal to the teeth. The palate forms the roof of the mouth, separating the oral and nasal cavities. The floor of the mouth is formed by the mylohyoid muscles and is occupied mainly by the tongue. The lateral walls of the mouth are defined by the cheeks and retromolar regions.

The mouth is concerned primarily with the ingestion and mastication of food, and secondarily with phonation and ventilation.

The *lips* (5.1) have a muscular skeleton, the orbicularis oris muscle, and are covered externally by skin and internally by mucous membrane. The orbicularis oris muscle is a muscle of facial expression (see page 108) and passes circumferentially through both the upper and lower lips. The red zone of the lip (the vermilion) is a feature characteristic of man. The sharp junction between the vermilion and the skin is called the vermilion border. The vermilion of the upper lip protrudes in the midline to form the tubercle. The lower lip shows a slight depression corresponding to the tubercle. Both the upper and lower lips widen and then narrow as they pass from the midline to the corners of the lips. The upper lip is separated from the cheeks by nasolabial grooves. Similar grooves appear with age to delineate the lower lip. These are called the labiomarginal sulci. A labiomental groove separates the lower lip from the chin. In the midline of the upper lip is situated the philtrum. The corners of the lips (the labial commissures) are usually located adjacent to the maxillary canine and mandibular first premolar teeth. The lips exhibit sexual dimorphism. The skin of the male is hirsute and is generally thicker and firmer, but less mobile.

The *oral vestibule* (5.2) is a slit-like space between the lips or cheeks and the teeth. When the teeth occlude, the vestibule is a closed space which only communicates with the oral cavity proper in the retromolar regions. Where the mucosa covering the alveolus of the jaw is reflected onto the lips and cheeks, a trough or sulcus is formed which is called the fornix vestibuli. A variable number of sickle-shaped folds containing loose connective tissue run across the fornix vestibuli. The upper and lower labial frena (or frenula) are such folds in the midline. Other folds may traverse the fornix near the canines or premolars. The folds in the lower fornix are said to be more pronounced than those in the upper fornix.

The *cheeks* extend from the labial commissures anteriorly to the ridges of mucosa overlying the ascending rami of the mandible posteriorly. They are bounded superiorly and inferiorly by the upper and the lower fornix vestibuli.

Within the cheek is the buccinator muscle which is a muscle of facial expression (see page 112). The mucosa of the cheek is tightly adherent to the buccinator muscle and is thus stretched when the mouth is opened and wrinkled when closed. Ectopic sebaceous glands may be evident as yellow patches (Fordyce's spots). Few structural landmarks are visible: the parotid duct drains into the cheek opposite the maxillary second molar tooth and a hyperkeratinised line (the linea alba) may be seen at a position related to the occlusal plane of the teeth. In the retromolar region, a fold of mucosa containing the pterygomandibular raphe extends from the upper to the lower alveolus. The pterygomandibular space (in which the lingual and inferior alveolar nerves run; see page 188) lies lateral to this fold and medial to the ridge produced by the mandibular ramus.

5.1 The external appearance of the lips (the anterior boundary of the mouth)

1	The vermilion zone of the lower lip
2	The labial commissure (corner of lips)
3	The tubercle of the upper lip
4	The philtrum of the upper lip
5	Nasolabial groove
6	Labiomarginal sulcus
7	Labiomental groove

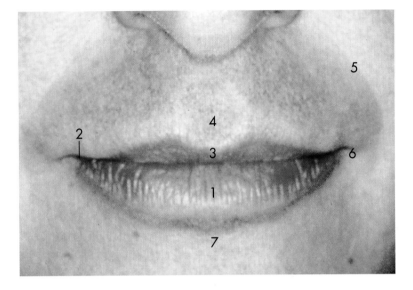

5.2 The oral vestibule

1	The vestibular sulcus (fornix vestibuli)
2	Midline frenum from upper lip
3	Lateral frena associated with upper lip
4	Labial mucosa (non-keratinised)
5	Alveolar mucosa (non-keratinised)
6	Attached gingiva (gum) (keratinised)

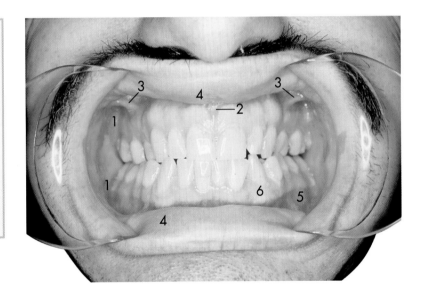

The *floor of the mouth* (5.3) is a small horseshoe-shaped region beneath the movable part of the tongue and above the muscular diaphragm produced by the mylohyoid muscles. In the midline, near the base of the tongue, a fold of tissue called the lingual frenum extends onto the inferior surface of the tongue. Rarely, the lingual frenum extends across the floor of the mouth to be attached onto the mandibular alveolus. The sublingual papilla is a large centrally positioned protuberance at the base of the tongue. The submandibular salivary ducts open into the mouth at this papilla. On either side of the sublingual papilla are the sublingual folds. Beneath these folds lie the submandibular ducts and sublingual salivary glands.

The inferior surface of the tongue is covered by a thin lining of non-keratinised mucous membrane which is tightly bound to the underlying muscles. In the midline, extending onto the floor of the mouth, lies the lingual frenum. Lateral to the frenum lie irregular, fringed folds of mucous membrane called the fimbriated folds. Visible through the mucosa are the deep lingual veins.

The dorsum of the tongue may be subdivided into an anterior two-thirds (palatal part) and a posterior third (pharyngeal part) (5.4). The junction between these two parts is marked by a shallow V-shaped groove called the sulcus terminalis. The angle (or V) of the sulcus terminalis is directed posteriorly. Near the angle may be seen a small pit called the foramen caecum. This is the primordial site of development of the thyroid gland. The mucosa of the palatal part of the tongue is partly keratinised and is characterised by the presence of numerous papillae. The most conspicuous papillae are the circumvallate papillae which lie immediately in front of the sulcus terminalis. Also found are filiform, fungiform and foliate papillae. The pharyngeal surface of the tongue is covered with large rounded nodules called lingual follicles. These are composed of lymphatic tissue (the lingual tonsil). The posterior part of the tongue slopes towards the epiglottis where folds of mucous membrane, the glosso-epiglottic folds, join the two. The anterior pillars of the fauces (the palatoglossal arches) extend from the soft palate to the sides of the tongue near the circumvallate papillae.

The *palate* is divided into the immovable hard palate anteriorly and the movable soft palate posteriorly. As their names indicate, the skeleton of the hard palate is bony, whereas that of the soft palate is fibrous.

The hard palate (5.5) is formed by the two palatine processes of the maxillary bones and the two horizontal plates of the palatine bones. It is bounded anteriorly and laterally by the alveolus of the upper jaw which supports the teeth. A cross-shaped set of sutures traverses the palate. Running anteroposteriorly and dividing the palate into right and left halves is the median palatine suture. This suture is continuous with the intermaxillary suture between the maxillary central incisor teeth. Behind the central incisors, the junction between the palatine processes of the maxillary bones is incomplete, thus forming the incisive fossa. Incisive foramina (two lateral or one anterior and one posterior) pass into this fossa and transmit the nasopalatine nerves and the terminal parts of the greater palatine vessels. Running transversely across the palate between the maxillary and the palatine bones is the transverse palatine suture. This suture is incomplete on each side at the greater palatine foramina. Through the greater palatine foramen pass the greater (anterior) palatine nerve and vessels. Behind the foramen lie one or more lesser palatine foramina through which pass the lesser (posterior) palatine nerves and vessels.

The posterior borders of the horizontal plates of the palatine bones are concave and in the midline form a sharp ridge of bone, the posterior nasal spine. To the posterior edge of the hard palate is attached the fibrous aponeurosis of the soft palate, which is formed by the tendons of the tensor veli palatini muscles (see page 170).

5.3 The ventral surface (inferior surface) of the tongue, related to the floor of the mouth

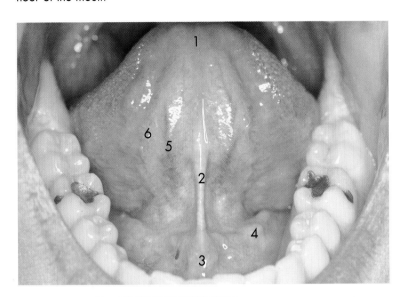

1	Tip of tongue
2	Lingual frenum
3	Sublingual papilla
4	Sublingual fold
5	Deep lingual vein
6	Fimbriated fold

5.4 The dorsum of the tongue

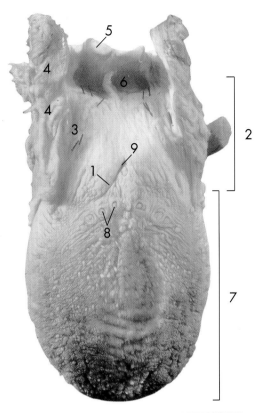

1	Sulcus terminalis
2	Posterior third (pharyngeal part)
3	Lingual follicles
4	Pillars of fauces
5	Epiglottis
6	Vallecula defined by median and lateral glosso-epiglottic folds
7	Anterior two-thirds (palatal part)
8	Circumvallate papillae
9	Foramen caecum

5.5 Osteology of the hard palate

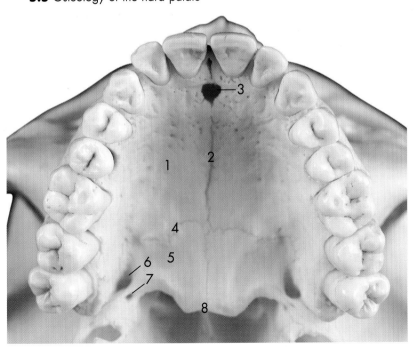

1	Palatine process of maxillary bone
2	Median palatine suture
3	Incisive fossa
4	Transverse palatine suture
5	Horizontal plate of palatine bone
6	Greater (anterior) palatine foramen
7	Lesser (posterior) palatine foramen
8	Posterior nasal spine

The shape and size of the dome of the palate varies considerably (5.6). The mucosa covering the hard palate shows an incisive papilla immediately behind the maxillary central incisors. This covers the nasopalatine nerves as they emerge from the incisive fossa. Extending back from the incisive papilla is a ridge termed the palatine raphe. The palatine rugae are irregular folds which radiate transversely from the incisive papilla and the anterior part of the palatine raphe. The hard palate is covered by a mucoperiosteum (except at the junction with the alveolus, where a submucosa is present in which run the greater palatine nerves and vessels).

The boundary between the hard and soft palate is readily palpable and may be distinguished by a contrast in colour, the soft palate being a darker red with a yellowish tint. Extending from each side of the free border of the soft palate are two prominent folds called the pillars of the fauces. The anterior pillar is the palatoglossal arch; the posterior pillar is the palatopharyngeal arch. These arches cover the palatoglossus and palatopharyngeus muscles. Between the anterior and posterior pillars of the fauces is located the tonsillar fossa which houses the palatine tonsil. Extending backwards and downwards from the free edge of the soft palate in the midline is the uvula (5.7).

THE TEETH (5.8)

A strict definition of a tooth is difficult to construct because of the great diversity in its structure and function. A suitable definition for a human tooth might be: a hard body in the mouth, attached to, but not forming part of the jaws, which is primarily concerned with the comminution of food.

Man has two generations of teeth, the deciduous (primary) dentition and the permanent (secondary) dentition. There are no teeth in the mouth at birth but by the age of 3 years the deciduous dentition is complete. By 6 years, the first permanent teeth appear and thence the deciduous teeth are exfoliated one by one to be replaced by their permanent successors. There is thus a period where there is a mixed dentition. A complete permanent dentition is present at about the age of 18 years.

There are 20 teeth in the deciduous dentition — 10 in each jaw. There are 32 teeth in the permanent dentition — 16 in each jaw. In both dentitions, there are three basic tooth forms: incisiform, caniniform and molariform. Incisiform teeth (incisors) are cutting teeth, having thin, blade-like crowns. Caniniform teeth (canines) are piercing or tearing teeth, having stout, pointed, cone-shaped crowns. Molariform teeth (molars and premolars) are grinding teeth, possessing several cusps on otherwise flattened biting surfaces. Premolars are bicuspid teeth which are peculiar to the permanent dentition and which replace the deciduous molars.

Identification of teeth is made not only according to the dentition to which they belong and to the basic tooth form, but also according to their anatomical location within the jaws. The tooth-bearing regions can be divided into four quadrants, the right and left maxillary and mandibular quadrants. A tooth may therefore be identified according to the quadrant in which it is located (e.g. a right maxillary deciduous incisor or a left mandibular permanent molar). In both the permanent and deciduous dentitions, the incisors may be distinguished according to their relationship to the midline. The incisor nearest the midline is the central or first incisor, the incisor which is more laterally positioned being called the lateral or second incisor. The permanent premolars and the permanent and deciduous molars can also be distinguished according to their anteroposterior relationships. The anterior premolar is the first premolar, the premolar behind it being the second premolar. Likewise, the molar most anteriorly positioned is designated the first molar, the one behind it being the second molar. In the permanent dentition, the tooth most posteriorly positioned is the third molar.

5.6 The hard palate

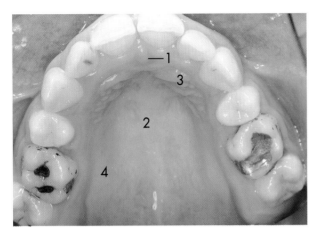

1 Incisive papilla
2 Palatine raphe
3 Palatine rugae
4 Area of palatine submucosa associated
   with the pathway of the greater palatine
   nerves and vessels

5.7 The soft palate

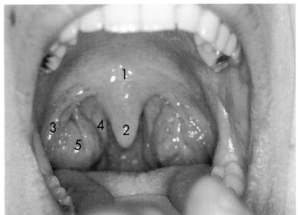

1 Soft palate
2 Uvula
3 Anterior pillar of fauces (palatoglossal arch)
4 Posterior pillar of fauces (palatopharyngeal
   arch)
5 Tonsillar fossa with palatal tonsil

5.8 The permanent teeth within the skull

1 Central (first) incisor
2 Lateral (second) incisor
3 Canine
4 First premolar
5 Second premolar
6 First molar
7 Second molar
Note: the third molars are absent

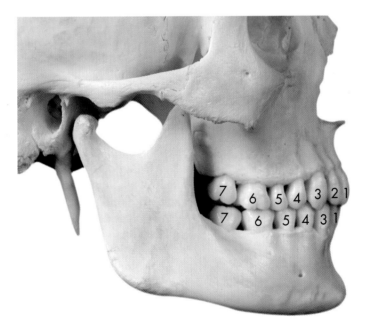

THE SALIVARY GLANDS

Salivary glands are compound, tubular, acinous, merocrine glands whose ducts open into the oral cavity. They secrete a fluid, the saliva, which among its many functions aids in the mastication, digestion and deglutition of food.

There are three pairs of major salivary glands: the parotid, the submandibular and the sublingual glands. Numerous minor salivary glands are also scattered throughout the oral mucosa.

THE PAROTID GLAND (5.9)

The parotid gland is the largest salivary gland. It is almost entirely serous. The parotid duct runs through the cheek and drains into the mouth opposite the maxillary second permanent molar tooth. The parotid gland is situated in front of the external ear and consequently is described in detail in relation to the face (see pages 124–127).

THE SUBMANDIBULAR GLAND (5.10–5.12)

This gland is intermediate in size between the parotid and sublingual glands. The submandibular gland is a mixed gland, serous cells predominating over the mucous cells in the ratio of approximately 3:2.

The submandibular gland is found in the floor of the mouth and in the suprahyoid region of the neck. A large part of the gland is visible just beneath the inferior border of the mandible. There is a prominent depression in the mandible on its inner surface below the mylohyoid line for the gland (the submandibular fossa). The gland has an important relationship with the mylohyoid muscle, wrapping around the posterior free edge of the muscle (not unlike a letter C). Thus, the gland is divided into a superficial and a deep part.

The superficial part of the submandibular gland is located in the digastric triangle of the neck. Indeed, it occupies most of this region and often extends to overlap the digastric muscle. Posteriorly, it comes to lie close to the apex of the parotid gland, with only the stylomandibular ligament intervening. Superiorly, the superficial part of the submandibular gland lies under the inferior border of the mandible. Inferiorly, it is partially enclosed by the investing layer of deep cervical fascia. The medial surface lies on the mylohyoid muscle and hooks round the posterior free edge of this muscle to link with the deep part of the submandibular gland.

The superficial part of the submandibular gland is related to the facial artery, the facial vein, the cervical branch of the facial nerve, the mylohyoid nerve, and the submandibular lymph nodes. The facial artery passes across the upper surface of the gland and often produces a distinct groove. The artery then runs between the gland and the inferior border of the mandible before crossing onto the face. The facial vein and the cervical branch of the facial nerve (sometimes also the marginal mandibular branch of the facial nerve) cross the gland superficially. The submandibular lymph nodes are usually located close to the superficial part of the gland, beneath the inferior border of the mandible. Indeed, some lymph nodes are embedded in the substance of the gland. The mylohyoid nerve and the mylohyoid and submental vessels are found between the gland and the mylohyoid muscle.

The deep part of the submandibular gland is situated on the superficial surface of the hyoglossus muscle in the floor of the mouth. It extends forward to reach the posterior end of the sublingual salivary gland. Indeed, the two glands may merge to form a sublingual–submandibular complex. It is from the deep part of the submandibular gland that the submandibular duct emerges. The submandibular gland on the hyoglossus muscle is closely related to the lingual and hypoglossal nerves.

Where the submandibular gland folds around the posterior border of the mylohyoid muscle, it lies close to the styloglossus muscle, stylohyoid ligament and the glossopharyngeal nerve. These structures separate the gland from the wall of the pharynx.

5.9 The parotid salivary gland

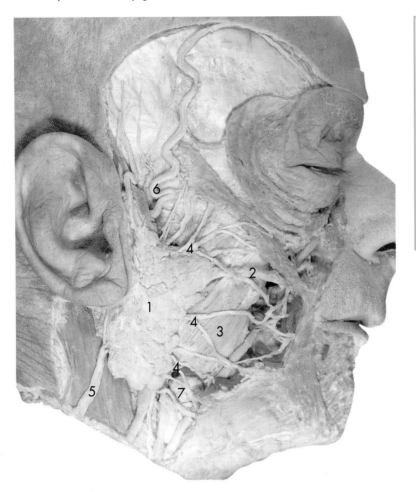

1   Superficial surface of the parotid gland
2   Parotid duct (Stensens duct)
3   Masseter muscle
4   Branches of facial nerve emerging from parotid gland
5   Great auricular nerve
6   Superficial temporal artery emerging from parotid gland
7   Superficial part of submandibular salivary gland

5.10 The submandibular salivary gland seen in the upper part of the neck

1   Superficial part of the submandibular gland
2   Inferior border of mandible
3   Anterior belly of digastric muscle
4   Posterior belly of digastric muscle
5   Facial artery
6   Hypoglossal nerve
7   Sternocleidomastoid muscle

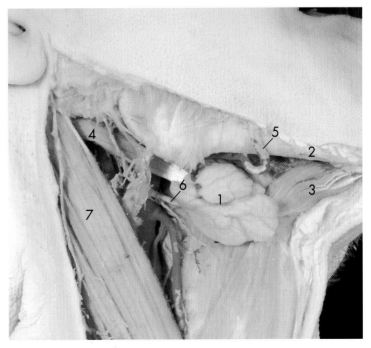

The *submandibular duct* (Wharton's duct) commences in the superficial part of the submandibular gland but emerges from the deep part. The duct is approximately 5 cm long. It runs forwards towards the floor of the mouth between the mylohyoid and the hyoglossus muscles. In the floor of the mouth, the duct initially lies below the lingual nerve. As these structures pass behind the sublingual gland, the duct is crossed twice by the lingual nerve, first on its lateral side then on its medial side. The duct now continues forward to empty at the sublingual papilla in the floor of the mouth. The terminal part of the submandibular duct lies just beneath the oral mucosa on the sublingual fold. Just before it opens into the mouth, the submandibular duct may receive a duct(s) from the anterior part of the sublingual gland.

THE SUBLINGUAL GLAND (5.11, 5.12)

The sublingual salivary gland is the smallest of the major salivary glands. It is located in the floor of the mouth, above the mylohyoid muscle and below the oral mucosa. The sublingual gland produces a distinct ridge under the tongue, the sublingual fold. The gland is narrow and flat and can be described as almond-shaped.

The sublingual gland is a mixed gland. It differs from the submandibular gland, however, because the mucous elements predominate over the serous in the ratio of approximately 3:1.

The sublingual gland lies adjacent to the sublingual fossa of the mandible. The genioglossus muscle runs medial to the gland. The two sublingual glands almost meet in the midline. Between the sublingual gland and the genioglossus muscle lie the submandibular duct (near the upper border of the gland), the lingual and hypoglossal nerves (as they run into the substance of the tongue) and the sublingual artery.

The sublingual gland can be subdivided into anterior and posterior parts. Each part differs according to the method of drainage. Unlike the other major salivary glands, there is not a single main salivary duct, but as many as 20 small ducts. The ducts from the posterior part of the sublingual gland empty at the sublingual fold in the floor of the mouth. The ducts from the anterior part of the gland may unite to form a larger duct which either joins the submandibular duct or drains directly into the floor of the mouth at the sublingual papilla. This larger duct is sometimes referred to as Bartholin's duct.

THE MINOR SALIVARY GLANDS

The minor salivary glands include the labial, buccal, palatoglossal, palatal and lingual glands. The labial and buccal glands contain both mucous and serous elements. The palatoglossal glands are mucous glands and are located around the pharyngeal isthmus. The palatal glands are also mucous glands. They are located in both the soft and hard palate. The anterior and posterior lingual glands are mainly mucous. The anterior glands are embedded within muscle near the ventral surface of the tongue and open by means of four or five ducts near the lingual frenum. The posterior glands are located in the root of the tongue. Around the circumvallate papillae are serous glands (of Von Ebner).

THE INNERVATION OF THE SALIVARY GLANDS

The salivary glands are innervated by way of cranial parasympathetic ganglia. The secretomotor supply for the parotid gland is derived from the glossopharyngeal nerve via the otic ganglion (see page 126). The secretomotor supply for the submandibular and sublingual glands is provided by the facial nerve via the submandibular ganglion (see page 182). The minor salivary glands are innervated by parasympathetic fibres travelling with sensory branches of the trigeminal nerve (e.g. palatine glands by the greater and lesser palatine nerves via the pterygopalatine ganglion).

5.11 Medial view of floor of mouth

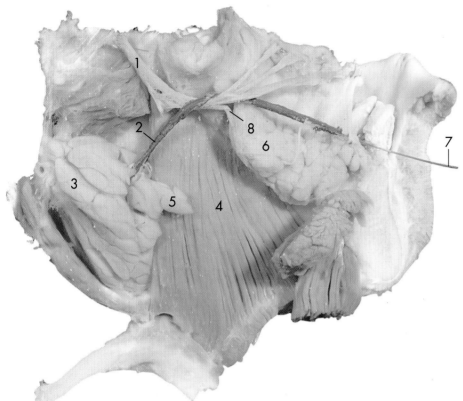

1 Lingual nerve
2 Submandibular duct
3 Submandibular gland
4 Mylohyoid muscle
5 Deep part of submandibular gland behind posterior border of mylohyoid muscle
6 Sublingual gland
7 Bristle in opening of submandibular duct at sublingual papilla
8 Branch of lingual nerve to sublingual gland carrying parasympathetic fibres

5.12 Coronal section through the tongue and floor of mouth

1 Superior longitudinal intrinsic muscles
2 Body of tongue with vertical and transverse intrinsic muscles
3 Lingual septum
4 Genioglossus muscle
5 Geniohyoid muscle
6 Mylohyoid muscle
7 Sublingual salivary gland
8 Anterior belly of digastric muscle

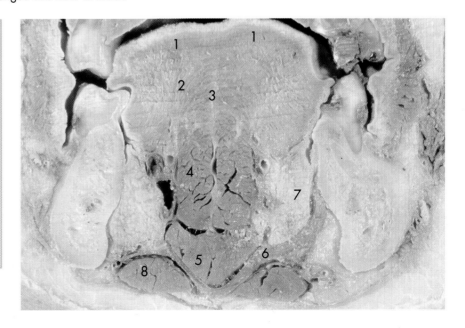

THE ORAL MUSCULATURE

THE MUSCLES OF THE LIPS AND THE CHEEK

Within the lips is the orbicularis oris muscle and within the cheek is the buccinator muscle. These muscles belong to the group of muscles termed the muscles of facial expression, and are consequently described with the face (see pages 104–113). The orbicularis oris muscle is innervated by the buccal and marginal mandibular branches of the facial nerve. The buccinator muscle is supplied by the buccal branch of the facial nerve.

THE MUSCLES OF THE TONGUE

The tongue is comprised of intrinsic and extrinsic muscles. The intrinsic muscles are restricted to the substance of the tongue, whereas the extrinsic muscles arise outside the tongue.

The *intrinsic muscles* of the tongue can be divided into three fibre groups: the transverse, longitudinal and vertical groups (5.12, 5.13). However, these groups cannot readily be distinguished because their fibres intercalate. The transverse fibres pass laterally from a sheet of connective tissue which runs longitudinally through the midline of the tongue (the lingual septum). The longitudinal fibres are subdivided into the superior and inferior longitudinal muscles of the tongue. The vertical fibres pass directly between the upper and lower surfaces of the tongue. They are particularly prominent at the lateral borders of the tongue. The intrinsic musculature is responsible for changing the shape of the tongue. The muscles receive their motor innervation from the hypoglossal nerve.

The *extrinsic muscles* of the tongue arise from the skull and hyoid bone and thence spread into the body of the tongue. The extrinsic musculature is composed of four pairs of muscles: genioglossus, hyoglossus, styloglossus and palatoglossus.

The genioglossus muscle (5.12, 5.14–5.16)

Attachments: This muscle lies anteriorly near the median plane. It originates from the superior genial tubercle (mental spine) on the medial surface of the body of the mandible. The genioglossus muscle fans out into the substance of the tongue. The two genioglossus muscles cannot easily be separated near their origins. As the muscles enter the tongue, however, a thin strip of connective tissue intervenes. The superior fibres of the genioglossus muscle pass upwards and anteriorly towards the tip of the tongue. Some of the inferior fibres insert onto the body of the hyoid bone.

Innervation: Genioglossus receives its motor innervation from the hypoglossal nerve.

Vasculature: The lingual artery (sublingual branch) and the facial artery (submental branch) supply this muscle.

Actions: The genioglossus muscle is a protractor and depressor of the tongue.

The hyoglossus muscle (5.14, 5.15)

Attachments: This is a thin, quadrilateral muscle which provides an important landmark in the floor of the mouth. It originates from the superior border of the greater horn of the hyoid bone. It passes vertically upwards to insert into the side of the tongue. A part of the muscle is attached to the base of the lesser horn of the hyoid bone and has been called chondroglossus. At its origin, the hyoglossus muscle is separated from the attachment of the middle constrictor muscle of the pharynx by the lingual artery.

Innervation: The hypoglossal nerve supplies the hyoglossus muscle.

Vasculature: The lingual artery (sublingual branch) and the facial artery (submental branch) supply hyoglossus.

Actions: The muscle depresses the tongue.

5.13 Coronal section of the tongue to show the intrinsic musculature

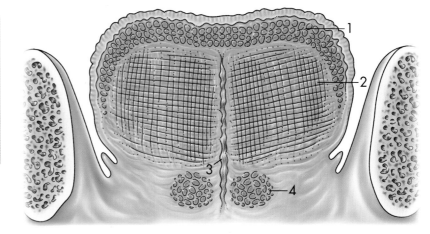

1 Superior longitudinal muscle
2 Vertical and transverse muscles
3 Lingual septum
4 Inferior longitudinal muscle

5.14 The tongue and floor of the mouth, seen in sagittal section

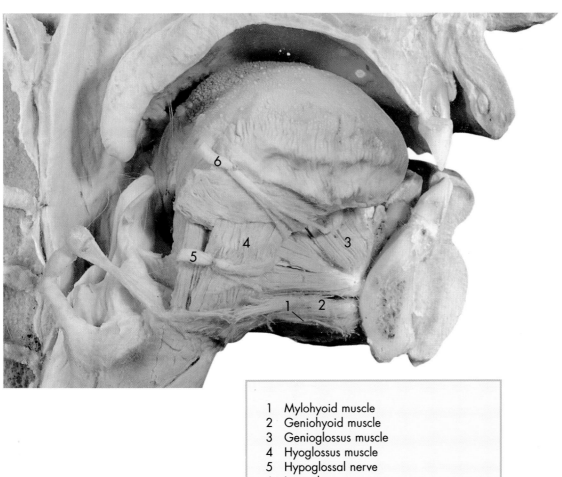

1 Mylohyoid muscle
2 Geniohyoid muscle
3 Genioglossus muscle
4 Hyoglossus muscle
5 Hypoglossal nerve
6 Lingual nerve

The styloglossus muscle (5.15, 5.17)

Attachments: Styloglossus arises from the tip of the styloid process of the temporal bone and from the upper end of the stylomandibular ligament. It passes downwards and forwards to enter the tongue below the insertion of the palatoglossus muscle. At this point, its fibres intercalate with the fibres of the hyoglossus muscle. The muscle then continues forwards towards the tip of the tongue.

Innervation: The muscle is supplied by the hypoglossal nerve.

Vasculature: The sublingual branch of the lingual artery supplies the styloglossus muscle.

Actions: Styloglossus retracts and elevates the tongue.

The palatoglossus muscle

Palatoglossus is more closely associated with the palate than to the tongue. It is therefore described with the muscles of the palate (see page 172).

THE MUSCLES IN THE FLOOR OF THE MOUTH

The floor of the mouth is the region located between the medial surface of the mandible, the inferior surface of the tongue, and the mylohyoid muscles. The mylohyoid muscles are attached to the mylohyoid lines of the mandible and consequently structures above these lines are related to the floor of the mouth whereas structures below the lines are related to the upper part of the neck.

The two mylohyoid muscles form a muscular diaphragm for the floor of the mouth. Above this diaphragm are found the genioglossus and geniohyoid muscles medially and the hyoglossus muscle laterally. Below the diaphragm lie the digastric and stylohyoid muscles.

The mylohyoid muscle (5.11, 5.12, 5.16)

Attachments: The mylohyoid muscle arises from the mylohyoid line (internal oblique line) on the medial surface of the body of the mandible. Its fibres slope downwards, forwards and inwards. The anterior fibres of the mylohyoid muscle interdigitate with the corresponding fibres on the opposite side to form a median raphe. This raphe is attached above to the symphysis menti of the mandible and below to the hyoid bone. The posterior fibres of the mylohyoid muscle are inserted onto the anterior surface of the body of the hyoid bone (near its lower border).

Innervation: The muscle is supplied by the mylohyoid branch of the mandibular division of the trigeminal nerve.

Vasculature: The mylohyoid muscle receives its arterial supply from three sources: the lingual artery (sublingual branch), the maxillary artery (the mylohyoid branch of the inferior alveolar artery), and the facial artery (submental branch).

Actions: The muscle raises the floor of the mouth during the first stages of swallowing. It also helps to depress the mandible when the hyoid bone is fixed. Conversely, it aids in elevation of the hyoid bone.

The geniohyoid muscle (5.12, 5.14–5.16)

Attachments: This muscle originates from the inferior genial tubercle (mental spine). It passes backwards and slightly downwards to insert onto the body of the hyoid bone (anterior surface).

Innervation: The innervation is shared with the thyrohyoid muscle, namely the first cervical spinal nerve travelling with the hypoglossal nerve.

Vasculature: The blood supply is derived from the lingual artery (sublingual branch).

Actions: The geniohyoid muscle elevates the hyoid bone and is a weak depressor of the mandible.

The main structures found above the mylohyoid muscle (i.e. in the floor of the mouth) are: the lingual, glossopharyngeal and hypoglossal nerves, the sublingual gland and the deep part of the submandibular gland, the lingual artery and the submandibular parasympathetic ganglion.

The structures related to the inferior surface of the mylohyoid muscle (i.e. the digastric and submental triangles of the neck; see pages 324–326) include: the superficial part of the submandibular gland, the facial, submental and mylohyoid blood vessels, the submandibular and submental lymph nodes, the mylohyoid nerve and the veins that form the anterior jugular veins in the submental triangle.

5.15 Structures on the hyoglossus muscle in the floor of the mouth

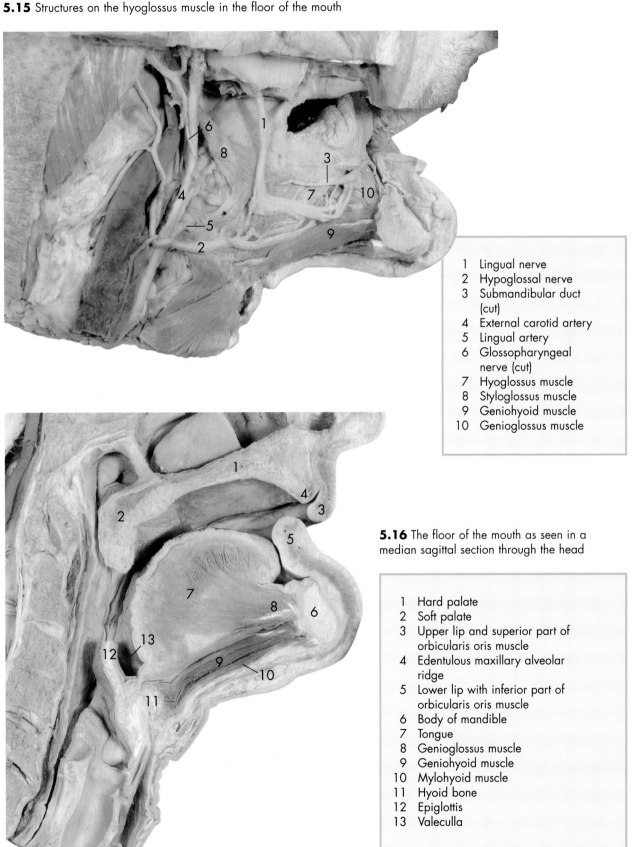

1	Lingual nerve
2	Hypoglossal nerve
3	Submandibular duct (cut)
4	External carotid artery
5	Lingual artery
6	Glossopharyngeal nerve (cut)
7	Hyoglossus muscle
8	Styloglossus muscle
9	Geniohyoid muscle
10	Genioglossus muscle

5.16 The floor of the mouth as seen in a median sagittal section through the head

1	Hard palate
2	Soft palate
3	Upper lip and superior part of orbicularis oris muscle
4	Edentulous maxillary alveolar ridge
5	Lower lip with inferior part of orbicularis oris muscle
6	Body of mandible
7	Tongue
8	Genioglossus muscle
9	Geniohyoid muscle
10	Mylohyoid muscle
11	Hyoid bone
12	Epiglottis
13	Valeculla

THE MUSCLES OF THE PALATE

The soft palate has a fibrous aponeurosis whose shape and position is altered by the tensor veli palatini, the levator veli palatini, the palatoglossus, and the palatopharyngeus muscles. The musculature of the soft palate also includes the musculus uvulae.

The tensor veli palatini muscle (5.17–5.21)

Attachments: This muscle arises from the scaphoid fossa of the sphenoid bone (at the root of the pterygoid plates) and from the lateral side of the cartilaginous part of the auditory tube. The fibres converge towards the pterygoid hamulus, where the muscle becomes tendinous. The tendon bends at right angles around the hamulus to become the palatine aponeurosis. The aponeurosis is attached to the posterior border of the hard palate. Medially, it merges with the aponeurosis of the other side. Posteriorly, it becomes indistinct and merges with the submucosa at the posterior edge of the soft palate.

Innervation: The motor innervation of the muscle is derived from the mandibular nerve via the nerve to the medial pterygoid muscle.

Vasculature: The arterial blood supply is derived from the facial artery (ascending palatine branch) and the maxillary artery (descending palatine branch).

Actions: When the tensor veli palatini muscles act together, the palatine aponeurosis becomes taut and horizontal and provides a platform upon which other palatine muscles may act to change the position of the soft palate. Acting singly, the muscle pulls the soft palate laterally.

The levator veli palatini muscle (5.17–5.21)

Attachments: This muscle originates from the base of the skull at the apex of the petrous part of the temporal bone, and from the medial side of the cartilaginous part of the auditory tube. The muscle curves downwards, medially and forwards to enter the palate immediately below the opening of the auditory tube. In its course, the muscle passes between the base of the skull and the superior margin of the superior constrictor muscle of the pharynx.

Innervation: The nerve supply to the muscle is derived from the cranial part of the accessory nerve via the pharyngeal plexus.

Vasculature: The blood supply is derived from the facial artery (ascending palatine branch) and the maxillary artery (descending palatine branch).

Actions: The levator muscles of the palate form a U-shaped muscular sling. When the palatine aponeurosis is stiffened by the tensor muscles, contraction of the levator muscles produces an upwards and backwards movement of the soft palate. In this way, the nasopharynx is shut off from the oropharynx by the apposition of the soft palate onto the posterior wall of the pharynx.

5.17 Deep dissection of infratemporal fossa to show tensor palati muscle

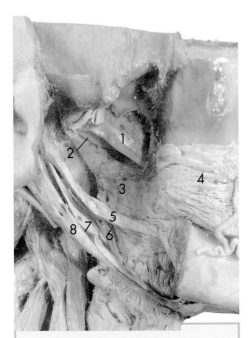

1 Tensor palati muscle
2 Levator palati muscle
  (partially hidden)
3 Superior constrictor muscle
4 Buccinator muscle
5 Styloglossus muscle
6 Stylopharyngeus muscle
7 Stylohyoid muscle
8 Posterior belly of digastric muscle

5.18 Deep dissection of infratemporal fossa with tensor palati muscle removed to reveal levator palati muscle

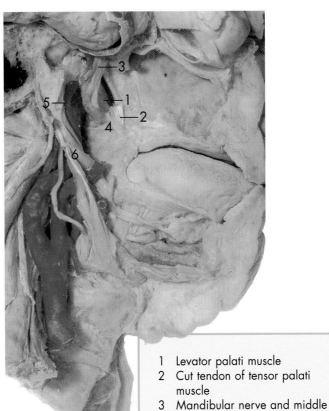

1 Levator palati muscle
2 Cut tendon of tensor palati muscle
3 Mandibular nerve and middle meningeal artery
4 Buccinator muscle
5 Internal carotid artery
6 Styloid group of muscles

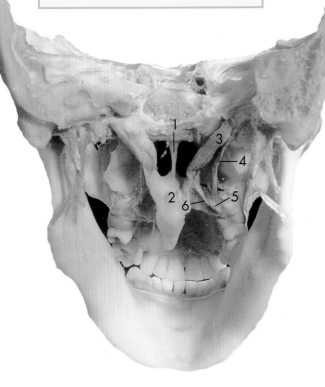

5.19 Soft palate viewed posteriarly showing the tensor and levator palati muscles

1 Nasal septum
2 Soft palate
3 Levator palati muscle
4 Tensor palati muscle
5 Pterygoid hamulus
6 Tendon of tensor palati muscle

The palatoglossus muscle (5.20, 5.21, 11.3)
This muscle can be classified as either a muscle of the palate or as an extrinsic muscle of the tongue.

Attachments: The palatoglossus muscle arises from the palatine aponeurosis and runs to the tongue as the anterior pillar of the fauces. Its fibres intercalate with the transverse muscle fibres of the tongue.

Innervation: Unlike the extrinsic muscles of the tongue, which are innervated by the hypoglossal nerve, the palatoglossus muscle is supplied by the cranial part of the accessory nerve via the pharyngeal plexus.

Vasculature: The muscle receives its blood supply from the facial artery (ascending palatine branch) and the ascending pharyngeal artery.

Actions: The palatoglossus muscles acting together raise the tongue and narrow the oropharyngeal isthmus.

The palatopharyngeus muscle (5.20, 5.21, 11.3)
Although this muscle arises from the soft palate, it is described as a longitudinal muscle of the pharynx (see page 404).

Musculus uvulae arises from the posterior nasal spine at the back of the hard palate and from the palatine aponeurosis. It passes backwards and downwards to insert into the mucosa of the uvula. Its innervation and vasculature is similar to that of the levator veli palatini muscle. It moves the uvula upwards and laterally.

INNERVATION OF THE ORO-DENTAL TISSUES

The oral mucosa receives its sensory innervation primarily from the maxillary and mandibular divisions of the trigeminal nerve. The trigeminal nerve also supplies the teeth and their supporting tissues. The salivary glands are supplied by secretomotor, parasympathetic fibres from the facial and glossopharyngeal nerves. The motor innervation of the oral musculature is derived mainly from the mandibular, facial, accessory and hypoglossal nerves.

THE INNERVATION OF THE TEETH AND GINGIVAE

The dentition in the lower jaw is innervated by the mandibular nerve. The teeth receive their nerve supply from the molar and incisive branches of the inferior alveolar nerve. The lingual gingivae are supplied mainly by the lingual branch of the mandibular nerve. The labial gingivae are innervated by the mental branch of the inferior alveolar nerve and the buccal gingivae by the buccal branch of the mandibular nerve.

The innervation of the dentition in the upper jaw is derived almost entirely from the maxillary nerve. The teeth are supplied by the anterior, middle and posterior superior alveolar branches. The palatal gingivae are innervated by the nasopalatine and greater (anterior) palatine branches via the pterygopalatine ganglion. The labial and buccal gingivae are supplied by the infra-orbital and the posterior superior alveolar branches.

Table 5.1 summarises the nerve supply to the teeth and gingivae.

5.20 Muscles of the soft palate viewed from behind

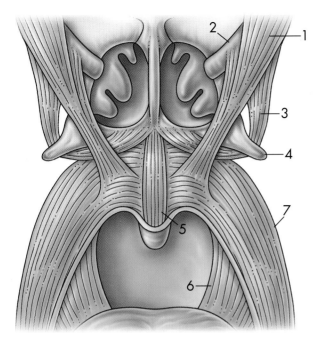

5.21 Muscles of the soft palate viewed from the side at the oropharyngeal isthmus

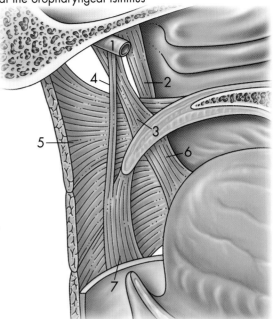

1 Levator veli palatini muscle
2 Auditory tube
3 Tensor veli palatini muscle
4 Pterygoid hamulus
5 Musculus uvulae
6 Palatopharyngeus muscle
7 Palatoglossus muscle

1 Auditory tube
2 Tensor veli palatini muscle
3 Levator veli palatini muscle
4 Salpingopharyngeus muscle
5 Superior constrictor muscle
6 Palatoglossus muscle
7 Palatopharyngeus muscle

Table 5.1 Sensory innervation of the teeth and gingivae. The teeth are numbered according to their position along the tooth row.

Maxilla	Nasopalatine nerve	Greater palatine nerve			Palatal gingiva
	Anterior superior dental nerve	Middle superior alveolar nerve		Posterior superior alveolar nerve	Teeth
	Infra-orbital nerve	Posterior superior alveolar nerve and buccal nerve			Buccal gingiva
	1 2 3	4 5	6 7	8	
Mandible	Mental nerve	Buccal nerve and perforating branches of inferior alveolar nerve			Buccal gingiva
	Incisive nerve	Inferior alveolar nerve			Teeth
	Lingual nerve and perforating branches of inferior alveolar nerve				Lingual gingiva

The inferior alveolar nerve (5.22, 5.23, 5.25–5.27)

The inferior alveolar nerve is the terminal branch of the posterior trunk of the mandibular nerve. It arises in the infratemporal fossa, deep to the lower head of the lateral pterygoid muscle. On emerging from beneath this muscle, the inferior alveolar nerve lies within the pterygomandibular space. Here, it gives off a mylohyoid branch which is a motor nerve to the anterior belly of the digastric muscle and the mylohyoid muscle (it may also have sensory fibres which enter the mandible in the mental region to participate in the nerve supply to the lower incisors). The inferior alveolar nerve enters the mandible through the mandibular foramen.

The course of the inferior alveolar nerve through the mandible is variable. The molar branches to the premolar and molar teeth come either directly from the inferior alveolar nerve in the mandibular canal by short or long branches, or indirectly from the nerve outside the mandibular canal by a series of alveolar branches. The mandibular canal may be closely related to the roots of the mandibular molars, even to the extent of occasionally perforating a root.

The main trunk of the inferior alveolar nerve divides near the premolars into mental and incisive nerves. The mental nerve runs for a short distance in a mental canal before leaving the body of the mandible at the mental foramen to emerge onto the face. It supplies the skin and mucosa of the lower lip, and the labial gingivae of the mandibular anterior teeth. The incisive nerve runs forwards in an incisive canal. This nerve usually innervates only the incisor and canine teeth, but occasionally it supplies the first premolar.

5.22 Infratemporal fossa showing mandibular nerve branches

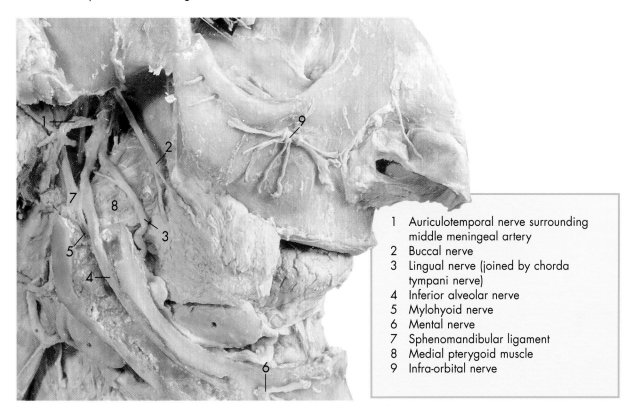

1 Auriculotemporal nerve surrounding middle meningeal artery
2 Buccal nerve
3 Lingual nerve (joined by chorda tympani nerve)
4 Inferior alveolar nerve
5 Mylohyoid nerve
6 Mental nerve
7 Sphenomandibular ligament
8 Medial pterygoid muscle
9 Infra-orbital nerve

5.23 Medial view of infratemporal fossa showing inferior alveolar nerve

1 Mandibular nerve trunk
2 Auriculotemporal nerve
3 Inferior alveolar nerve
4 Mylohyoid nerve
5 Lingual nerve
6 Nerve to medial pterygoid muscle
7 Medial pterygoid muscle
8 Buccal nerve

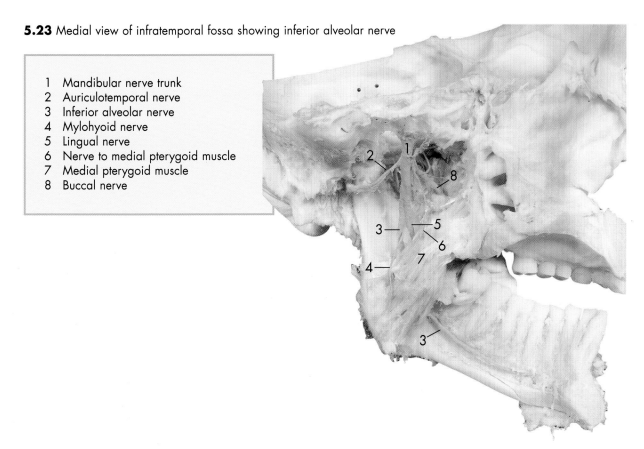

The superior alveolar nerves (5.24, 6.25, 7.33)
There are usually three superior alveolar nerves supplying the maxillary dentition: the posterior, middle and anterior superior alveolar nerves.

The *posterior superior alveolar nerve* arises from the maxillary nerve in the pterygopalatine fossa (see page 214). It descends onto the posterior wall of the maxilla, passing through the pterygomaxillary fissure, and divides into dental and gingival branches. The dental branches enter the maxilla and run in narrow canals above the roots of the molar teeth. The gingival branch does not enter the bone but runs along the outer surface of the maxillary tuberosity to supply the buccal gingivae of the maxillary molar teeth.

The *middle superior alveolar nerve* is found in about 70 per cent of individuals. The nerve generally arises in the floor of the orbit from the infra-orbital branch of the maxillary nerve. It can also arise directly from the maxillary nerve in the pterygopalatine fossa. The middle superior alveolar nerve runs in the posterior, lateral or anterior wall of the maxillary air sinus. It terminates above the roots of the premolar teeth.

The *anterior superior alveolar nerve* arises from the infra-orbital nerve within the infra-orbital canal. It generally appears as a single nerve, occasionally as two or three branches. The nerve runs in the anterior wall of the maxillary sinus and terminates near the anterior nasal spine after giving off a small nasal branch.

The three superior alveolar nerves form a plexus just above the roots of the maxillary teeth. Indeed, it is difficult to trace the precise innervation of the teeth from a specific superior alveolar nerve. As a general rule, however, the incisors and canine are supplied by the anterior nerve, the molars by the posterior nerve and the premolars by the middle nerve.

THE SENSORY INNERVATION OF THE LIPS AND CHEEKS

The mucosa of the upper lip is supplied by the infra-orbital branch of the maxillary nerve. The lower lip is innervated by the mental branch of the mandibular nerve.

The mucosa of the cheeks is innervated by the buccal branch of the mandibular nerve.

The buccal nerve (5.25, 5.27)
The buccal nerve is the terminal branch of the anterior trunk of the mandibular nerve. It arises in the infratemporal fossa (see page 140), behind the upper head of the lateral pterygoid muscle. The buccal nerve passes between the two heads of the lateral pterygoid muscle and crosses the infratemporal fossa. It runs into the upper part of the retromolar fossa at the anterior border of the ramus of the mandible. The buccal nerve breaks up into several branches within the buccinator muscle. It innervates both the mucosa and the skin of the cheek and the buccal gingivae of the mandibular cheek teeth (perhaps even of the maxillary cheek teeth).

5.24 Frontal aspect of face showing maxillary nerve

1 Orbit
2 Maxillary nerve
3 Posterior superior alveolar nerve
4 Maxillary nerve becoming infra-orbital nerve in floor of orbit
5 Infra-orbital nerve entering face at infra-orbital foramen

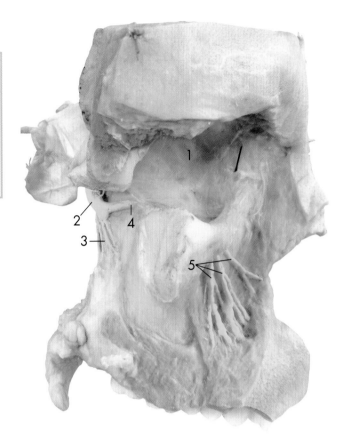

5.25 Demonstration of sensory branches of the mandibular nerve in the infratemporal fossa (some of the nerves and branches have been thickened for demonstration purposes)

1 Lateral pterygoid muscle
2 Buccal branch of mandibular nerve
3 Lingual nerve
4 Inferior alveolar nerve
5 Mental nerve
6 Infra-orbital nerve
7 Medial pterygoid muscle

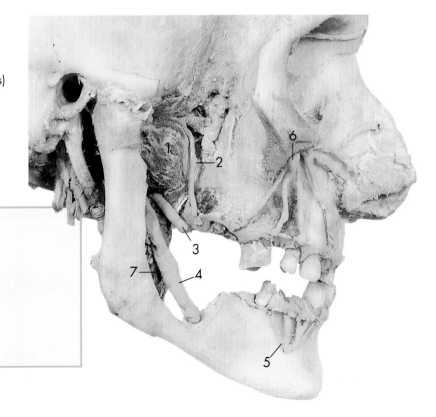

THE SENSORY INNERVATION OF THE TONGUE AND THE FLOOR OF THE MOUTH (5.26)

Concerning general sensation (i.e. excluding taste), three distinct nerve fields can be recognised on the dorsum of the tongue. The anterior part of the tongue in front of the circumvallate papillae is supplied by the lingual branches of the mandibular nerves. Behind, and including, the circumvallate papillae, the tongue is innervated primarily by the glossopharyngeal nerves. Small areas on the posterior part of the tongue around the epiglottis are supplied by the superior laryngeal branches (internal branches) of the vagus nerves. Concerning taste, the anterior part of the tongue is innervated by the chorda tympani branches of the facial nerves. These are distributed through the lingual nerves. The posterior part of the tongue, including the circumvallate papillae, has a similar innervation for taste as that for general sensation.

The mucosa on the ventral surface of the tongue and on the floor of the mouth is supplied by the lingual branches of the mandibular nerves.

The lingual nerve (5.22, 5.23, 5.25, 5.27, 5.28, 5.30)

The lingual nerve is derived from the posterior trunk of the mandibular nerve within the infratemporal fossa (see page 142). It receives the chorda tympani branch of the facial nerve beneath the lateral pterygoid muscle. At the level of the mandibular foramen, the lingual nerve lies on the medial pterygoid muscle and is anterior to the inferior alveolar nerve. The lingual nerve then leaves the infratemporal fossa, passing downwards and forwards to lie close to the lingual alveolar plate of the mandibular third molar tooth. Before curving forwards into the tongue, the nerve is found above the origin of the mylohyoid muscle and lateral to the hyoglossus muscle. On the superficial surface of the hyoglossus muscle, the lingual nerve twists twice around the submandibular salivary duct, first on the lateral side of the duct and then on the medial side. It enters the tongue behind the sublingual salivary gland. Suspended from the lingual nerve as it runs across the hyoglossus muscle is the submandibular parasympathetic ganglion.

The lingual nerve itself supplies the mucosa covering the anterior two-thirds of the dorsum of the tongue, the ventral surface of the tongue, the floor of the mouth, and the lingual gingivae of the mandibular teeth.

The chorda tympani fibres travelling with the lingual nerve are of two types: sensory and parasympathetic. The sensory fibres are associated with taste for the anterior two-thirds of the dorsum of the tongue. The parasympathetic fibres are preganglionic fibres that pass to the submandibular ganglion. Postganglionic fibres are distributed to the submandibular and sublingual salivary glands (see page 182).

THE SENSORY INNERVATION OF THE PALATE

The sensory supply to the palate is derived mainly from branches of the maxillary nerve via the pterygopalatine ganglion. A small area behind the incisor teeth is supplied by the nasopalatine nerves. The remainder of the hard palate is innervated by the greater palatine nerves. The soft palate is supplied by the lesser palatine nerves. There is evidence to suggest that some areas supplied by the lesser palatine nerves may also be innervated from the facial nerves. The posterior part of the soft palate and the uvula may be supplied by the glossopharyngeal nerves.

The nasopalatine nerve (5.29)

This nerve runs along the nasal septum from the pterygopalatine ganglion and emerges onto the hard palate at the incisive fossa behind the maxillary first incisor teeth. The nasopalatine nerve innervates the gingivae behind the maxillary incisor teeth.

5.26 Sensory innervation of the dorsum of the tongue

| 1 | Vagus nerve | 3 | Lingual nerve (chorda |
| 2 | Glossopharyngeal nerve | | tympani nerve for taste) |

1
2
3

5.27 Lateral view of infratemporal fossa showing the lingual nerve

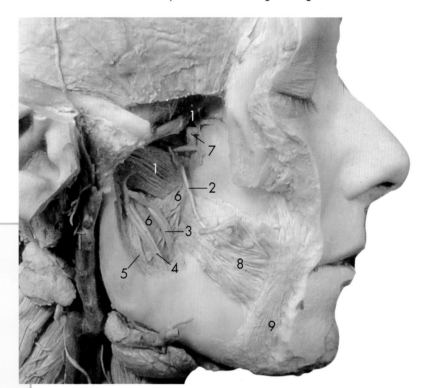

1	Lateral pterygoid muscle (two heads)
2	Buccal nerve
3	Lingual nerve with accompanying branch from maxillary artery
4	Inferior alveolar nerve and artery
5	Mylohyoid nerve
6	Medial pterygoid muscle (two heads)
7	Maxillary artery
8	Buccinator muscle
9	Depressor anguli oris

5.28 Infratemporal fossa viewed medially showing sensory branches of the mandibular nerve

1	Ophthalmic nerve
2	Sphenoidal sinus
3	Trochlear nerve
4	Internal carotid artery
5	Middle meningeal artery
6	Auriculotemporal nerve
7	Maxillary artery
8	Chorda tympani
9	Lingual nerve
10	Inferior alveolar nerve
11	Nerve to medial pterygoid muscle
12	Tensor vali palatini muscle
13	Medial pterygoid muscle
14	External carotid artery
15	Submandibular duct
16	Sublingual gland
17	Otic ganglion

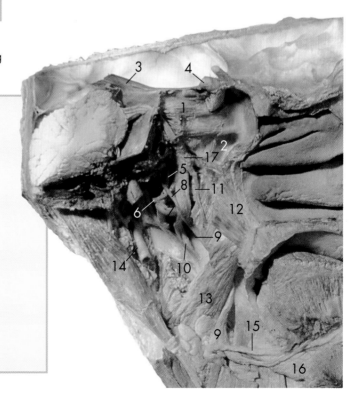

The greater and lesser palatine nerves (5.29, 5.30)

These nerves pass from the pterygopalatine ganglion, down the greater palatine canal at the back of the lateral wall of the nose. The greater palatine nerve runs through the greater palatine foramen and onto the back of the hard palate. It passes towards the front of the hard palate at the interface between the palatine and alveolar processes of the maxilla. In addition to supplying the mucosa of the palate, the greater palatine nerve innervates the palatal gingivae for the maxillary cheek teeth. The lesser palatine nerve emerges onto the palate at the lesser palatine foramen. It runs backwards into the soft palate.

THE SENSORY INNERVATION AT THE OROPHARYNGEAL ISTHMUS

The mucosa over the pillars of the fauces is supplied by the glossopharyngeal nerve.

INNERVATION OF THE ORAL MUSCULATURE

The innervation of the various muscles associated with the mouth is derived from the mandibular division of the trigeminal, the facial, the cranial part of the accessory and the hypoglossal cranial nerves and the first cervical spinal nerves. The innervation is summarised in Table 5.2.

THE INNERVATION OF THE SALIVARY GLANDS

The lesser petrosal branch of the glossopharyngeal nerve supplies the parotid gland via the otic parasympathetic ganglion (see 5.30 and page 126). Postganglionic fibres pass to the gland through the auriculotemporal branch of the mandibular nerve.

The greater petrosal branch of the facial nerve probably supplies palatal and pharyngeal glands via the pterygopalatine parasympathetic ganglion (see page 216). Postganglionic fibres reach the palate with the nasopalatine, greater palatine and lesser palatine branches of the maxillary nerve.

The chorda tympani branch of the facial nerve provides secretomotor fibres via the submandibular parasympathetic ganglion to the submandibular and sublingual salivary glands via the submandibular ganglion (see 5.30, 5.33 and page 182). It probably also provides the innervation of minor salivary glands in the lips, cheeks and tongue.

Table 5.2 Innervation of the oral musculature.

Region	Muscle	Nerve
Lips	Orbicularis oris	Facial
Cheeks	Buccinator	Facial
Tongue (intrinsic musculature)	Transverse Longitudinal Vertical	Hypoglossal
Tongue (extrinsic musculature)	Genioglossus Hyoglossus Styloglossus	Hypoglossal
	Palatoglossus	Accessory (cranial part)
Floor of mouth	Mylohyoid	Mandibular division of trigeminal
	Geniohyoid	First cervical spinal nerve (via hypoglossal)
Palate	Tensor veli palatini	Mandibular division of trigeminal
	Levator veli palatini Palatoglossus Palatopharyngeus Salpingopharyngeus Musculus uvulae	Accessory (cranial part)

5.29 Innervation of the nose and palate via the pterygopalatine ganglion

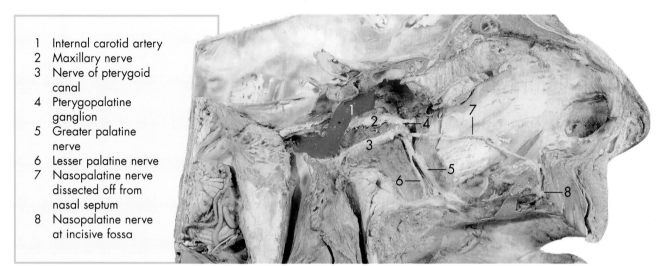

1 Internal carotid artery
2 Maxillary nerve
3 Nerve of pterygoid canal
4 Pterygopalatine ganglion
5 Greater palatine nerve
6 Lesser palatine nerve
7 Nasopalatine nerve dissected off from nasal septum
8 Nasopalatine nerve at incisive fossa

5.30 The pterygopalatine ganglion and the greater and lesser palatine nerves

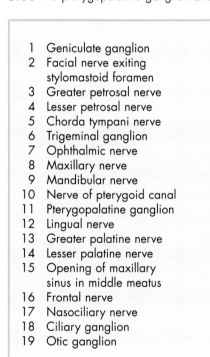

1 Geniculate ganglion
2 Facial nerve exiting stylomastoid foramen
3 Greater petrosal nerve
4 Lesser petrosal nerve
5 Chorda tympani nerve
6 Trigeminal ganglion
7 Ophthalmic nerve
8 Maxillary nerve
9 Mandibular nerve
10 Nerve of pterygoid canal
11 Pterygopalatine ganglion
12 Lingual nerve
13 Greater palatine nerve
14 Lesser palatine nerve
15 Opening of maxillary sinus in middle meatus
16 Frontal nerve
17 Nasociliary nerve
18 Ciliary ganglion
19 Otic ganglion

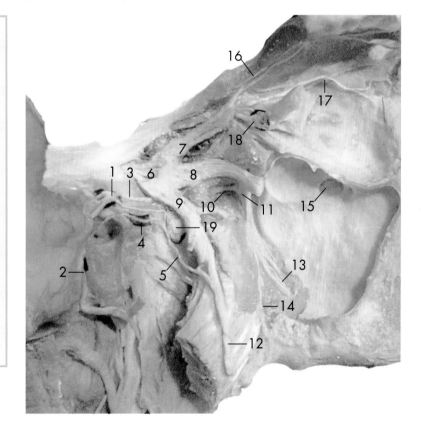

The submandibular ganglion (5.32, 5.33)

This parasympathetic ganglion is found in the floor of the mouth, on the superficial surface of the hyoglossus muscle and under cover of the mylohyoid muscle. The ganglion lies between the lingual nerve and the deep part of the submandibular gland. Indeed, it is suspended by two roots from the lingual nerve. The prime function of the submandibular ganglion is to supply the submandibular and sublingual salivary glands.

In common with the other parasympathetic ganglia in the head, the submandibular ganglion has a parasympathetic, a sympathetic and a sensory supply. Only the parasympathetic fibres synapse within the ganglion.

Preganglionic parasympathetic fibres originate from the superior salivatory nucleus in the brain stem. The fibres pass with the nervus intermedius of the facial nerve into the internal acoustic meatus and exit the skull with the chorda tympani nerve at the petrotympanic fissure. The chorda tympani nerve joins the lingual nerve in the infratemporal fossa and by this route the parasympathetic fibres reach the submandibular ganglion. It is claimed that the preganglionic parasympathetic fibres pass via the posterior root linking the ganglion to the lingual nerve.

The sympathetic supply to the ganglion is derived from the superior cervical ganglion. It reaches the submandibular ganglion via the sympathetic nerve plexus surrounding the facial artery.

The sensory supply arises from the adjacent lingual nerve.

Branches from the ganglion pass directly to the submandibular gland. The sublingual gland however is supplied by fibres which re-enter the lingual nerve by the anterior connecting root (5.11).

THE BLOOD SUPPLY OF THE ORO-DENTAL TISSUES

THE BLOOD SUPPLY OF THE TEETH

The main arteries to the teeth and jaws are derived from the maxillary artery, a terminal branch of the external carotid. The alveolar arteries (the superior and inferior alveolar arteries) follow approximately the same course as the alveolar nerves.

The *inferior alveolar artery* supplies the mandibular teeth. It is derived from the maxillary artery before it crosses the lateral pterygoid muscle in the infratemporal fossa (5.31). A mylohyoid branch is given off before the inferior alveolar artery passes through the mandibular foramen to enter the mandibular canal. The inferior alveolar artery terminates within the body of the mandible as the mental and incisive arteries. The mental artery emerges onto the face at the mental foramen. The incisive artery continues forwards within the incisive canal to supply the mandibular anterior teeth.

There are three superior alveolar arteries which supply the maxillary dentition: the posterior, middle and anterior superior alveolar arteries. The superior alveolar arteries form plexuses just above the root apices of the teeth.

The *posterior superior alveolar artery* usually arises from the maxillary artery in the pterygopalatine fossa. It courses tortuously over the maxillary tuberosity before entering the upper jaw to supply the molar and premolar teeth (3.34).

The *middle superior alveolar artery*, when present, arises from the infra-orbital artery (a branch of the maxillary artery in the pterygopalatine fossa). The middle superior alveolar artery runs down the lateral wall of the maxillary sinus, terminating near the canine tooth.

5.31 Infratemporal fossa showing maxillary artery

1 Maxillary artery
2 Inferior alveolar artery
3 Inferior alveolar nerve
4 Medial pterygoid mucsle
5 Facial artery and vein
6 Buccinator muscle
7 Buccal nerve
8 Lateral pterygoid muscle
9 Posterior superior alveolar artery

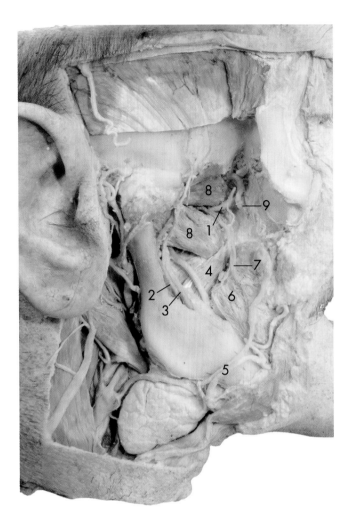

5.32 The submandibular parasympathetic ganglion

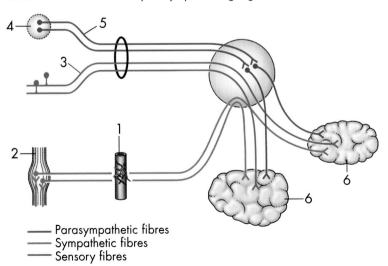

Parasympathetic fibres
Sympathetic fibres
Sensory fibres

1 Facial artery
2 Superior cervical ganglion
3 Lingual nerve
4 Superior salivatory nucleus in brainstem
5 Chorda tympani nerve
6 Submandibular and sublingual glands

The *anterior superior alveolar artery* also arises from the infra-orbital artery. It runs down the anterior wall of the maxillary sinus towards the anterior teeth.

The gingival tissues derive their blood supply from the maxillary and lingual arteries.

The buccal gingivae associated with the mandibular cheek teeth are supplied by the buccal branch of the maxillary artery and by perforating branches from the inferior alveolar artery. The labial gingivae around the anterior teeth are supplied by the mental artery and by perforating branches of the incisive artery. The lingual gingivae are supplied by perforating branches from the inferior alveolar artery and by the lingual artery of the external carotid.

The buccal gingivae around the maxillary cheek teeth are supplied by gingival and perforating branches from the posterior superior alveolar artery and by the buccal artery. The labial gingivae of anterior teeth are supplied by labial branches of the infra-orbital artery and by perforating branches of the anterior superior alveolar artery. The palatal gingivae are supplied primarily by branches of the greater palatine artery.

THE BLOOD SUPPLY OF OTHER ORAL STRUCTURES

The palate derives its blood supply from the greater and lesser palatine branches of the maxillary artery. (The nasopalatine artery does not reach the palate, the greater palatine artery passing through the incisive foramen.)

The cheek is supplied by the buccal branch of the maxillary artery, the floor of the mouth and tongue by the lingual arteries. The lips are mainly supplied by superior and inferior labial branches of the facial arteries.

The lingual artery (5.33–5.35) is the third branch of the external carotid artery. It reaches the floor of the mouth by passing between the hyoglossus muscle and the middle constrictor of the pharynx. The artery here crosses the stylohyoid ligament and is accompanied by the lingual veins and the glossopharyngeal nerve. At the anterior border of the hyoglossus muscle, the lingual artery (with the lingual nerve) bends sharply upwards towards the genioglossus muscle of the tongue. The branches of the lingual artery in the floor of the mouth are: the dorsal lingual branches, the sublingual artery and the deep lingual artery. The dorsal lingual branches supply the back of the dorsum of the tongue and the region around the pillars of the fauces. The sublingual artery supplies the sublingual gland and other structures in the floor of the mouth. The deep lingual artery is the terminal part of the lingual artery, which is found on the inferior surface of the tongue near the lingual frenum.

THE VENOUS DRAINAGE OF THE ORO-DENTAL TISSUES

The veins from the teeth are collected into inferior alveolar veins for the lower jaw and superior alveolar veins for the upper jaw. These may drain anteriorly to the facial veins (through the mental foramina for the inferior alveolar veins) or posteriorly to the pterygoid plexuses in the infratemporal fossae (through the mandibular foramina for the inferior alveolar veins).

No accurate description is available concerning the venous drainage of the gingivae, although it may be assumed that buccal, lingual, greater palatine and nasopalatine veins are involved. These veins run into the pterygoid plexuses, apart from the lingual veins which pass directly into the internal jugular veins.

The lingual veins are variable, but they usually follow two routes. The dorsal lingual vein drains the dorsum of the tongue. It passes with the lingual artery deep to the hyoglossus muscle, where it becomes known as the lingual vein. The lingual vein joins the internal jugular vein at the level of the greater horn of the hyoid bone. The deep lingual vein is visible through the mucosa of the ventral surface of the tongue. It joins the sublingual vein (from the sublingual salivary gland) to become the vein accompanying the hypoglossal nerve on the hyoglossus muscle. This terminates by either joining the lingual vein or by draining directly into the internal jugular vein.

The veins of the hard palate generally pass into the pterygoid plexus, those of the soft palate into the pharyngeal plexus.

Venous blood from the lips drains into the facial veins via superior and inferior labial veins.

5.33 Neck viewed medially showing origin of lingual artery

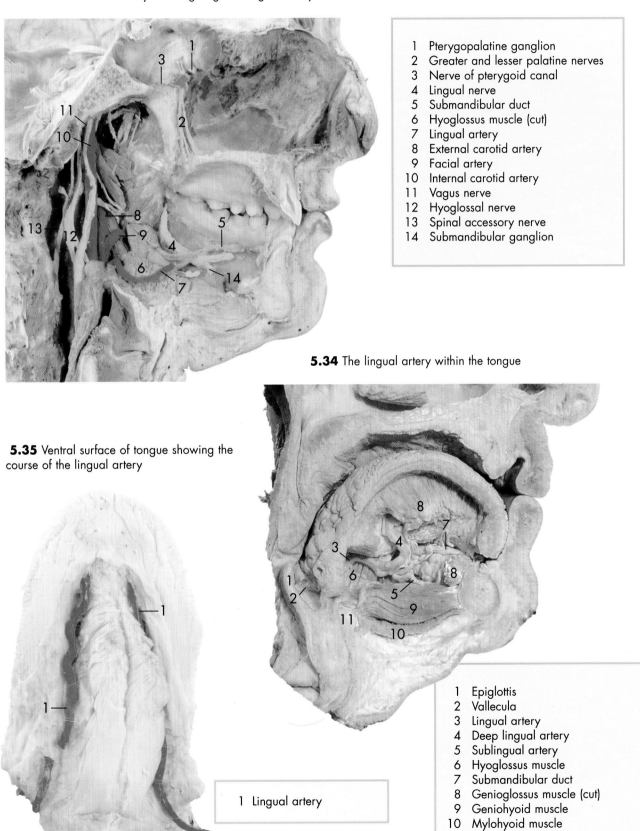

1	Pterygopalatine ganglion
2	Greater and lesser palatine nerves
3	Nerve of pterygoid canal
4	Lingual nerve
5	Submandibular duct
6	Hyoglossus muscle (cut)
7	Lingual artery
8	External carotid artery
9	Facial artery
10	Internal carotid artery
11	Vagus nerve
12	Hyoglossal nerve
13	Spinal accessory nerve
14	Submandibular ganglion

5.34 The lingual artery within the tongue

5.35 Ventral surface of tongue showing the course of the lingual artery

1	Lingual artery

1	Epiglottis
2	Vallecula
3	Lingual artery
4	Deep lingual artery
5	Sublingual artery
6	Hyoglossus muscle
7	Submandibular duct
8	Genioglossus muscle (cut)
9	Geniohyoid muscle
10	Mylohyoid muscle
11	Hyoid bone

THE LYMPHATIC DRAINAGE OF THE MOUTH

The principal sites of drainage of lymphatic vessels from oro-dental tissues are: the submental, submandibular, and jugulodigastric lymph nodes. The manner of drainage is however so variable that there is no precise and accurate description.

The lymph vessels from the teeth usually run directly into the submandibular lymph nodes on the same side. Lymph from the mandibular incisors, however, drains into the submental lymph nodes. Occasionally, lymph from the molars may pass directly into the jugulodigastric group of nodes.

The lymph vessels of the labial and buccal gingivae of the maxillary and mandibular teeth unite to drain into the submandibular nodes, though in the labial region of the mandibular incisors they may drain into the submental lymph nodes. The lingual and palatal gingivae drain into the jugulodigastric group of nodes, either directly or indirectly through the submandibular nodes.

Lymphatics from the bulk of the palate terminate in the jugulodigastric group of nodes. Vessels from the posterior part of the soft palate terminate in pharyngeal lymph nodes.

Lymphatics from the anterior two-thirds of the tongue may be subdivided into two groups of vessels, marginal and central vessels. The marginal lymphatics drain the lateral third of the upper surface of the tongue and the lateral margin of its lower surface. The remaining regions drain into the central vessels. The marginal vessels pass to the submandibular lymph nodes of the same side. The vessels at the tip of the tongue pass to the submental lymph nodes. Central vessels behind the tip drain into ipsilateral and contralateral submandibular lymph nodes. Some marginal and central lymph vessels pass directly to the jugulodigastric group of nodes (or even the jugulo-omohyoid nodes). Lymphatics from the posterior third of the tongue drain into the deep cervical group of nodes, vessels centrally draining both ipsilaterally and contralaterally.

At the oropharyngeal isthmus lie the palatine tonsils between the pillars of the fauces, and the lingual tonsils on the pharyngeal surface of the tongue. These tonsils form part of a ring of lymphoid tissue known as Waldeyer's tonsillar ring. The other components are the tubal tonsils and adenoid tissue (pharyngeal tonsils) in the nasopharynx (see page 400).

THE TISSUE SPACES AROUND THE JAWS

The dissemination of infection in soft tissues is influenced by the natural barriers presented by bone, muscle and fascia. Around the jaws, however, the tissue spaces are primarily defined by muscles, principally the mylohyoid, buccinator, masseter, medial pterygoid, superior constrictor and orbicularis oris muscles. None of the 'spaces' are actually empty and they should merely be regarded as potential spaces which are normally occupied by loose connective tissue. It is only when inflammatory products destroy the loose connective tissue that a definable space is produced.

The important potential tissue spaces are:

Lower jaw:

- Submental
- Submandibular
- Sublingual
- Buccal
- Submasseteric
- Parotid
- Pterygomandibular
- Parapharyngeal
- Peritonsillar

Upper jaw:

- Palatal
- Facial
- Infratemporal

(The spaces are paired except for the submental, sublingual and palatal spaces.)

5.37 The lymphatic drainage of the oro-dental tissues

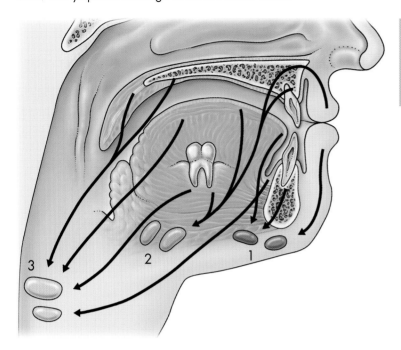

1	Submental lymph nodes
2	Submandibular lymph nodes
3	Jugulodigastric lymph nodes

5.37 Tissue spaces in the retromandibular region

1 Fornix vestibuli
2 Peritonsillar space
3 Buccal space (filled with buccal pad fat)
4 Submasseteric spaces
5 Pterygomandibular space
6 Parapharyngeal space
7 Parotid space

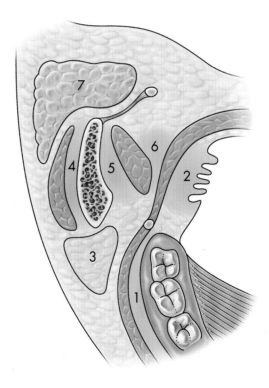

The submental and submandibular spaces are located below the inferior border of the mandible, beneath the mylohyoid muscle, in the suprahyoid region of the neck. The submental space lies beneath the chin in the midline, between the mylohyoid muscles and the investing layer of deep cervical fascia. It is bounded laterally by the two anterior bellies of the digastric muscles. The submental space communicates posteriorly with the two submandibular spaces. The submandibular space is situated between the anterior and posterior bellies of the digastric muscle. It communicates with the sublingual space around the posterior free border of the mylohyoid muscle.

The sublingual space lies in the floor of the mouth, above the mylohyoid muscles. It is continuous across the midline and communicates with the submandibular spaces over the posterior free borders of the mylohyoid muscles.

The buccal space is located in the cheek, on the lateral side of the buccinator muscle.

Between the lateral surface of the ramus of the mandible and the masseter muscle is a series of spaces called the submasseteric spaces. These spaces are formed because the fibres of the masseter muscle have multiple insertions on to most of the lateral surface of the ramus.

Between the medial surface of the ramus of the mandible and the medial pterygoid muscle lies the pterygomandibular space.

Behind the ramus of the mandible is located the parotid space, in and around the parotid gland.

The parapharyngeal space is bounded by the superior constrictor of the pharynx and the medial surface of the medial pterygoid muscle. This space is restricted to the infratemporal region of the head and the suprahyoid region of the neck. It communicates with the retropharyngeal space which itself extends into the retrovisceral space in the lower part of the neck (see pages 334–344) for a description of the tissue spaces in the neck).

The peritonsillar space lies around the palatine tonsil between the pillars of the fauces. It is part of the intrapharyngeal space and is bounded by the medial surface of the superior constrictor of the pharynx and its mucosa.

In the upper jaw, the muscles of facial expression define a number of very small tissue spaces in the face. One such space is the canine fossa, between the levator labii superioris and zygomaticus muscles.

There is not truly a tissue space in the hard palate, as the mucosa there is firmly bound to the periosteum. However, inflammation can strip away some of this periosteum to produce a well-circumscribed abscess.

The infratemporal space is the upper extremity of the pterygomandibular space. It is closely related to the maxillary tuberosity and therefore the upper molars.

5.38 Coronal section through floor of mouth showing tissue spaces

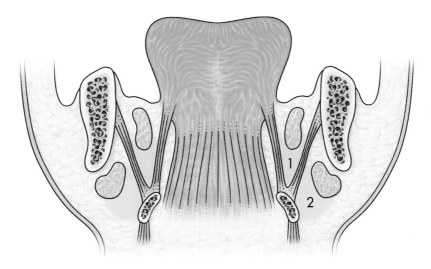

1 Sublingual tissue space
2 Submandibular tissue space

5.39 Inferior view of floor of mouth (suprahyoid region of neck) showing tissue space

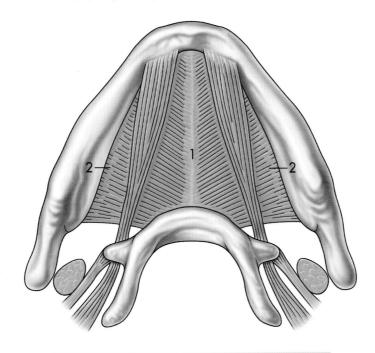

1 Submental tissue space
2 Submandibular tissue spaces

chapter 6
THE NOSE

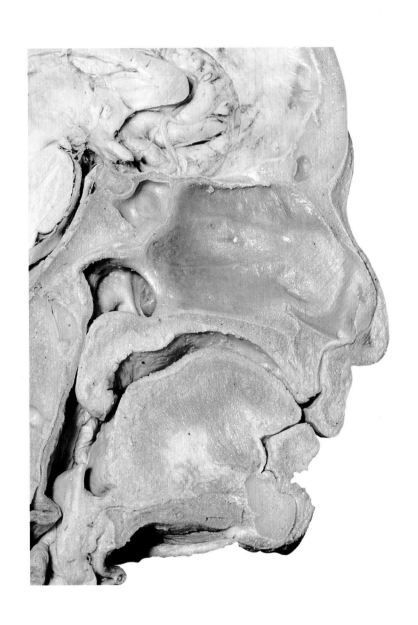

Chapter 6 THE NOSE

The nose is the upper part of the respiratory tract. It occupies the midline region of the head between the oral cavity and the cranial cavity. The nose opens on the face at the nostrils (anterior nares). Behind, it opens into the nasopharynx through the choanae (posterior nares).

That part of the nose which projects from the face is termed the external nose. The nasal cavity internally is divided into two nasal fossae by the nasal septum. Prominent processes project from the lateral walls of the nasal cavity (the superior, middle and inferior nasal conchae). The lateral walls are also significant for being the sites of drainage of the ethmoid, frontal, maxillary and sphenoidal air sinuses and of the nasolacrimal ducts.

The functions of the nose are primarily those concerned with ventilation and olfaction. Inspired air is filtered and debris is removed in a film of mucus. The air is also warmed and humidified at the nose. Another function of the nose is to act as a resonating chamber and thus to play a role in speech.

At the back of the nose, and below the apex of each orbit, lie the pterygopalatine fossae.

THE EXTERNAL NOSE

The external nose is essentially pyramidal in shape. Superiorly, it is confluent with the forehead at the root of the nose where it is supported by the nasal bone at the bridge. This part of the external nose is immobile. Inferiorly, the tip of the nose is termed the apex. The ridge connecting the root and apex is referred to as the dorsum of the nose. The apex and the dorsum are supported by cartilage and are mobile. The anterior nares are separated by a septum which joins the apex of the nose to the philtrum of the upper lip. The anterior nares lead into the nasal vestibule. Here, the skin is characterised by having coarse hairs. The flared lateral margins of the external nose are known as the alae. The nasolabial grooves of the upper lip continue around the alae to form alar grooves.

The *skeleton of the external nose* (6.1) comprises both bony and cartilaginous elements. The bony elements lie near the bridge of the nose and consist of the frontal processes of the maxillae, the nasal part of the frontal bone and the nasal bones. The cartilaginous elements form the lower part of the external nose. In the midline is the septal cartilage. This is quadrangular and fits posteriorly into the notch between the perpendicular plate of the ethmoid and the vomer. The septal cartilage is also attached to the nasal crest of the maxilla and to the anterior nasal spine. The septal cartilage at the apex of the external nose is termed the columella. The columella can also be defined as the tip of the mobile part of the septum. The lateral surfaces of the external nose are supported by the lateral (upper) nasal cartilages and the greater (lower) nasal cartilages. The lateral nasal cartilages are triangular plates. They are united in the midline with each other and with the septal cartilage. The greater nasal cartilages are thin and C-shaped; the medial and lateral edges are termed crura. These cartilages extend from the apex of the nose into the alae to maintain the patency of the anterior nares. The greater nasal cartilages are joined to each other, and to the septal and lateral nasal cartilages, by fibrous tissue. Fibrous tissue also joins the back of the greater nasal cartilage to the maxilla. Some lesser alar cartilages may be found here.

The *muscles of the external nose* (6.2) belong to the muscles of facial expression. They comprise procerus, compressor naris, dilator naris, and depressor septi. The levator labii superioris alaeque nasi muscle can also be included in this group, although it is usually considered with the oral group of facial muscles. The nasal group of facial muscles is described fully on pages 106–107.

6.1a Skeleton of external nose

6.1b Septum of now showing nasal cartilage

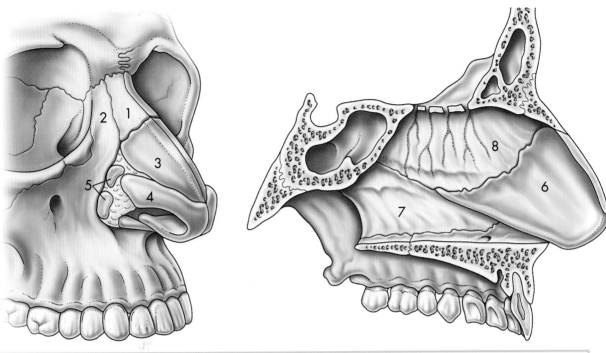

1 Nasal bone	5 Lesser alar cartilage
2 Frontal process of maxilla	6 Septal cartilage
3 Lateral nasal cartilage	7 Vomer
4 Greater nasal cartilage	8 Perpendicular plate of ethmoid bone

6.2 Muscles of external nose

1 Levator labil superioris alaeque nasi
2 Procerus
3 Fascia of procerus
4 Fascia between opposite compressor nares muscles
5 Depressor septi

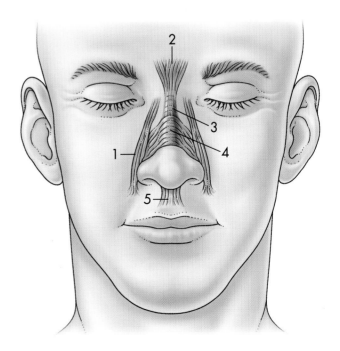

The *cutaneous innervation of the external nose* (see page 116) is derived from branches of the ophthalmic and maxillary divisions of the trigeminal nerve. Supratrochlear and infratrochlear branches of the ophthalmic nerve supply skin in the region of the root, bridge and upper part of the side of the nose. The external nasal branch of the ophthalmic nerve runs in a groove on the internal surface of the nasal bone to supply skin in the lower part of the nose around the midline (including the apex). The infra-orbital branch of the maxillary nerve (nasal branch) supplies the side of the lower part of the external nose (6.3).

The *blood supply to the external nose* is derived from three sources, the facial, ophthalmic and maxillary arteries. The facial artery gives off a lateral nasal branch (from the angular artery) and a septal branch (from the superior labial artery). The ophthalmic artery provides a dorsal nasal artery which, appearing above the medial palpebral ligament of the eyelid, supplies skin on the dorsum of the nose. An additional branch from the ophthalmic artery is the anterior ethmoidal artery. This terminates as the external nasal artery. The maxillary artery gives off an infra-orbital artery which provides nasal branches. Venous blood drains into the distal part of the facial vein (the angular vein) and into the ophthalmic veins. The lymphatics of the external nose drain into the submandibular group of lymph nodes.

THE NASAL CAVITY

The nasal cavity is divided in the midline by the nasal septum, forming two nasal fossae. Because the septum often deviates to one side at the vomero-ethmoidal suture, the nasal fossae are frequently of unequal size. The floor of the nasal fossa is wider than its roof, giving the fossa a pear-shaped outline in cross-section.

THE OSTEOLOGY OF THE NASAL CAVITY (1.49, 6.4, 6.5)

The anterior nasal aperture (piriform aperture) is bounded mainly by the maxillary bones. The nasal bones form the superior margin of the aperture.

The nasal fossa must remain patent for ventilation. The patency is maintained by the rigidity of the bony walls. Each nasal fossa has a roof, a floor, a lateral wall and a medial wall.

The medial wall is formed by the nasal septum. It is composed of the septal cartilage anteriorly, the perpendicular plate of the ethmoid bone postero-superiorly and the vomer postero-inferiorly. At the base of the nasal septum is the nasal crest formed by the maxillary and palatine bones.

The bones which comprise the remaining walls of the nasal fossa are the ethmoid, frontal, lacrimal, maxillary, nasal, palatine, sphenoid, and vomer bones and the bone of the inferior concha.

The roof of the nasal fossa is formed centrally by the cribriform plate of the ethmoid bone. Anteriorly lies the nasal bone and the nasal spine of the frontal bone. Posteriorly is located the body of the sphenoid overlapped by the ala of the vomer and the sphenoidal process of the palatine bone. The cribriform plate transmits olfactory nerves into the roof of the nasal cavity and also the anterior ethmoidal nerves and vessels.

The floor of the nasal fossa is formed by the palatine process of the maxilla anteriorly and the horizontal plate of the palatine bone posteriorly.

6.3a Lateral wall of the nose showing some of the innervation and the pterygopalatine ganglion

1	Anterior ethmoidal nerve
2	Olfactory nerve
3	Pterygopalatine ganglion
4	Greater palatine nerve
5	Lesser palatine nerve
6	Nasopalatine nerve on nasal septum

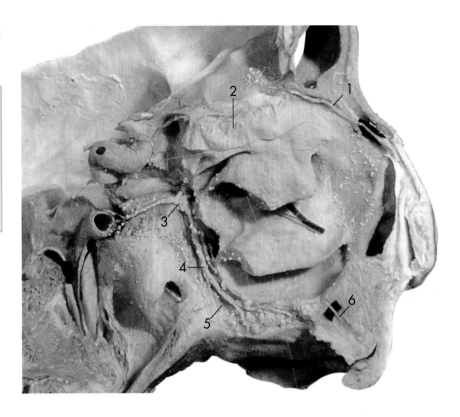

6.3b Frontal view of orbit showing nerves which help innervate the external nose

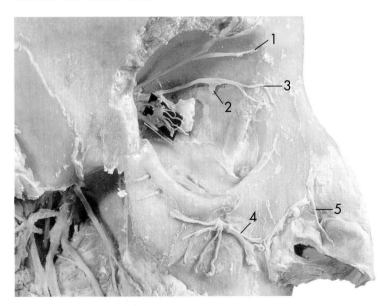

1	Supratrochlear nerve
2	Anterior ethmoidal nerve
3	Infratrochlear nerve
4	Nasal branch of infra-orbital nerve
5	External nasal nerve

6.4 Frontal view of skull showing osteology of nose

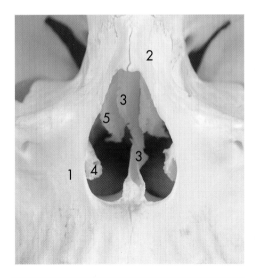

1	Maxilla
2	Nasal bone
3	Nasal septum
4	Inferior nasal concha
5	Middle nasal concha

The lateral wall of the nasal fossa consists mainly of the medial surface of the maxilla, with the large maxillary hiatus being reduced in size by the overlapping of the lacrimal and ethmoid bones above, the palatine bone behind and the inferior concha below. From the lateral wall project the three nasal conchae. The superior and middle conchae are part of the labyrinth of the ethmoid bone. The inferior concha is a separate bone. The region above and behind the superior nasal concha is called the spheno-ethmoidal recess. The region between the superior and middle nasal conchae is the superior meatus. Between the middle and inferior conchae is located the middle meatus. Below the inferior nasal concha is the inferior meatus.

The nasolacrimal canal on the lateral wall of the nasal fossa is formed by the lacrimal groove of the maxilla articulating with the descending process of the lacrimal bone and the lacrimal process of the inferior concha.

The sphenopalatine foramen, which links the nasal cavity with the pterygopalatine fossa, lies high up in the posterior part of the lateral wall. It is formed by the notch between the orbital and sphenoidal processes of the perpendicular plate of the palatine bone articulating with the body of the sphenoid bone. This foramen transmits the nasopalatine and posterior superior nasal nerves and the sphenopalatine vessels.

The lateral wall of the nose is noted for being the site of drainage of the paranasal air sinuses. The sphenoidal sinus drains into the spheno-ethmoidal recess. The posterior ethmoidal air cells drain into the superior meatus. The frontal and maxillary air sinuses and the anterior and middle ethmoidal air cells drain into the middle meatus. The opening of the nasolacrimal canal lies in the inferior meatus.

The posterior nasal apertures (choanae) link the nasal fossae with the nasopharynx. The bones which contribute to this region are the palatine, sphenoid and vomer bones. The posterior border of the vomer separates the two posterior nasal apertures. Each aperture is bounded below by the posterior border of

the horizontal plate of the palatine bone, laterally by the medial pterygoid plate, and above by the body and vaginal process of the sphenoid bone and the ala of the vomer. A groove on the lower surface of the vaginal process of the sphenoid bone is converted into the palatovaginal canal by articulation with the upper surface of the sphenoidal process of the palatine bone. This canal transmits the pharyngeal branch of the pterygopalatine ganglion and the pharyngeal branch of the maxillary artery. The vomerovaginal canal lies between the upper surface of the vaginal process of the sphenoid bone and the ala of the vomer. The pharyngeal branch of the sphenopalatine artery passes through this occasional canal.

The appearance of the lateral wall of the nasal fossa (6.6–6.8)

Many of the important features of the nose are found on the lateral walls of the nasal fossae.

The inferior margin of the lateral wall is horizontal. The upper margin is curved, being highest at its middle (beneath the cribriform plate of the ethmoid) and sloping downwards anteriorly and posteriorly.

Corresponding to the ala of the external nose is a small recess termed the vestibule. This area is lined with skin which has coarse hairs (the vibrissae). The vestibule is bounded above by a ridge (the limen nasi) which represents the upper border of the greater nasal cartilage. Beyond the ridge, the mucosa of the nose is of the respiratory type. Above the vestibule, level with the middle meatus, is a shallow depression called the atrium. A curved ridge called the agger nasi may be found above the atrium. This ridge overlies the anterior part of the ethmoidal crest of the maxilla.

Behind the vestibule and atrium are the nasal conchae. The superior nasal concha is the smallest and lies posteriorly in the upper part of the lateral wall. The middle nasal concha is joined anteriorly to the superior nasal concha and is approximately twice its length. The inferior nasal concha is the longest, extending forwards in front of the middle nasal concha.

6.5 Osteology of the lateral wall of the nose

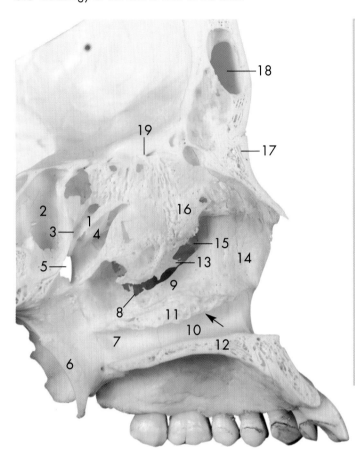

1 Superior concha
2 Sphenoidal sinus
3 Spheno-ethmoidal recess
4 Superior meatus
5 Sphenopalatine foramen
6 Medial pterygoid plate of sphenoid
7 Perpendicular plate of palatine bone
8 Opening of maxillary sinus
9 Middle meatus
10 Inferior meatus
11 Inferior concha
12 Hard palate
13 Uncinate process of ethmoid
14 Medial surface of maxilla
15 Hiatus semilinaris
16 Middle concha
17 Nasal bone
18 Frontal sinus
19 Cribriform plate of ethmoid

Arrow indicates position of opening of nasolacrimal canal

6.6 Lateral wall of the nose

1 Vestibule
2 Frontal sinus
3 Ethmoidal sinus
4 Superior concha
5 Middle concha
6 Inferior concha
7 Levator palati muscle
8 Tensor palati muscle

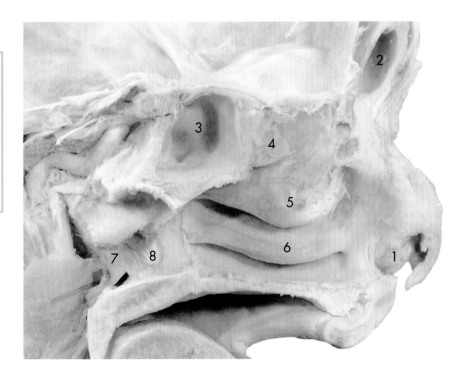

Below the conchae lie regions called the superior, middle and inferior meatuses. The area above and behind the superior nasal concha is called the spheno-ethmoidal recess.

The superior meatus is the narrow region below the superior nasal concha and above the posterior part of the middle nasal concha. Posterior ethmoidal air cells drain by one or more openings into the anterior part of the superior meatus.

The middle meatus lies between the middle and inferior conchae. There is a prominent bulge in its upper part called the ethmoidal bulla. The bulla represents the site of the middle ethmoidal air cells, their opening being found on or above the bulla. The bulla forms the upper boundary of a groove, the hiatus semilunaris. The groove is bounded below by a ridge related to the uncinate process of the ethmoid bone. The hiatus semilunaris runs forwards and upwards as a curved channel with a funnel-shaped extremity (the ethmoidal infundibulum). The frontal sinus may drain through a simple opening or into a more obvious channel called the frontonasal duct. The point of drainage may then be either in front of, above, or directly into the ethmoidal infundibulum. The anterior ethmoidal air cells drain separately into the ethmoidal infundibulum or into the frontonasal duct. The maxillary sinus drains further back in the hiatus semilunaris and may have one or two openings.

The inferior meatus lies below the inferior concha. Because the concha is arched, the meatus is highest in its middle. The anterior portion of the inferior meatus is the site of drainage of the nasolacrimal duct. The opening may vary from being rounded to slit-like. When slit-like, the opening is bounded above and in front by a fold of mucosa called the plica lacrimalis.

The spheno-ethmoidal recess is a small triangular region above the superior concha. It is closely related to the cribriform plate of the ethmoid and thus the olfactory nerves. The recess receives the opening of the sphenoidal air sinus.

A small fold called the supreme nasal concha is found above the superior nasal concha in about 60% of cases. The area between this fold and the superior

Figure 6.7 (opposite)
1 Middle ethimoidal sinus opening
2 Bulla ethmoidalis
3 Hiatus semilunaris
4 Opening of maxillary sinus
5 Middle meatus
6 Inferior concha
7 Inferior meatus
8 Bristle in nasolacrimal duct opening
9 Greater palatine nerve
10 Pterygopalatine ganglion
11 Nerve of pterygoid canal
12 Maxillary nerve

nasal concha is called the supreme meatus. It receives an opening from a posterior ethmoidal air cell.

The appearance of the medial wall of the nasal fossa (6.9)

This wall is formed by the nasal septum. The septum is relatively featureless, although a small opening may be visible anteriorly on each side close to the inferior border. This opening leads backwards into a small recess called the vomeronasal organ. This is vestigial in man but has an olfactory function in some animals. A small cartilage, the vomeronasal cartilage, may sometimes be found in association with the vomeronasal organ.

The appearance of the roof and floor of the nasal fossa (6.8)

The roof is highest centrally, where it is related to the cribiform plate of the ethmoid. The roof slopes downwards anteriorly beneath the frontal bone and posteriorly beneath the sphenoid bone.

The floor of the nasal cavity is related to the hard palate and is relatively flat and horizontal. A slight depression of the mucosa may be seen overlying the incisive canal.

The nasal mucosa

Above the superior concha, the mucosa is termed olfactory mucosa because it contains the olfactory cells. In vivo, this mucosa has a distinct yellowish colour. In contrast, the remaining nasal mucosa is of the respiratory type (ciliated columnar) and appears pink. This is particularly thick and well vascularised at the free margins of the nasal conchae.

6.7 Lateral wall of nose showing middle and inferior meatuses

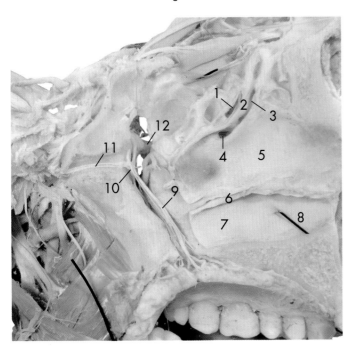

6.8 Coronal section through nose

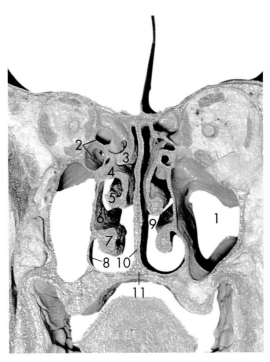

6.9 The nasal septum

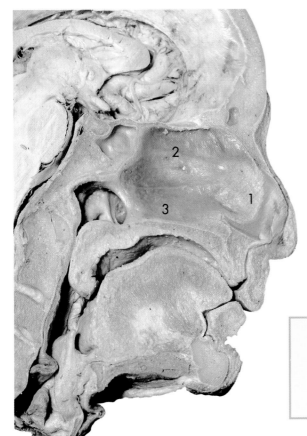

1	Maxillary sinus
2	Ethmoidal sinus
3	Superior nasal concha
4	Superior meatus
5	Middle nasal concha
6	Middle meatus
7	Inferior concha
8	Inferior meatus
9	Nasal cavity
10	Nasal septum
11	Palate

1	Mucosa covering nasal septum
2	Mucosa covering perpendicular plate of ethmoid bone
3	Mucosa covering vomer bone

THE INNERVATION OF THE NASAL CAVITY (5.30, 6.10, 6.11)

Special sensation related to olfaction is associated with the olfactory nerves (i.e. the first cranial nerves). General sensation to the nasal mucosa is related to branches from the ophthalmic and maxillary divisions of the trigeminal nerves (i.e. the fifth cranial nerves).

The olfactory epithelium is located in the roof of the nasal cavity, extending onto the lateral walls of the nasal fossae (above the superior nasal conchae) and the uppermost part of the nasal septum. Filaments of the olfactory nerves (about 20 on each side) pass upwards through the cribiform plate of the ethmoid bone into the cranial cavity to synapse in the olfactory bulbs. Each filament is ensheathed by the meninges. Thus, a potential pathway exists for the spread of infection from the nose to the cranial cavity.

The anterior ethmoidal nerve is the only branch of the ophthalmic nerve which supplies the nasal mucosa. It arises from the nasociliary nerve and mainly supplies an area in front of the nasal conchae (it also innervates the anterior extremities of the middle and inferior conchae). After leaving the orbit through the anterior ethmoidal foramen, the anterior ethmoidal nerve enters the cranial cavity onto the cribiform plate of the ethmoid. It leaves the cranial cavity through a small slit near the crista galli and enters the roof of the nasal cavity. Here, the nerve runs in a groove on the inner surface of the nasal bone. The anterior ethmoidal nerve passes downwards and forwards and gives rise to lateral and medial internal nasal branches. The lateral internal nasal branches pass to the lateral wall of the nose whereas the medial internal nasal branches run to the nasal septum. When the anterior ethmoidal nerve emerges at the inferior margin of the nasal bone it becomes the external nasal nerve (see page 116).

The maxillary nerve contributes many branches which supply the nasal mucosa. The infra-orbital and the posterior superior alveolar nerves arise directly from the maxillary nerve. The posterior superior nasal, greater palatine and nasopalatine nerves arise indirectly by way of the pterygopalatine ganglion.

The infra-orbital nerve is the terminal branch of the maxillary nerve. After passing onto the face at the infra-orbital foramen, it provides a nasal branch which supplies the skin of the vestibule and the mobile part of the nasal septum. The anterior superior alveolar branch of the infra-orbital nerve also supplies nasal mucosa. Its nasal branch passes through a small canal in the lateral wall of the nose (below the level of the inferior concha) to innervate the anterior part of the inferior meatus and the adjacent part of the floor of the nose and adjoining nasal septum.

The posterior superior nasal nerve originates at the pterygopalatine ganglion. It enters the back of the nasal cavity through the sphenopalatine foramen and gives off lateral and medial branches. The lateral branches supply the posterosuperior part of the lateral wall of the nose around the superior and middle nasal conchae. The medial branches cross the roof of the nasal cavity to supply the septum overlying the posterior part of the perpendicular plate of the ethmoid.

The greater (anterior) palatine nerve also arises from the pterygopalatine ganglion. It descends in the greater palatine canal where it gives off posterior inferior nasal branches. These branches pass through small openings in the perpendicular plate of the palatine bone to supply the postero-inferior portion of the lateral wall of the nose (below and including the middle meatus).

The nasopalatine nerve passes from the pterygopalatine ganglion into the nasal cavity through the sphenopalatine foramen. It runs across the roof of the nasal cavity to reach the back of the nasal septum. It then passes downwards and forwards, lying in a groove on the vomer, to supply the postero-inferior part of the septum. The floor of the nose is supplied anteriorly by the nasal branch of the anterior superior alveolar nerve and posteriorly by the nasal branches of the greater (anterior) palatine and by the nasopalatine nerves. Autonomic fibres to glands and vessels in the nose are distributed with the above mentioned branches of the maxillary nerve via the pterygopalatine ganglion. In addition, autonomic fibres are presumed to be distributed with the anterior ethmoidal nerve via the ciliary ganglion.

6.10 View of orbit showing nerves innervating the nose

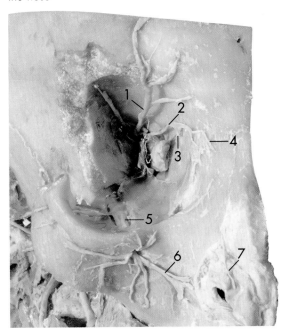

6.11a Lateral wall of nose showing sensory innervation

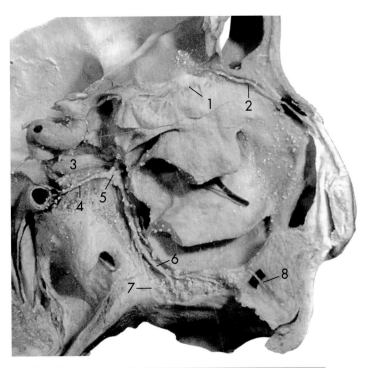

1 Frontal nerve
2 Nasociliary nerve
3 Anterior ethmoidal nerve
4 Infratrochlear nerve
5 Infra-orbital branch of maxillary
   nerve
6 Nasal branch of infra-orbital
   nerve
7 External nasal nerve

1 Olfactory nerve
2 Anterior ethmoidal nerve
3 Maxillary nerve
4 Nerve of pterygoid canal
5 Pterygopalatine ganglion
6 Greater palatine nerve
7 Lesser palatine nerve
8 Nasopalatine nerve on nasal septum

6.11b The innervation of the lateral wall of the nose (excluding the olfactory nerve)

1 Greater palatine nerve
2 Posterior superior nasal nerve
   (lateral branch)
3 Anterior ethmoidal nerve
4 Infra-orbital nerve (nasal branch)
5 Anterior superior alveolar nerve

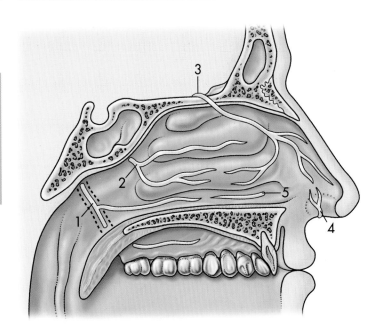

THE ARTERIES OF THE NASAL CAVITY (6.12, 6.13)

The general distribution of the arteries is similar to that of the nerves. The main vessels arise from the ophthalmic and maxillary arteries, with small contributions from the facial artery.

The ophthalmic artery (see pages 260–264) provides anterior and posterior ethmoidal branches to the nasal cavity. The anterior ethmoidal artery accompanies the anterior ethmoidal nerve and supplies the anterior parts of the lateral wall and the nasal septum. Its terminal branch is the external nasal artery. The posterior ethmoidal artery supplies a small part of the lateral wall of the nose around the superior nasal concha and the posterosuperior region of the nasal septum.

The sphenopalatine artery is the terminal branch of the maxillary artery in the pterygopalatine fossa. It enters the lateral wall of the nose through the sphenopalatine foramen. The artery accompanies the posterior superior nasal nerve and gives off branches to supply much of the posterior part of the lateral wall of the nose. These branches for part of their course lie within the middle and inferior nasal conchae. The sphenopalatine artery crosses the roof of the nasal cavity to supply the postero-inferior part of the nasal septum.

The greater palatine artery is also a branch of the maxillary artery in the pterygopalatine fossa. It accompanies the greater palatine nerve in the greater palatine canal and gives branches supplying the inferior meatus. After passing onto the hard palate through the greater palatine foramen, the greater palatine artery gives a branch that passes up through the incisive canal to supply the anterior part of the nasal septum.

The superior labial branch of the facial artery is the main source of supply of the anterior part of the nasal septum.

THE VEINS AND LYMPHATICS OF THE NASAL CAVITY

There are conspicuous venous plexuses in the lateral walls of the nasal fossae and in the nasal septum (particularly inferiorly). Indeed, the plexuses are said to resemble plexuses in erectile tissue. Consequently, the nasal cavity is susceptible to blockage should the plexuses become engorged.

The veins draining the nose essentially correspond to the arteries. Veins from the posterior part of the nose generally pass to the sphenopalatine vein which runs back through the sphenopalatine foramen to drain into the pterygoid venous plexus. The anterior part of the nose is drained mainly by veins accompanying the anterior ethmoidal arteries, these veins passing to the ophthalmic or the facial veins.

Lymphatics in the anterior part of the nose drain into the submandibular lymph nodes. The lymphatics posteriorly drain into the upper deep cervical nodes.

6.12 The vasculature of the lateral wall of the nose

1	Greater palatine artery
2	Sphenopalatine artery
3	Posterior ethmoidal artery
4	Anterior ethmoidal artery
5	Branches from facial artery

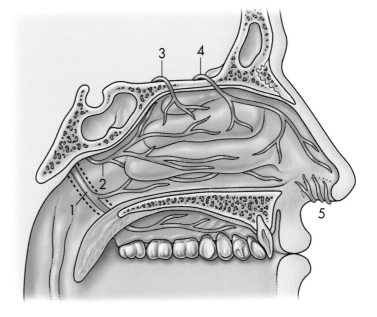

6.13 The vasculature of the nasal septum

1	Greater palatine artery
2	Sphenopalatine artery
3	Posterior ethmoidal artery
4	Anterior ethmoidal artery
5	Superior labial artery (septal branch)

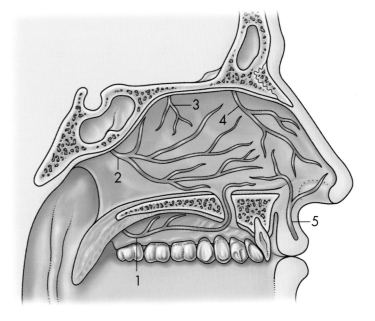

THE PARANASAL AIR SINUSES

The paranasal air sinuses are invaginations from the lateral wall of the nose extending into the surrounding bones. There are four sets of paired sinuses, frontal, ethmoidal, sphenoidal and maxillary. The sinuses are lined by respiratory epithelium. There is considerable variation in the morphology of the sinuses from individual to individual and between the sinuses of each side. The precise function of the paranasal sinuses is unknown, although some believe that the sinuses lighten the skull and add resonance to the voice. It is conceivable, however, that they simply reflect the considerable growth of the bones in which they are situated.

THE FRONTAL AIR SINUSES (6.14, 6.17)

The frontal sinuses lie in the frontal bone above and behind the superciliary arches. A sinus can extend into the medial part of the roof of the orbit. In such cases, a thin layer of bone often separates the sinus from the floor of the cranial cavity and from the roof of the orbit. The frontal sinuses frequently are of unequal size, the larger sinus sometimes extending across the midline. The bony septum separating the frontal sinuses is also often asymmetrically positioned. Each sinus may be partially subdivided by additional septa. The anterior ethmoidal air cells may encroach into the frontal sinuses.

The frontal sinus drains into the middle meatus of the lateral wall of the nasal fossa, either through a simple opening or as a channel termed the frontonasal duct. The point of drainage varies. The frontal sinus can drain directly into the ethmoidal infundibulum of the hiatus semilunaris. More commonly, however, the ethmoidal infundibulum is blind-ended and the frontal sinus drains in front of or above the infundibulum.

The frontal sinus is innervated by the supra-orbital branch of the ophthalmic nerve. The arteries supplying the sinus are the supra-orbital and anterior ethmoidal branches of the ophthalmic artery. Venous drainage is into adjacent veins, including an anastomotic vein joining the supra-orbital and superior ophthalmic veins. Lymph vessels drain into the submandibular group of nodes.

THE ETHMOIDAL AIR SINUSES (6.15, 6.16)

The ethmoidal air sinuses occupy the two lateral masses (labyrinths) of the ethmoid bone between the lateral wall of the nose and the medial wall of the orbit. The orbital wall is particularly thin.

The walls of the ethmoidal air sinuses are incomplete and are covered by adjacent bones (i.e. frontal, lacrimal, maxillary, sphenoidal and palatine bones). Furthermore, the sinuses may not be restricted to the ethmoid bone but may encroach into the frontal, maxillary and sphenoidal air sinuses and into the middle nasal concha, unicate process and agger nasi of the nose.

Each sinus is subdivided into a number of air cells (between three and eighteen). The air cells are separated from each other by thin, incomplete, bony septa. Three groups of air cells are usually found: anterior, middle, and posterior. However, some anatomists combine the anterior and middle air cells as a single anterior group.

The anterior ethmoidal cells occupy the anterior portion of the lateral mass of the ethmoid bone. There are approximately eleven air cells in this group. They drain into the middle meatus of the lateral wall of the nose via the frontonasal duct or the ethmoidal infundibulum.

6.14 Lateral wall of the nose showing air sinuses and their points of drainage

1	Olfactory nerve
2	Frontal sinus
3	Superior concha
4	Sphenoidal sinus
5	Middle concha
6	Opening of frontal sinus in middle meatus
7	Opening of middle ethmoidal sinus
8	Opening of nasolacrimal duct
9	Opening of eustachian tube

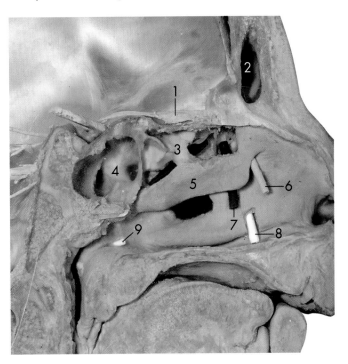

6.15 Coronal section through nose showing sphenoidal and maxillary air sinuses

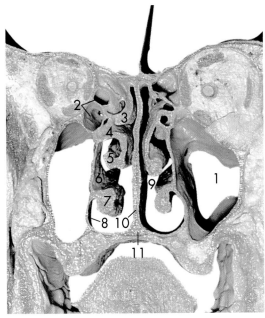

6.16 Horizontal section of head showing the ethmoid and sphenoidal sinuses

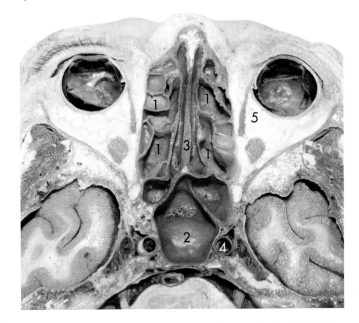

1	Maxillary sinus
2	Ethmoidal sinus
3	Superior nasal concha
4	Superior meatus
5	Middle nasal concha
6	Middle meatus
7	Inferior concha
8	Inferior meatus
9	Nasal cavity
10	Nasal septum
11	Palate

1	Ethmoid sinuses
2	Sphenoidal sinus
3	Nasal septum
4	Internal carotid artery
5	Orbit

The middle ethmoidal cells produce the ethmoidal bulla in the middle meatus of the lateral wall of the nose. There are usually three middle ethmoidal air cells. They drain on or above the bulla.

There are about six posterior ethmoidal cells. They lie in the posterior portion of the lateral mass of the ethmoid bone and drain into the superior meatus of the lateral wall of the nose.

The anterior and middle ethmoidal cells are innervated by the anterior ethmoidal branch of the ophthalmic nerve. The posterior ethmoidal cells are supplied by lateral branches of the posterior superior nasal nerve from the pterygopalatine ganglion and by the posterior ethmoidal branch of the ophthalmic nerve.

The ethmoidal air sinus is supplied by the lateral posterior nasal branches of the sphenopalatine artery. In addition, the anterior and posterior ethmoidal air cells are supplied respectively by the anterior and posterior ethmoidal branches of the ophthalmic artery. The veins that drain the sinuses correspond to the arteries. The sphenopalatine vein passes to the pterygoid venous plexus. The anterior and posterior ethmoidal veins join the superior ophthalmic vein. Lymphatics from the anterior and middle air cells drain into the submandibular nodes, whereas those from the posterior cells drain into the retropharyngeal nodes.

The ethmoidal vessels and nerves cross the roof of the ethmoidal air sinus and the posterior ethmoidal cells are closely related to the optic canal.

THE SPHENOIDAL AIR SINUSES (6.14, 6.16–6.18)

These two sinuses lie within the body of the sphenoid bone at the back of the nasal cavity. They are separated by a bony septum which is usually positioned asymmetrically. The size of the sinuses varies considerably. Although usually limited to the body of the sphenoid, the sinuses can be found within the greater wings and pterygoid processes of the sphenoid, and even within the basilar part of the occipital bone. Occasionally, a posterior ethmoidal air cell may be found extending into the body of the sphenoid bone.

The sphenoidal sinuses drain into the posterior walls of the spheno-ethmoidal recesses.

The sphenoidal sinuses are situated almost centrally within the cranium and have important relationships (8.11). The optic chiasma and the pituitary gland in the sella turcica lie above the sinuses. Laterally is the cavernous sinus. The oculomotor, trochlear, ophthalmic and maxillary nerves invaginate the lateral dura wall of the cavernous sinus. The internal carotid artery and the abducent nerve lie within the cavernous sinus itself. The basilar artery and the pons lie posteriorly and the nasopharynx inferiorly. The pterygoid canals are situated just beneath the sphenoidal sinuses.

The sphenoidal sinus is innervated by the posterior ethmoidal branch of the ophthalmic nerve and by the orbital branch from the pterygopalatine ganglion. The arterial supply is derived from the posterior ethmoidal branch of the ophthalmic artery and from nasal branches of the sphenopalatine artery. Veins pass into those draining the nasal cavity or into the superior ophthalmic vein (via the posterior ethmoidal vein). Lymphatics from the sphenoidal sinus pass to the retropharyngeal nodes.

6.17 Lateral wall of the nose showing drainage sites of some air sinuses

1 Bristle in frontal sinus
2 Crista galli
3 Superior concha
4 Middle concha
5 Middle meatus
6 Inferior concha
7 Inferior meatus
8 Bristle in opening of frontal sinus in middle meatus
9 Sphenoidal sinus
10 Bristle in opening of sphenoidal sinus in sphenoethmoidal recess
11 Bristle in opening of nasolacrismal duct
12 Bristle in opening of auditory tube

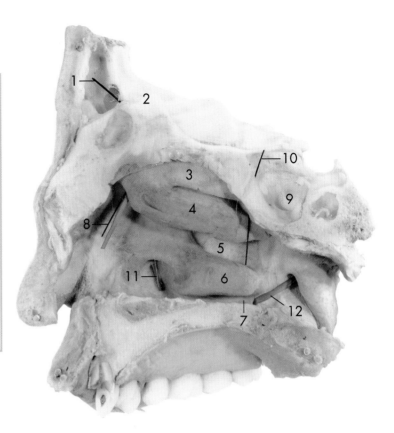

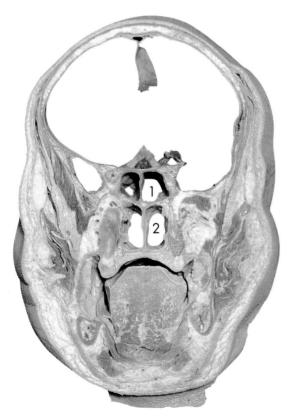

6.18 Coronal section of head showing sphenoidal sinus

1 Sphenoidal sinus
2 Nasal cavity

THE MAXILLARY AIR SINUSES (5.30, 6.8, 6.19, 6.20)

These are the largest of the paranasal sinuses. They are situated in the bodies of the maxillary bones.

The maxillary sinus is pyramidal in shape. The base (medial wall) forms part of the lateral wall of the nose. The apex extends into the zygomatic process of the maxilla. The roof of the sinus is part of the floor of the orbit. The floor of the sinus is formed by the alveolar process and part of the palatine process of the maxilla. The anterior wall of the maxillary sinus is the facial surface of the maxilla and the posterior wall is the infratemporal surface of the maxilla. The sinus may be partially divided by incomplete bony septa.

The medial wall of the maxillary sinus has the opening (ostium) of the sinus. The roof has the infra-orbital nerve and vessels within the infra-orbital canal. The floor of the sinus lies below the level of the floor of the nose and is related to the roots of the cheek teeth. As the size of the sinus varies considerably, this relationship will also vary. Usually, at least the second premolar and first molar are related to the floor of the sinus. However, the sinus may extend anteriorly to the first premolar (and sometimes even to the canine) and posteriorly to the third molar tooth. The anterior superior alveolar nerve and vessels (which arise from the infra-orbital nerve and vessels near the midpoint of the infra-orbital canal) pass downwards in a fine canal (canalis sinuosus) in the anterior wall of the maxillary sinus, to be distributed to the anterior teeth. The posterior superior alveolar nerve and vessels pass through canals in the posterior surface of the sinus.

In an isolated maxillary bone, the ostium of the maxillary sinus is large. However, the ostium in an intact specimen is considerably reduced by portions of the adjacent bones (namely the perpendicular plate of the palatine bone, the uncinate process of the ethmoid bone, the inferior nasal concha and the lacrimal bone) and by the overlying nasal mucosa. The ostium lies high up at the back of the medial wall of the maxillary sinus, being unfavourably situated for drainage. It usually opens into the posterior part of the ethmoidal infundibulum, and hence into the hiatus semilunaris of the middle meatus of the lateral wall of the nose. An accessory ostium is sometimes present behind the major ostium.

The innervation of the maxillary sinus is derived from the maxillary nerve via its infra-orbital and posterior, middle and anterior superior alveolar branches. The arterial supply to the sinus is derived chiefly from the maxillary artery via its posterior superior alveolar, anterior superior alveolar, infra-orbital and greater palatine branches. The veins draining the sinus correspond to the arteries and pass to the facial vein or the pterygoid venous plexus. The lymphatics pass to the submandibular nodes.

6.19 Horizontal section of head showing maxillary sinus

1 External naris
2 Nasal septum
3 Middle nasal concha
4 Maxillary sinus

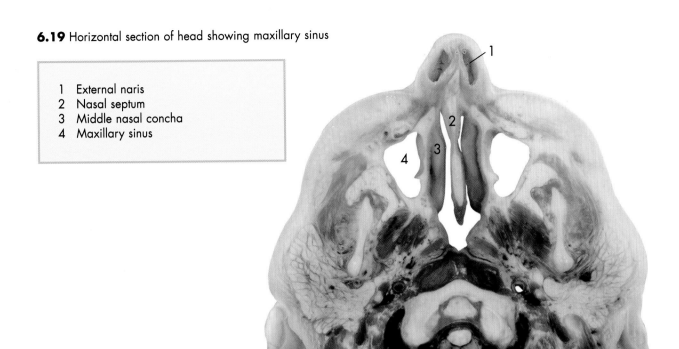

6.20 Parasagittal section of maxillary sinus showing its drainage position high up on its wall

1 Maxillary sinus
2 Opening (ostium) of
   maxillary sinus into lateral
   wall of nose

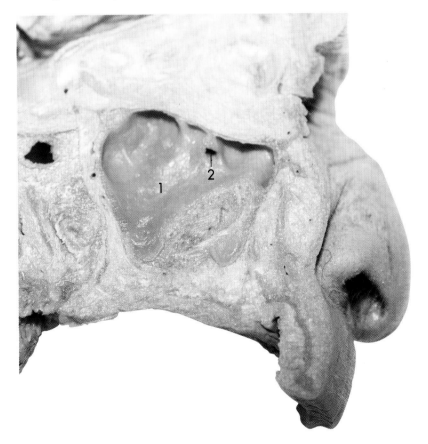

THE PTERYGOPALATINE FOSSA (6.21–6.23)

The pterygopalatine fossa is situated on the lateral side of the skull, between the infratemporal (posterior) surface of the maxilla and the pterygoid process of the sphenoid bone. It is an important region because it contains blood vessels and nerves supplying the nose, palate and upper jaw; the maxillary division of the trigeminal nerve, the pterygopalatine parasympathetic ganglion, and the terminal part of the maxillary artery.

The pterygopalatine fossa communicates with the infratemporal fossa through the pterygomaxillary fissure. The anterior wall of the fossa is the infratemporal surface of the maxilla. The posterior wall of the fossa is the pterygoid process. The medial wall is formed by the perpendicular plate of the palatine bone. The lateral wall shows the pterygomaxillary fissure. The pyramidal process of the palatine bone is situated inferiorly and articulates with the tuberosity of the maxilla. It fills the triangular gap between the lower ends of the medial and lateral pterygoid plates.

The pterygomaxillary fissure transmits the maxillary artery from the infratemporal fossa, the posterior superior alveolar branches of the maxillary division of the trigeminal nerve, and the sphenopalatine veins.

The fissure continues above with the posterior end of the inferior orbital fissure in the floor of the orbit. Passing through the inferior orbital fissure from the pterygopalatine fossa are the infra-orbital and zygomatic branches of the maxillary nerve, the orbital branches of the pterygopalatine ganglion and the infra-orbital blood vessels.

Opening into the pterygopalatine fossa posteriorly are the foramen rotundum from the middle cranial fossa and the pterygoid canal from the region of the foramen lacerum at the base of the skull. The maxillary division of the trigeminal nerve passes through the foramen rotundum. The pterygoid canal transmits the nerve of the pterygoid canal (greater petrosal plus deep petrosal nerves, see page 216) and an accompanying artery.

On the medial wall of the pterygopalatine fossa lies the sphenopalatine foramen. This foramen communicates with the nasal cavity. It transmits the nasopalatine and posterior superior nasal nerves (from the pterygopalatine ganglion) and the sphenopalatine vessels.

At the base of the pterygopalatine fossa, the greater and lesser palatine nerves (from the pterygopalatine ganglion), together with accompanying vessels, pass into the hard palate to emerge at the greater and lesser palatine foramina.

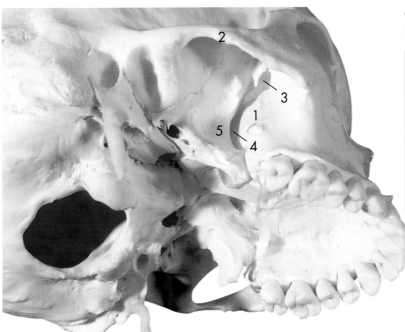

6.21 Bony landmarks of the pterygopalatine fossa

1 Posterior surface of maxilla
2 Zygomatic arch
3 Inferior orbital fissure
4 Pterygomaxillary fissure leading into pterygopalatine fossa
5 Lateral pterygoid plate

6.22 Anterior view of sphenoid bone showing foramen opening into posterior part of pterygopalatine fossa

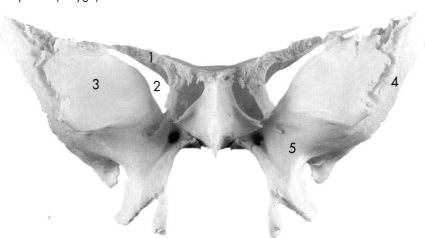

1 Lesser wing
2 Superior orbital fissure
3 Orbital surface of greater wing
4 Temporal surface of greater wing
5 Maxillary surface of greater wing

6.23 Lateral view of palatine bone showing the sphenopalatine notch

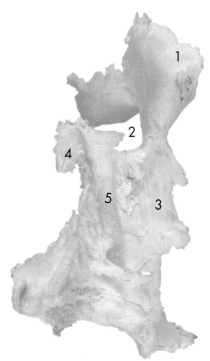

1 Orbital process
2 Sphenopalatine notch
3 Perpendicular plate
4 Sphenoidal process
5 Greater palatine groove

THE MAXILLARY NERVE (6.24–6.27)

This division of the trigeminal nerve (the fifth cranial nerve) contains only sensory fibres. Developmentally, it is the nerve of the maxillary process on the embryonic face. Functionally, it supplies the maxillary teeth and their supporting structures, the hard and soft palate, the maxillary air sinus, much of the nasal cavity, and skin overlying the middle part of the face.

The maxillary nerve arises from the trigeminal ganglion on the floor of the middle cranial fossa. The nerve passes along the lateral dural wall of the cavernous sinus to exit the cranial cavity at the foramen rotundum. It emerges into the upper part of the pterygopalatine fossa, where most of its branches are derived. These branches can be classified into those which come directly from the maxillary nerve, and those which are associated with the pterygopalatine parasympathetic ganglion.

The branches of the maxillary nerve include:

- Branches from the main nerve trunk:
  Meningeal nerve
  Ganglionic branches
  Zygomatic nerve
  Zygomaticotemporal nerve
  Zygomaticofacial nerve
  Posterior superior alveolar nerve
  Infra-orbital nerve
  Middle superior alveolar nerve
  Anterior superior alveolar nerve

- Branches from the pterygopalatine ganglion:
  Orbital nerve
  Nasopalatine nerve
  Posterior superior nasal branches
  Greater (anterior) palatine nerve
  Lesser (posterior) palatine nerve
  Pharyngeal branch

The *meningeal nerve* is the only branch from the main trunk of the maxillary nerve that does not originate in the pterygopalatine fossa: it arises within the middle cranial fossa before the foramen rotundum. It runs with the middle meningeal artery and innervates the dura mater lining the middle cranial fossa.

The *ganglionic branches*, usually two in number, connect the maxillary nerve to the pterygopalatine ganglion. These branches contain sensory fibres which pass through the pterygopalatine ganglion without synapsing (see page 216), and postganglionic autonomic fibres from the ganglion, which are destined for the lacrimal gland in the orbit.

The *zygomatic nerve* leaves the pterygopalatine fossa through the inferior orbital fissure. It passes along the lateral wall of the orbit before dividing into zygomaticotemporal and zygomaticofacial branches. These pass through the zygomatic bone to supply overlying skin. The zygomaticotemporal nerve also gives a branch to the lacrimal nerve, which carries autonomic fibres to the lacrimal gland.

6.24 Branches of the pterygopalatine ganglion

1 Greater palatine nerve
2 Lesser palatine nerve
3 Palatine nerves in greater palatine canal
4 Pharyngeal nerve
5 Pterygopalatine ganglion
6 Posterior superior nasal nerve
7 Nasopalatine nerve

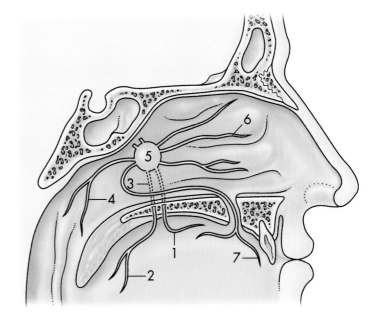

6. 25 The course of the maxillary nerve

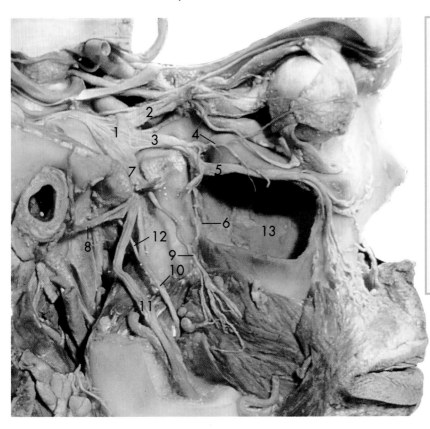

1 Trigeminal ganglion
2 Ophthalmic nerve
3 Maxillary nerve
4 Zygomatic nerve dividing into zygomaticofacial and zygomaticotemporal divisions
5 Infra-orbital nerve
6 Posterior superior alveolar nerve
7 Mandibular nerve
8 Auriculotemporal nerve
9 Buccal nerve
10 Lingual nerve
11 Inferior alveolar nerve
12 Chorda typani nerve
13 Maxillary sinus

The *posterior superior alveolar nerve(s)* is one of three superior alveolar nerves that supply the maxillary teeth. The middle and anterior superior alveolar nerves are branches of the infra-orbital nerve (see below). The posterior superior alveolar nerve(s) leaves the pterygopalatine fossa through the pterygomaxillary fissure. Thence, it runs on the tuberosity of the maxilla and eventually pierces the bone to supply the maxillary molar teeth and the maxillary sinus. Before entering the maxilla, the nerve provides a gingival branch which innervates the buccal gingivae around the maxillary molars. The extra-bony course of the posterior superior alveolar nerve is variable. The nerve can subdivide into several branches just before or just after it enters the maxilla. Alternatively, it may arise as several distinct branches at the main trunk of the maxillary nerve.

The *infra-orbital nerve* can be regarded as the terminal branch of the maxillary nerve proper. It leaves the pterygopalatine fossa to enter the orbit at the inferior orbital fissure. Initially lying in a groove in the floor of the orbit (the infra-orbital groove), the infra-orbital nerve runs into a canal (the infra-orbital canal) and passes onto the face at the infra-orbital foramen.

The middle and anterior superior alveolar nerves arise from the infra-orbital nerve in the orbit. The middle superior alveolar nerve is found in about 70% of subjects. Occasionally, it arises from the maxillary nerve in the pterygopalatine fossa. The nerve may run in the posterior, lateral or anterior walls of the maxillary air sinus to terminate at the premolar teeth. The anterior superior alveolar nerve arises within the infra-orbital canal generally as a single nerve but sometimes as two or three small branches. The nerve runs down the anterior wall of the maxillary sinus in a narrow, sinuous canal (the canalis sinuosus) to reach the maxillary incisor teeth. Near the anterior nasal spine, the anterior superior alveolar nerve gives off a small nasal branch which innervates the nasal mucosa around the anterior naris.

The terminal branches of the infra-orbital nerve arise as the nerve emerges through the infra-orbital foramen onto the face. Palpebral branches supply skin of the lower eyelid. Nasal branches innervate skin overlying the side of the external nose (also part of the septum between the anterior nares). Labial branches supply the skin and oral mucosa of the upper lip, the labial gingivae of the anterior teeth in the upper jaw, and the skin overlying the anterior part of the cheek covering the body of the maxilla.

The branches of the maxillary nerve that arise with the pterygopalatine ganglion contain not only sensory fibres from the maxillary nerve, but also autonomic fibres from the ganglion, which are mainly distributed to glands and blood vessels.

The *orbital nerve* passes from the pterygopalatine ganglion into the orbit through the inferior orbital fissure. It supplies periosteum and, via sympathetic fibres, the orbitalis muscle. The orbital nerve can also pass through the posterior ethmoidal foramen to innervate posterior ethmoidal air cells and the sphenoidal air sinus.

The *nasopalatine nerve* runs from the pterygopalatine ganglion into the nasal cavity through the sphenopalatine foramen. It passes across the roof of the nasal cavity to reach the back of the nasal septum. The nasopalatine nerve then passes downwards and forwards within a groove on the vomer to supply the postero-inferior part of the nasal septum. It terminates by passing through the incisive canal onto the hard palate to supply oral mucosa around the incisive papilla.

The *posterior superior nasal nerve* enters the back of the nasal cavity through the sphenopalatine foramen. It divides into lateral and medial branches. The lateral branches supply the posterosuperior part of the lateral wall of the nasal fossa. The medial branches cross the roof of the nasal cavity to supply the nasal septum overlying the posterior part of the perpendicular plate of the ethmoid.

The *greater (anterior) palatine nerve* passes downwards from the pterygopalatine ganglion, through the greater palatine canal, and onto the hard palate at the greater palatine foramen. Within the greater palatine canal, it gives off nasal branches that innervate the postero-inferior part of the lateral wall of the nasal fossa. On the palate, it runs forwards at the interface between the palatine process and the alveolar process of the maxilla to supply much of the mucosa of the hard palate and palatal gingivae (except around the incisive papilla).

The *lesser (posterior) palatine nerve(s)* passes downwards from the pterygopalatine ganglion, through the greater palatine canal, and onto the palate at the lesser palatine foramen (or foramina). It runs backwards to supply the soft palate.

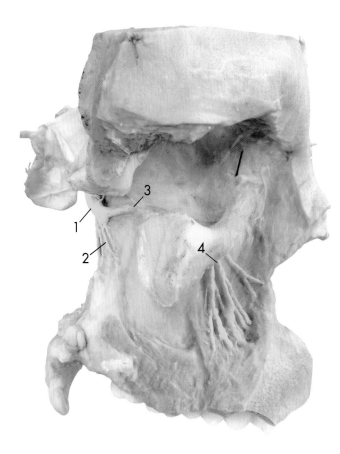

6.26 The course of the maxillary nerve

1 Maxillary nerve at the inferior orbital fissure
2 Posterior superior alveolar nerves
3 Infra-orbital nerve entering infra-orbital canal
4 Terminal branches of infra-orbital nerve passing through the infra-orbital foramen

1 Maxillary nerve
2 Pterygopalatine ganglion
3 Nerve of pterygoid canal
4 Nasopalatine nerve dissected from nasal septum
5 Nasopalatine nerve at incisive fossa
6 Greater palatine nerve
7 Lesser palatine nerve

6.27 The maxillary nerve and the pterygopalatine ganglion

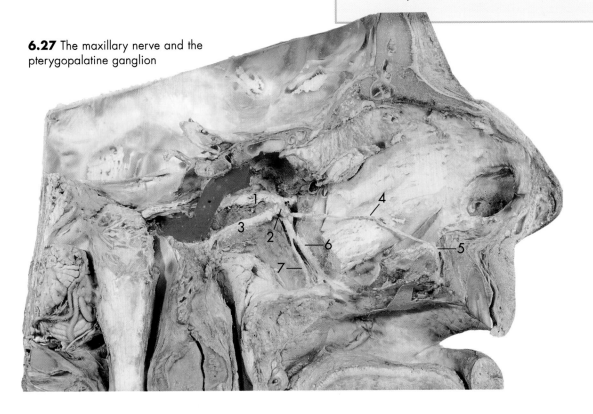

The pharyngeal branch from the pterygopalatine ganglion passes through the palatovaginal canal to supply mucosa of the nasopharynx.

THE PTERYGOPALATINE GANGLION (5.30, 6.7, 6.24, 6.27–6.29)

This parasympathetic ganglion is situated below the maxillary nerve in the pterygopalatine fossa, connected by two ganglionic branches. It is concerned primarily with supplying the nose, palate, and lacrimal gland. Indeed, it can be thought of as 'the hay fever ganglion', as it is responsible for the symptoms of 'running nose and eyes'.

Like other parasympathetic ganglia in the head, three types of fibres enter the pterygopalatine ganglion: parasympathetic, sympathetic, and sensory fibres. However, only the parasympathetic fibres synapse in the ganglion. The preganglionic parasympathetic fibres originate from the superior salivatory nucleus in the brain stem. The fibres pass with the nervus intermedius of the facial nerve. They subsequently emerge as the greater (superficial) petrosal nerve. This occurs within the facial canal of the temporal bone, close to the geniculate ganglion of the facial nerve. The greater petrosal nerve then passes through the bone to appear on the floor of the middle cranial fossa. It then runs medially in a shallow groove to the foramen lacerum. Passing within the foramen lacerum, the greater petrosal nerve enters the pterygoid canal which lies at the base of the pterygoid process. On leaving the pterygoid canal, the nerve emerges into the pterygopalatine fossa and joins the pterygopalatine ganglion. Postganglionic sympathetic fibres run to the pterygopalatine ganglion by a complex course. From the superior cervical ganglion, sympathetic fibres pass to the internal carotid plexus and appear as the deep petrosal nerve. This enters the pterygoid canal to reach the pterygopalatine ganglion. The greater petrosal nerve and the deep petrosal nerve join within the pterygoid canal to become known as the nerve of the pterygoid canal. The sensory fibres to the ganglion run in the ganglionic branches of the maxillary nerve.

The nerves leaving the pterygopalatine ganglion are the orbital nerve, the nasopalatine nerve, the greater and lesser palatine nerves, the posterior superior nasal nerves, and the pharyngeal nerve. These are described above with the maxillary nerve. The fibres supplying the lacrimal gland first pass from the ganglion in one of the ganglionic branches to the maxillary nerve. They then travel with the zygomatic and zygomaticotemporal branches. Within the orbit, they pass from the zygomaticotemporal nerve to the lacrimal nerve (of the ophthalmic nerve) to attain the lacrimal gland.

6.28 The pterygopalatine parasympathetic ganglion

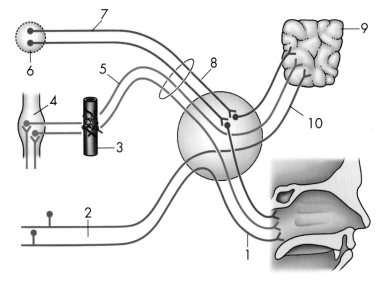

1 Pharyngeal, nasal and palatine branches of pterygopalatine ganglion
2 Maxillary nerve
3 Internal carotid artery
4 Superior cervical ganglion
5 Deep petrosal nerve
6 Superior salivatory nucleus in brainstem
7 Greater petrosal nerve
8 Nerve of pterygoid canal
9 Lacrimal gland
10 Zygomatic and lacrimal nerves

— Parasympathetic fibres
— Sympathetic fibres
— Sensory fibres

6.29 The pterygopalatine ganglion

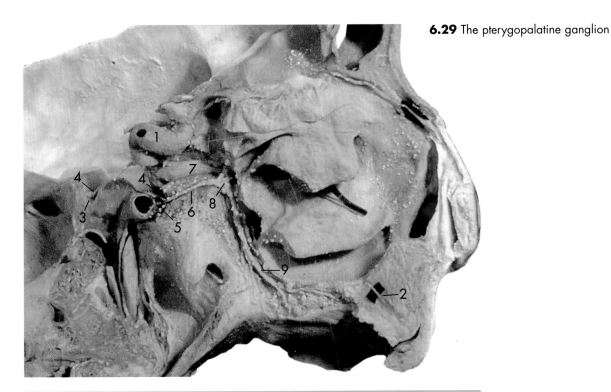

1 Internal carotid artery
2 Nasopalatine nerve on nasal septum
3 Facial nerve in middle ear
4 Greater petrosal nerve
5 Deep petrosal nerve
6 Nerve of pterygoid canal
7 Maxillary nerve
8 Pterygopalatine ganglion
9 Greater and lesser palatine nerves

THE MAXILLARY ARTERY (6.30, 6.31)

The maxillary artery continues from the infratemporal fossa into the pterygopalatine fossa through the pterygomaxillary fissure. It terminates within the pterygopalatine fossa, where it is called the third part of the maxillary artery. The first and second parts of the maxillary artery in the infratemporal fossa are described on page 144.

The third part of the maxillary artery gives branches which accompany the branches of the maxillary nerve (including those associated with the pterygo-palatine ganglion).

The posterior superior alveolar artery runs through the pterygomaxillary fissure onto the maxillary tuberosity. It supplies the maxillary molar and premolar teeth, their buccal gingivae, and the maxillary air sinus.

The infra-orbital artery enters the orbit through the inferior orbital fissure. It runs on the floor of the orbit in the infra-orbital groove and infra-orbital canal to emerge onto the face at the infra-orbital foramen. The infra-orbital artery gives off the anterior superior alveolar artery within the infra-orbital canal. This branch runs downwards to supply the anterior teeth and the anterior part of the maxillary sinus. The infra-orbital artery on the face supplies the lower eyelid, part of the cheek, the side of the external nose, and the upper lip.

The artery of the pterygoid canal passes through the canal to provide branches to part of the auditory tube and tympanic cavity of the ear, and the upper part of the pharynx. The maxillary artery also provides a pharyngeal branch which passes through the vomerovaginal canal to the nasopharynx.

The descending palatine artery leaves the pterygo-palatine fossa through the greater palatine canal. Within this canal, it divides into the greater and lesser palatine arteries. The greater palatine artery supplies the inferior meatus of the lateral wall of the nose before passing onto the roof of the palate at the greater palatine foramen. It runs forwards to supply the hard palate and the palatal gingivae of the maxillary teeth. It also provides a branch which runs up into the incisive canal to anastomose with the sphenopalatine artery, thereby contributing to the supply of the nasal septum. The lesser palatine artery (or arteries) emerges onto the palate at the lesser pala-tine foramen (or foramina). It supplies the soft palate.

The sphenopalatine artery enters the lateral wall of the nose through the sphenopalatine foramen. The artery initially accompanies the posterior superior nasal nerve and gives off branches to supply much of the posterior part of the lateral wall of the nose. The sphenopalatine artery then crosses the roof of the nose to accompany the nasopalatine nerve and to supply the postero-inferior part of the nasal septum.

VEINS OF THE PTERYGOPALATINE FOSSA

The veins are extremely variable but generally corres-pond to the branches of the maxillary artery. The main site of drainage is into the pterygoid venous plexus in the infratemporal fossa. For example, the sphenopalatine vein draining the back of the nose passes into the pterygopalatine fossa through the sphenopalatine foramen. It reaches the pterygoid venous plexus via the pterygomaxillary fissure.

The inferior ophthalmic vein in the floor of the orbit provides a connecting branch to the pterygoid venous plexus, which passes through the inferior orbital fissure in the region of the pterygopalatine fossa.

6.30 Lateral view of infratemporal fossa showing maxillary artery

1 Buccinator muscle
2 Inferior alveolar nerve and artery
3 External carotid artery
4 Medial pterygoid muscle
5 Lateral pterygoid muscle (lower head)
6 Maxillary artery
7 Lateral pterygoid muscle (upper head)

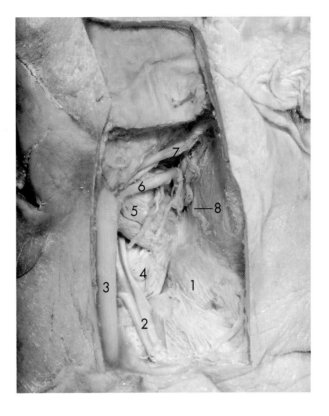

6.31 Lateral view of infratemporal fossa with pterygoid muscles removed to show course of maxillary artery

1 Posterior superior alveolar artery
2 Third part (pterygopalatine part) of maxillary artery
3 Second part (pterygoid part) of maxillary artery
4 Deep temporal artery
5 First part (mandibular part)
6 Inferior alveolar artery
7 Accessory meningeal artery
8 Middle meningeal artery
9 Superficial temporal artery
10 Posterior auricular artery
11 Posterior belly of digastric and stylohyoid muscles
12 Occipital artery
13 Spinal accessory nerve
14 Hypoglossal nerve
15 Facial artery

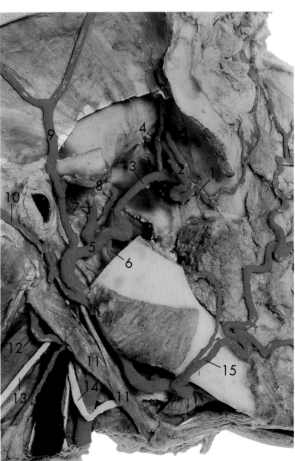

chapter 7
THE ORBIT

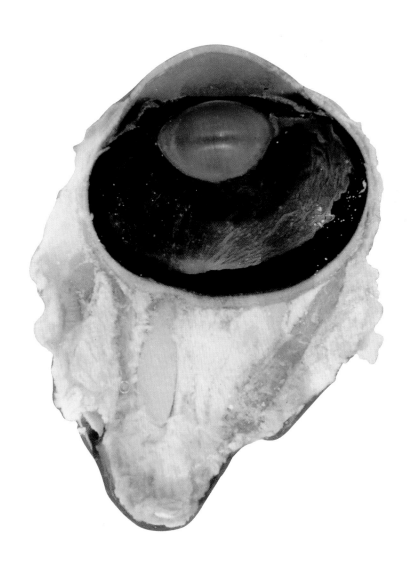

Chapter 7 THE ORBIT

The upper part of the facial skeleton shows two pyramidal-shaped cavities called the orbital cavities or orbits. They house and protect the eyes and thus should be regarded as part of the neurocranium. The eyes are the organs of special sense concerned with vision and can be thought of as extensions of the brain.

THE OSTEOLOGY OF THE ORBIT (7.1)

The orbital aperture (aditus of the orbit) is bounded above by the supra-orbital margin of the frontal bone, laterally by the zygomatic bone and the zygomatic process of the frontal bone, below by the zygomatic bone and the maxilla, and medially by the frontal bone and the anterior lacrimal crest of the frontal process of the maxilla.

The orbital cavity is pyramidal in shape, with the apex pointing posteriorly. It has a roof, a floor, and medial and lateral walls. The bones which comprise the orbital cavity are the ethmoid, frontal, lacrimal, maxillary, palatine, sphenoid, and zygomatic bones.

The roof of the orbit is formed mainly by the orbital part of the frontal bone. The lesser wing of the sphenoid bone is situated posteriorly at the apex.

The floor of the orbit is comprised of the orbital surfaces of the maxillary and the zygomatic bones, with a small contribution from the palatine bone near the apex (the orbital process of the palatine bone).

The medial wall of the orbit begins at the anterior lacrimal crest of the maxilla. Behind this lies the lacrimal bone. Most of the medial wall behind the lacrimal bone is formed by the orbital plate of the ethmoid bone. The body of the sphenoid bone contributes to the medial wall posteriorly. Between the anterior lacrimal crest of the maxilla and the posterior lacrimal crest of the lacrimal bone is the fossa for the lacrimal sac.

The lateral wall of the orbit is formed anteriorly by the orbital surface of the zygomatic bone and posteriorly by the orbital surface of the greater wing of the sphenoid bone.

There are several foramina and fissures within the orbit:

At the superior orbital margin are the supra-orbital notch (or foramen) and the frontal notch (or foramen). These transmit respectively the supra-orbital and the supratrochlear nerves and vessels.

In the floor of the orbit is found the infra-orbital groove and the infra-orbital canal for the infra-orbital nerve and vessels.

At the medial wall is situated the opening of the nasolacrimal canal, and the anterior and posterior ethmoidal foramina for the anterior and posterior ethmoidal nerves and vessels. The nasolacrimal canal is located antero-inferiorly, close to the orbital margin. The ethmoidal foramina lie at the junction with the roof of the orbital cavity.

At the lateral wall is the zygomatico-orbital foramen (occasionally foramina). Through this foramen pass the zygomatic branches of the maxillary division of the trigeminal nerve (with accompanying vessels).

Near the apex of the orbital cavity are the optic canal, the superior orbital fissure and the inferior orbital fissure. The optic canal lies within the lesser wing of the sphenoid bone. It transmits the optic nerve and the ophthalmic artery. The superior orbital fissure lies between the greater and lesser wings of the sphenoid at the junction of the roof and lateral wall of the orbit. It transmits the oculomotor, trochlear, ophthalmic and abducent nerves, together with the ophthalmic veins. The inferior orbital fissure lies at the junction of the lateral wall and floor of the orbit, between the greater wing of the sphenoid and the maxilla. Through this fissure pass the infra-orbital and zygomatic branches of the maxillary division of the trigeminal nerve (with accompanying vessels).

7.1a Osteology of orbit, especially the lateral wall

1 Orbital surface of greater wing of sphenoid
2 Orbital surface of zygomatic bone
3 Inferior orbital fissure
4 Infra-orbital groove
5 Infra-orbital foramen
6 Opening of nasolacrimal canal
7 Superior orbital fissure
8 Optic canal
9 Frontal notch
10 Supra-orbital notch

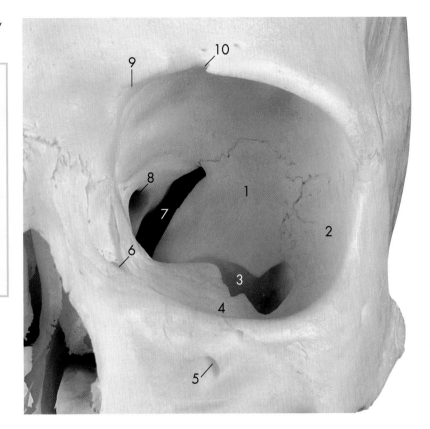

7.1b Osteology of orbit, especially the medial wall

1 Fossa for lacrimal sac
2 Posterior lacrimal crest
3 Lacrimal bone
4 Orbital plate of ethmoid bone
5 Anterior ethmoid foramen
6 Posterior ethmoid foramen
7 Orbital part of frontal bone
8 Orbital surface of maxilla
9 anterior lacrimal crest of maxilla

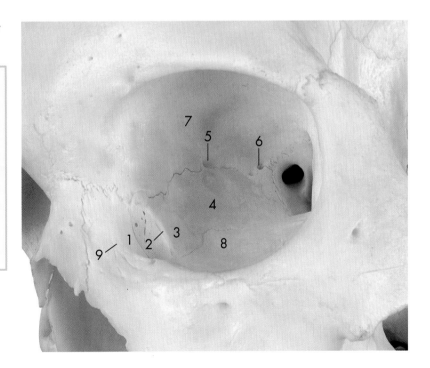

THE CONTENTS OF THE ORBIT (7.2, 7.3, 13.15)

The major structures which occupy the orbit are:

- Eye and optic nerve

- Extra-ocular muscles

- Oculomotor, trochlear and abducent nerves

- Ophthalmic and maxillary divisions of the trigeminal nerve

- Ciliary parasympathetic ganglion

- Ophthalmic vessels

- Lacrimal apparatus

Concerning the disposition of structures, the anterior part of the orbit is occupied chiefly by the eye and by the lacrimal apparatus which is responsible for the production and drainage of tears. The eyelids protect the exposed (anterior) surface of the eye. Running from the back of the eye to the brain is the optic nerve.

Many important structures pass through the apex of the orbit. Their disposition is best understood with respect to the origin of the four recti muscles from a fibrous ring called the common tendinous ring. This ring surrounds the optic canal and encloses part of the superior orbital fissure. Entering the orbit through the optic canal, and thus within the common tendinous ring, are the optic nerve and ophthalmic artery. Also entering the orbit within the common tendinous ring, but via the superior orbital fissure, are the superior and inferior divisions of the oculomotor nerve, the nasociliary branch of the ophthalmic nerve, and the abducent nerve. Entering the orbit through the superior orbital fissure outside the common tendinous ring are the trochlear nerve, and the frontal and lacrimal branches of the ophthalmic nerve.

The extra-ocular muscles which move the eyeball include the recti muscles and the superior and inferior oblique muscles. The superior oblique muscle is situated above the medial rectus muscle. The inferior oblique muscle lies in the floor of the orbit, beneath the inferior rectus muscle. The orbit also contains the levator palpebrae superioris muscle. This lies immediately above the superior rectus muscle. It runs against the roof of the orbit and is attached into the upper eyelid.

The orbit contains both motor and sensory nerves. The oculomotor, trochlear and abducent nerves supply the extra-ocular muscles. The optic nerve is the sensory nerve conveying visual information from the retina of the eye. Additional sensory branches pass with the ophthalmic and maxillary nerves through the orbit to supply skin of the face and scalp as well as some orbital structures. Another neural structure in the orbit is the ciliary parasympathetic ganglion. This ganglion is located at the apex of the orbit. It is concerned with the innervation of structures within the eye, including the intra-ocular muscles associated with the iris and the lens.

The main artery supplying the orbit is the ophthalmic artery, a branch of the internal carotid artery. Superior and inferior ophthalmic veins drain the orbit and pass back into the cavernous sinus.

Orbital fat fills the areas between the structures within the orbit, being particularly prominent around the optic nerve. The fat is said to play a role in stabilising the position of the eye.

7.2 Coronal section of orbit

1 Medial rectus muscle
2 Superior oblique muscle
3 Superior rectus and levator
  palpebrae superioris muscles
4 Lateral rectus muscle
5 Inferior rectus muscle
6 Inferior oblique muscle
7 Eyeball

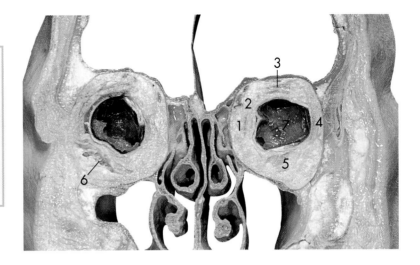

7.3a Relationships of structures at the apex of the orbit.
Note that the four recti muscles originate from a common
tendinous ring

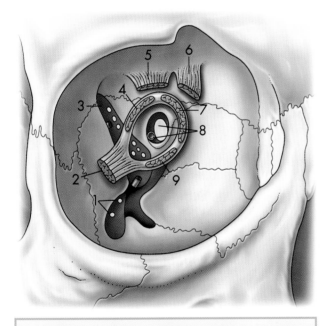

1 Zygomatic and infra-orbital nerves passing
  through the inferior orbital fissure
2 Lateral rectus muscle
3 Superior orbital fissure
4 Superior rectus muscle
5 Levator palpebrae superioris muscle
6 Superior oblique muscle
7 Medial rectus muscle
8 Optic nerve and ophthalmic artery emerging
  through the optic canal
9 Inferior rectus muscle

7.3b Relationships of structures at the apex of the
orbit. The enlargement shows the structures passing
through the superior orbital fissure

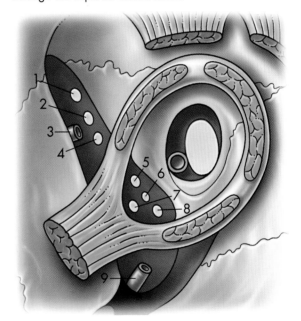

1 Lacrimal nerve
2 Frontal nerve
3 Superior ophthalmic vein
4 Trochlear nerve
5 Superior division of oculomotor
  nerve
6 Nasociliary nerve
7 Abducent nerve
8 Inferior division of oculomotor nerve
9 Inferior ophthalmic vein

THE EYE (7.4–7.10)

The eye is approximately spherical in shape, having a diameter of about 2.5 cm. It is not centrally positioned within the orbit but lies anteriorly. The eye is located closer to the roof than to the floor of the orbit. Furthermore, it is nearer the lateral wall than the medial wall.

The eye has three coats. The outer fibrous coat is the sclera. This continues anteriorly as the cornea. The middle coat is pigmented and is called the uveal tract. This layer is highly vascular and itself consists of three parts: the choroid, the ciliary body, the iris. The inner coat is the retina. This layer contains the photoreceptors and neurones.

The exposed surface (anterior surface) of the eye shows many features. The peripheral part forming the 'white of the eye' is the relatively avascular sclera. The sclera is seen through a thin, mucous membrane layer called the bulbar conjunctiva. This layer contains a fine vascular network. The sclera becomes transparent over the central portion of the eye as the cornea. The boundary between the sclera and the cornea is called the sclerocorneal junction or limbus. The dark, circular, central opening is the pupil. Surrounding the pupil is the iris.

The interior of the eye is divided into two segments by the lens. In front of the lens is a region termed the anterior segment. It is divisible into an anterior and a posterior chamber by the iris and is filled with a clear aqueous humour. The region behind the lens is the posterior segment. This contains a jelly-like substance referred to as the vitreous body.

Light entering the eye is refracted by the transparent cornea and the lens so that an image is brought to focus on the retina (the refractive indices of the aqueous humour and the vitreous body are similar to the refractive index of water). The iris acts as a diaphragm, controlling the amount of light passing into the eye. The ciliary body secretes the aqueous humour and contains muscle which controls the curvature of the lens.

The sclera and the cornea (7.4, 7.5)

The *sclera* comprises the posterior five-sixths of the external coat of the eye. It has a radius of curvature of approximately 12 mm. The sclera is white, opaque and relatively avascular. It meets the cornea at the limbus. The sclera is thick posteriorly but is especially thin immediately behind the sites of insertion of the extra-ocular muscles and at the entrance of the optic nerve. The sclera is referred to as the lamina cribrosa where it is pierced by the optic nerve. This region is so named because of the numerous perforations produced by nerve bundles.

Circumscribing the limbus is a sinus termed the sinus venosus sclerae or the canal of Schlemm. The sinus is essentially an endothelial-lined vessel indenting the deep surface of the sclera. The inner wall of the sinus is separated from the anterior chamber of the eye by a loose trabecular tissue called the trabecular meshwork. This tissue contains a series of endothelial-lined spaces. Aqueous fluid filters into the sinus through the trabecular meshwork. The fluid subsequently enters the bloodstream via an adjacent episcleral plexus of veins. This plexus drains into the anterior ciliary veins.

A particular feature of the sclera at the posterior end of the sinus venosus sclerae is the scleral spur. This flange of tissue gives attachment to the outer group of fibres of the ciliary muscle.

The sclera is pierced posteriorly around the optic nerve by the long and short ciliary nerves and vessels, anteriorly near the limbus by the anterior ciliary vessels, and just behind the equator of the eyeball by three or four vortex veins.

The *cornea* constitutes the anterior one-sixth of the external coat of the eye. Its radius of curvature is less than that of the sclera, being approximately 8 mm. Unlike the sclera, the cornea is transparent. This is due to its highly ordered structure, its lack of blood vessels, and its relative lack of fluid. The lack of a blood supply partly explains the reduced risk of early rejection of corneal grafts. The cornea is innervated by the long and short ciliary nerves (see page 256).

7.4 Surface features of the right eye

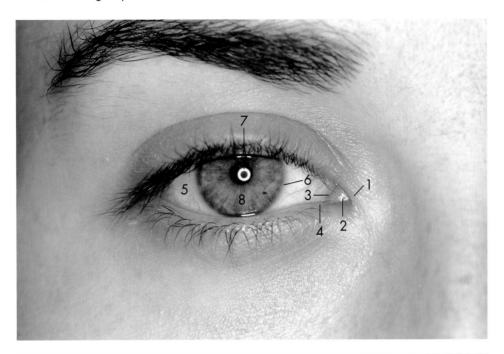

1	Medial canthus	5	Sclera
2	Lacrimal Caruncle	6	Sclerocorneal junction (limbus)
3	Plica semilunaris	7	Pupil
4	Lacrimal papilla	8	Iris

7.5 Sagittal section of eyeball

1	Cornea
2	Anterior chamber
3	Iris
4	Posterior chamber
5	Lens
6	Sclera
7	Choroid
8	Retina
9	Optic nerve
10	Superior rectus muscle
11	Inferior rectus muscle
12	Orbital fat

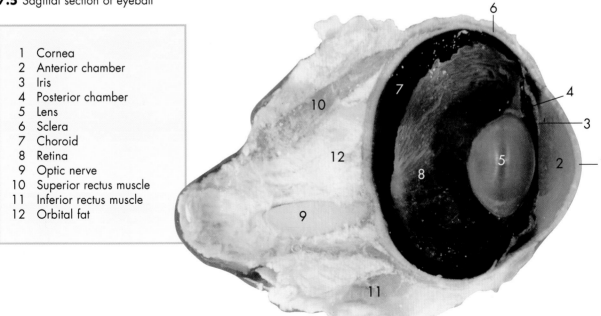

The uveal tract (7.5–7.7, 7.8)

This is comprised of three parts: the choroid, the ciliary body and the iris.

The *choroid* is the thin, vascular, pigmented layer between the sclera and the retina. It extends from the optic nerve to the anterior serrated margin of the retina (the ora serrata) where it is continuous with the ciliary body. The choroid is readily separated from the sclera, except around the optic nerve.

The numerous vessels in the choroid are arranged so that the larger ones are located externally and the smaller ones internally. Indeed, a distinct capillary layer called the choriocapillaris is found internally which supplies the outer portion of the retina.

The posterior part of the choroid is supplied by short posterior ciliary arteries (between 10 and 20 branches). These arise from the ophthalmic artery (beneath the optic nerve) and penetrate the sclera at the back of the eye. The anterior part of the choroid is supplied from three sources: the two long posterior ciliary arteries (which share a common origin from the ophthalmic artery with the short posterior ciliary arteries); the recurrent ciliary arteries (which are branches from the major arterial circle of the iris – see page 262); and the short posterior ciliary arteries. Many anastomoses exist between the vessels supplying the two parts of the choroid.

Venous blood from the choroid (indeed for most of the eyeball) passes into four large vortex veins (venae vorticosae). The vortex vein is so named because the veins which converge to form it display a characteristic whorled pattern. The vortex veins lie equidistant from each other and pierce the sclera midway between the optic nerve and the limbus. They lie on either side of the superior and inferior rectus muscles. The two superior vortex veins generally drain into the superior ophthalmic vein. The two inferior vortex veins usually drain into the inferior ophthalmic vein.

The *ciliary body* lies between the iris and the choroid. It is ring-like and is located about 6 mm behind the limbus. In cross-section, the ciliary body is approximately triangular, being thick in front and narrow behind where it blends with the choroid at the ora serrata. The iris is attached to the middle of the anterior surface of the ciliary body.

The posterior surface of the ciliary body can be divided into regions termed the pars plana and the pars plicata. The pars plana has a smooth, black appearance with faint lines (striae ciliaris) which radiate across from the elevations of the ora serrata. The pars plicata exhibits about 70 radial ridges (the ciliary processes). These ridges are lighter in colour than the grooves between them. Arising close to the surface of the epithelium of the pars plana, and having attachments throughout the entire posterior surface of the ciliary body, are a series of transparent, fine fibres which pass inwards to insert onto the lens. These form the suspensory ligament (zonule) of the lens. The muscle within the ciliary body will affect the degree of tension within the suspensory ligament and thereby regulate the convexity of the lens, allowing the eye to accommodate for near vision.

The ciliary body contains smooth muscle. The muscle is concentrated in the pars plicata and there are two distinct groups. There is an inner circular group which forms a sphincter around the ciliary body. An outer group has radially and longitudinally orientated fibres which are attached to the scleral spur. Contraction of the ciliary muscle relaxes the suspensory ligament with the result that the anterior surface of the lens bulges (thus focussing near objects on the retina). The muscle has no antagonist. Consequently, the suspensory ligament is tensed when the muscle relaxes. This results in the lens becoming flatter (thus focussing distant objects on the retina). The ciliary muscle is supplied by parasympathetic fibres which run with the oculomotor nerve. These relay in the ciliary ganglion and enter the eye via the short ciliary nerves.

7.6 The structure of the eye

1 Inferior rectus muscle
2 Retina
3 Fascia bulbi
4 Vitreous body
5 Hyaloid canal
6 Optic nerve
7 Superior rectus muscle
8 Ocular conjunctiva
9 Posterior chamber –
   containing aqueous
   humour
10 Anterior chamber –
   containing aqueous
   humour
11 Pupil
12 Lens
13 Cornea
14 Iris
15 Zonule
16 Ciliary body
17 Sclera
18 Choroid

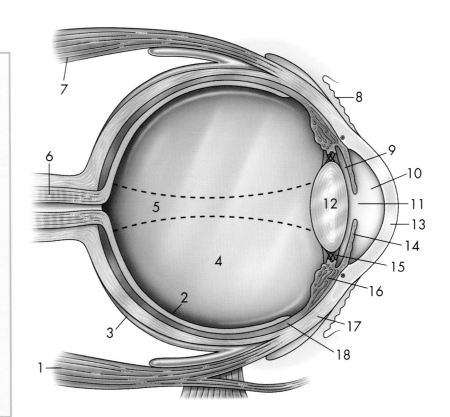

7.7 Section through the iris and
ciliary body

1 Pars plana
2 Ciliary muscle
3 Pars plicata with
   ciliary processes
4 Posterior chamber
5 Zonule
6 Lens
7 Pigmented epithelium
   of iris
8 Sphincter pupillae
   muscle
9 Iris
10 Dilator pupillae muscle
11 Anterior chamber
12 Cornea
13 Filtration angle
14 Trabecular meshwork
15 Sinus venosus sclerae
16 Scleral spur
17 Ocular conjunctiva

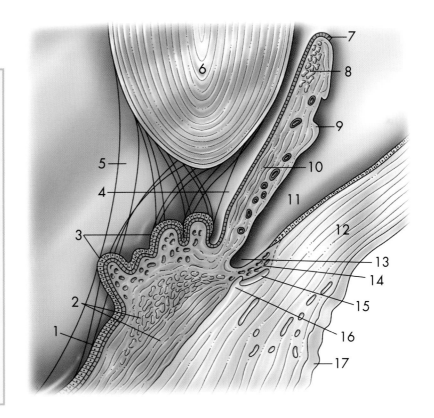

The arteries to the ciliary body are derived from the anterior ciliary arteries and the long posterior ciliary arteries before they unite to form the major arterial circle of the iris (see page 262). The anterior ciliary arteries originate from the muscular branches of the ophthalmic artery and enter the front of the eye. The long posterior ciliary arteries originate from branches of the ophthalmic artery at the back of the eye. The ciliary body receives additional branches from the major arterial circle of the iris. The arteries to the ciliary processes arise from the major arterial circle of the iris. Veins from the ciliary body drain into the vortex veins.

The *iris* is the most anterior part of the uveal tract. It is a thin disc which is perforated near the centre by the pupil. The iris meets the anterior surface of the ciliary body slightly behind the limbus.

The iris is separated from the cornea in front by the anterior chamber. Between the posterior surface of the iris and the lens is the shallow space of the posterior chamber. The anterior and posterior chambers are filled with aqueous humour and they communicate at the pupil.

The anterior surface of the iris is divided into two zones: the peripheral ring (the ciliary zone) and the central ring (pupillary zone). At the junction between the two zones is a circular ridge (the collarette). This ridge is a remnant of an embryonic vascular circle. Whereas the pupillary zone is relatively flat, the ciliary zone exhibits many radially-aligned, interlacing ridges. These ridges are wavy when the pupil is dilated and straight when the pupil is constricted. In contrast to the kaleidoscopic relief of the anterior surface of the iris, the posterior surface is smooth and dark (due to the presence of a deeply pigmented epithelium).

The connective tissue within the iris is termed the stroma. Between the stroma and the posterior epithelium of the iris lies some smooth muscle termed the dilator pupillae muscle. This thin layer of muscle extends from the base of the iris near the ciliary body to the margin of the pupil. Here, it meets the sphincter pupillae muscle. Contraction of the dilator pupillae muscle causes the pupillary zone of the iris to slide beneath the anterior portion of the ciliary zone, thereby dilating the pupil. The muscle is innervated by sympathetic fibres running with the long ciliary nerves. The sphincter pupillae muscle forms a ring around the margin of the pupil. Contraction of the muscle constricts the pupil. In common with the ciliary muscle, the sphincter pupillae is supplied by parasympathetic fibres which run with the oculomotor nerve. These enter the eye via the short ciliary nerves after relaying in the ciliary ganglion.

The iris is very vascular. Its blood supply is derived from the major arterial circle of the iris which, in spite of its name, lies in the ciliary body. This circle is formed by union of the long posterior ciliary and anterior ciliary arteries. The long posterior ciliary arteries arise from the ophthalmic artery at the back of the eye. The anterior ciliary arteries arise from muscular branches towards the front of the eye. Vessels pass radially from the major arterial circle through the iris, producing striations in the ciliary zone of the iris. At the collarette, near the margin of the pupil, these vessels anastomose to form the minor arterial circle of the iris. The veins accompany the arteries. They pass to the ciliary body and eventually drain into the vortex veins (7.8).

The variation in colour of the iris is related to the amount and distribution of pigment (melanin) in its stroma. Where there is little pigment the iris appears blue. Indeed, the blue coloration comes from light scattered from the deeply pigmented posterior epithelium of the iris. Where pigment is present in the stroma, this superimposes varying degrees of brown and mottled coloration. Most babies of ethnic groups with white skin initially have blue/cloudy grey eyes, the pigment in the stroma not appearing for some months.

7.8 The vasculature of the eye. The upper part of the diagram illustrates some ciliary arteries and the arterial circle of the iris. The lower part of the diagram illustrates one of the vortex veins

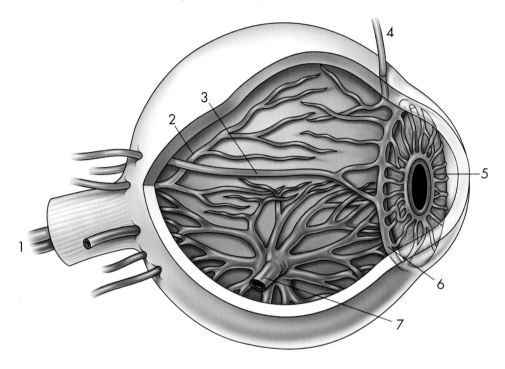

1 Central vessels of retina
2 Short ciliary artery
3 Long ciliary artery
4 Anterior ciliary artery
5 Minor arterial circle of iris
6 Major arterial circle of iris
7 A vortex vein

The retina (7.9, 7.10)

The retina is the inner coat of the eyeball. It is a thin layer and is light-sensitive. The retina extends forwards to about halfway between the limbus and the equator of the eye. This position corresponds to a serrated margin termed the ora serrata. The retina at the ora serrata is firmly attached to both the choroid and the vitreous body. The retina is transparent during life but becomes white and opaque soon after death.

Using an ophthalmoscope, three specialised areas can be identified at the back of the retina (the fundus of the retina): the optic disc, the macula lutea, the fovea centralis.

The optic disc is a pale circular area about 1.5 mm in diameter. It represents the site at which the optic nerve enters the retina. The retinal artery and vein also enter and leave at the optic disc. The depression within the optic disc is called the physiological cup. The disc is insensitive to light. Its projection in the lateral (temporal) visual field is consequently known as the blind spot.

The macula lutea is located about 3 mm lateral to the optic disc. It appears as a shallow depression which is approximately the same size as the optic disc. Unlike the disc, it has a yellowish coloration and lacks a well-defined border. The macula lutea has a capillary-free zone at its centre. In the very centre is a small pit called the fovea centralis.

The central artery of the retina is seen within the optic disc dividing into superior and inferior branches. Each branch gives off medial (nasal) and lateral (temporal) branches which continue to divide dichotomously. The central artery of the retina is an anatomical end artery as its capillaries do not anastomose with those of any other vessel. The artery supplies the inner region of the retina comprising the nerve fibres. The outer region containing the photoreceptors receives its nutrients by diffusion from the choroidal vessels. The retinal veins accompany the retinal arteries. Superior and inferior retinal veins join to form the central vein of the retina. This union occurs slightly proximal and lateral to the division of the companion artery. Through the ophthalmoscope, the retinal arteries characteristically appear narrower than the veins. They also appear a brighter red and, because of their convex walls, they usually reflect light and show a longitudinal streak.

The retina in most areas has a complex histology. It generally consists of 10 layers. The photoreceptors lie in the outer region (adjacent to the choroid) and the nerve fibres in the inner region. At the optic disc however are only found nerve fibres. At the macula lutea, the retinal vessels are absent and the elements comprising the inner layers are heaped up at the margin. This allows for the uninterrupted passage of light to the fovea centralis. The fovea is the most sensitive (and thinnest) part of the retina. It consists almost entirely of colour-sensitive photoreceptors (i.e. cones).

The lens (7.6, 7.7, 7.10)

The lens lies immediately behind the iris and the pupil. It is separated from the iris by the posterior chamber. The back of the lens is separated from the anterior surface of the vitreous body by a small fluid-filled space called the retrolenticular space.

The lens is a transparent, biconvex body which is surrounded by a highly elastic capsule. It has a gelatinous consistency, although the central part (the nucleus) is harder than the peripheral part (the cortex). The posterior surface of the lens is more convex than the anterior surface (radii of curvature 6 mm and 10 mm respectively). The most convex points on the anterior and posterior surfaces are termed the anterior and posterior poles. The anterior and posterior surfaces meet at the equator of the lens.

The lens is connected to the ciliary body by the suspensory ligament. The fibres of the suspensory ligament form a layer that extends about 1.5 mm onto the anterior surface of the lens capsule and about 1.3 mm onto the posterior surface of the capsule. The fibres that insert at the equator are usually smaller than those inserting anteriorly and posteriorly.

7.9 Fundus through ophthalmoscope

1	Optic disc
2	Macula lutea
3	Fovea centralis
4	Retinal artery
5	Retinal vein

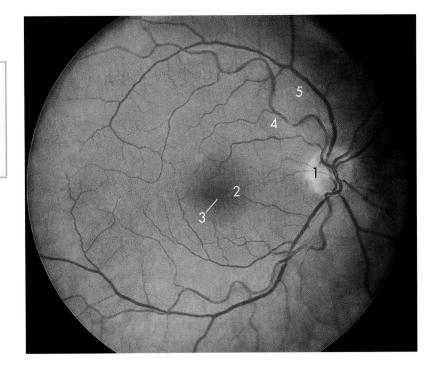

7.10 Sagittal section of eyeball

1	Cornea
2	Anterior chamber
3	Iris
4	Posterior chamber
5	Lens
6	Sclera
7	Choroid
8	Retina
9	Optic nerve
10	Superior rectus muscle
11	Inferior rectus muscle
12	Orbital fat

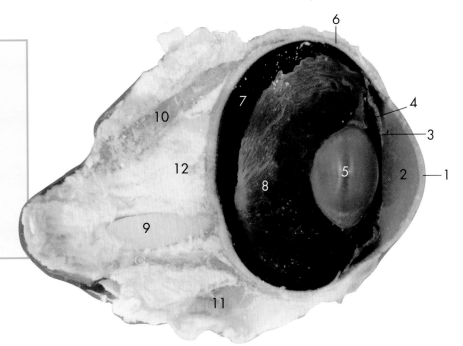

The chambers of the eye (7.5–7.7)
There are three spaces within the eye: the anterior chamber, the posterior chamber, the vitreous cavity. The anterior and posterior chambers (the anterior segment) lies in front of the lens. The vitreous cavity (the posterior segment) is located behind the lens.

The *anterior chamber* is bounded in front by the cornea and the limbus. Behind lies the iris and the ciliary body. Centrally, the anterior surface of the lens is seen through the pupil. The periphery of the anterior chamber, lying between the base of the iris and the limbus, is referred to as the filtration angle. This site is related to the trabecular meshwork and the sinus venosus sclerae at the limbus.

The *posterior chamber* is smaller than the anterior chamber. It is bounded in front by the posterior surface of the iris and behind by the lens and the suspensory ligament.

The *aqueous humour* is the fluid that occupies the anterior and posterior chambers. It is a colourless, transparent, protein-free fluid which is secreted continuously from the ciliary body. The anterior chamber has a capacity of about 0.2 ml and the posterior chamber of about 0.06 ml. The aqueous humour provides nutrients for the cornea and the lens. The fluid is drained from the eye through the trabecular meshwork at the limbus. It then passes through the sinus venosus sclerae into the adjacent episcleral venous plexus and eventually reaches the superior ophthalmic vein. The intra-ocular pressure is normally between 10 and 20 mmHg. Changes in the balance between the rate of formation and the rate of drainage of the aqueous humour will affect this pressure.

The *vitreous cavity* is the largest cavity, occupying the posterior four-fifths of the eye. It is bounded anteriorly by the lens, the suspensory ligament and the ciliary body. Behind and laterally, it is bounded by the retina. The vitreous cavity is filled by the vitreous body which is moulded to the shape of the cavity. Thus, the vitreous body is roughly spherical in outline, but is slightly concave anteriorly where it meets the posterior surface of the lens. This concavity is termed the lenticular fossa. The vitreous body is composed of a transparent, colourless, gel-like substance. It can be readily separated from the retina, except at the ora serrata and the optic disc. Condensation of some of the components of the vitreous body can give the impression of a surrounding membrane. A narrow canal (1–2 mm wide) may run from the lenticular fossa to the optic disc. This canal is called the hyaloid canal. It is slightly expanded at its ends and is filled with a more watery material. It represents the site of an embryonic artery (the hyaloid artery).

The fascia bulbi (7.11, 7.12)
The fascia bulbi (Tenon's capsule) is the thin, fibrous capsule which loosely covers the eye from the margin of the cornea anteriorly to the optic nerve posteriorly. Functionally, the eye fits into the fascia bulbi in a manner analogous to a ball and socket joint. Thus, the fascia supports the eye and allows for movement in all directions.

The inner surface of the fascia bulbi is smooth and is separated from the sclera by a fluid-filled space termed the episcleral space. Strands of the fascia however pass across the space to blend with the sclera.

The fascia bulbi is pierced by the tendons of the extra-ocular muscles and is reflected backwards around each muscle to provide a sheath. The fascia also projects to adjacent structures in the orbit to form check ligaments. These limit the actions of the extra-ocular muscles.

The most prominent check ligaments are the medial and lateral check ligaments. The medial check ligament extends from the sheath around the medial rectus muscle to the posterior lacrimal crest of the lacrimal bone on the medial wall of the orbit. The lateral check ligament extends from the sheath of the lateral rectus muscle to the marginal tubercle of the zygomatic bone on the lateral wall of the orbit.

7.11 Horizontal section through the orbit to show the fascia bulbi

1   Sheath around medial recus muscle
2   Medial check ligament
3   Lacrimal part of orbicularis oculi muscle
4   Lacrimal sac
5   Medial palpebral ligament
6   Orbital septum
7   Lateral palpebral ligament
8   Lateral check ligament
9   Fascia bulbi
10 Sheath around lateral recus muscle
11 Orbital periosteum
12 Meninges and subarachnoid space around optic nerve

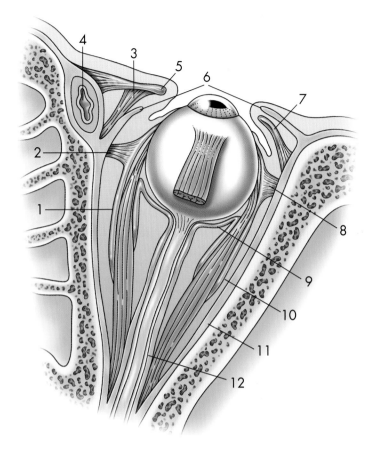

7.12 The eye viewed anteriorly showing ligaments and the extra-ocular muscles.

1   Inferior rectus muscle
2   Lateral check ligament
3   Lateral rectus muscle
4   Superior rectus muscle
5   Superior oblique muscle
6   Pulley (trochlea)
7   Medial rectus muscle
8   Medial check ligament
9   Suspensory ligament
10 Inferior oblique muscle

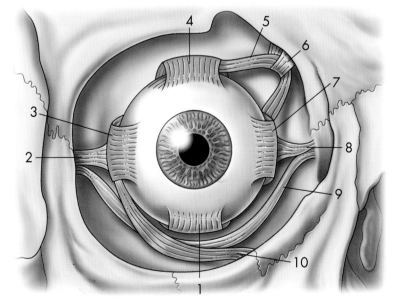

A check ligament from the sheath of the superior rectus muscle passes to the levator palpebrae superioris muscle. This ligament is responsible for the elevation of the upper eyelid when the gaze of the eye is directed upwards. From the sheath of the inferior rectus muscle is a ligament which projects forwards to insert into the lower eyelid between the orbicularis oculi muscle and the inferior tarsal plate. This ligament is thought to be responsible for depression of the lower eyelid when the gaze of the eye is directed downwards.

Check ligaments also project from the superior and inferior oblique muscles. The ligament from the superior oblique muscle passes to the trochlea; the ligament from the inferior oblique muscle extends to the lateral part of the floor of the orbit.

The fascia bulbi is thickened beneath the eye to form a suspensory ligament (the suspensory ligament of Lockwood). This is connected to the medial and lateral check ligaments. The suspensory ligament provides sufficient support for the eye such that, even when the maxilla forming the floor of the orbit is removed, the eye will retain its position.

The fascia bulbi is pierced towards the back of the eye by the optic nerve, the ciliary nerves and vessels, and the vortex veins. Some smooth muscle is associated with the fascia bulbi (see page 252).

THE EYELIDS (7.4, 7.13)

The eyelids (palpebrae) are two moveable folds which cover the anterior surface of the eye. They protect the eye from trauma or from excessive light. The act of blinking maintains a thin film of tears over the cornea.

The upper eyelid is larger and more mobile than the lower eyelid. When the eyelids are open, the upper lid just overlaps the upper part of the cornea, whereas the lower lid lies just below the cornea. The elliptical space between the eyelids is termed the palpebral fissure. When the eyelids are closed, the upper lid moves down to cover the whole of the cornea.

The eyelids are covered by skin externally and by conjunctiva internally. The skeletal framework of each eyelid is formed by fibrous tissue which is arranged as a tarsal plate and an orbital septum. The chief muscle within the eyelids is the orbicularis oculi muscle. This is a muscle of facial expression.

The skin of the eyelids is thin, elastic and almost translucent. The eyelids are demarcated from the adjacent facial skin by the superior and inferior palpebral furrows. Additional furrows appear with age just beyond the inferior orbital margins (e.g. a naso-jugal furrow medially and a malar furrow laterally).

Each lid margin exhibits a small elevation approximately one-sixth of the way along from the medial canthus of the eye. This is termed the lacrimal papilla. In the centre of the papilla is a small opening, the punctum lacrimale. The margin of each eyelid lateral to the lacrimal papilla is designated the ciliary part of the eyelid. From this part arise the eyelashes. These stiff hairs are arranged in two or three rows. The margin of each eyelid medial to the lacrimal papilla is termed the lacrimal part of the eyelid. It lacks eyelashes.

The lid margin for both the upper and lower eyelids exhibits a 'grey line' which corresponds to the muco-cutaneous junction. In front of this line are the eyelashes, behind it are the openings of the tarsal glands (meibomian glands). The tarsal glands are seen as a series of parallel, faint yellow lines.

7.13 Sagittal section through the orbit showing the structure of the eyelids

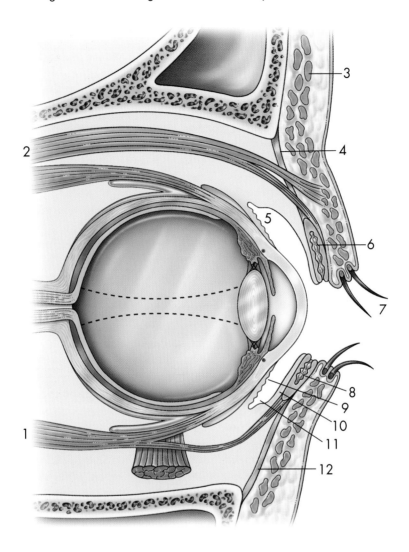

1 Inferior rectus muscle (note check ligament to inferior
   tarsal plate)
2 Levator palpebrae superioris muscle
3 Orbicularis oculi muscle
4 Orbital septum
5 Superior fornix
6 Superior tarsal plate containing meibomian glands
7 Eyelashes (cilia)
8 Inferior tarsal plate
9 Ocular conjunctiva
10 Palpebral conjunctiva
11 Inferior fornix
12 Orbital septum

The medial and lateral angles of the eye are referred to as the medial (inner) and lateral (outer) canthi. The medial canthus is about 2 mm lower than the lateral canthus, this distance being increased in Orientals. The lateral canthus is relatively featureless. The medial canthus shows several features. It is separated from the eyeball by a small triangular space, the lacrimal lake (lacus lacrimalis). Here also lies a small, reddish body called the lacrimal caruncle which contains sebaceous and sweat glands, and sometimes accessory lacrimal glands. The lacrimal caruncle represents an area of modified skin and contains some fine hairs. Lateral to the caruncle is the plica semilunaris, a fold of conjunctiva which is believed by some to be a vestige of the nictitating membrane of other animals. In Orientals, a semilunar fold of skin termed the epicanthus passes from the medial end of the upper eyelid to the lower eyelid and obscures the caruncle.

The lower eyelid can be everted to reveal its conjunctiva up to the point where it is reflected from the eyelid onto the sclera (i.e. at the inferior fornix). The upper eyelid is not easily everted.

The conjunctiva (7.13)
The conjunctiva is the thin, translucent, mucous membrane which lines the inner surface of the eyelids (palpebral conjunctiva) and which is reflected at the fornices to cover the anterior surface of the eye (ocular conjunctiva). The conjunctiva encloses a space called the conjunctival sac which opens to the exterior at the palpebral fissure. The superior fornix is level with the superior orbital margin whereas the inferior fornix is just above the inferior orbital margin. The lacrimal gland drains into the lateral portion of the superior fornix.

The palpebral conjunctiva is firmly attached to the underlying tarsal plates. Because it is translucent, the tarsal glands may be visualised through it as yellowish streaks. The palpebral conjunctiva is highly vascular and provides a readily accessible site for assessing signs of anaemia.

The ocular conjunctiva is loosely attached to the sclera. It is because this conjunctiva is translucent and relatively avascular that the white appearance of the sclera is visible. Over the cornea, the ocular conjunctiva consists only of a layer of epithelium.

The fibrous layer of the eyelids (7.13, 7.15)
This is comprised of the orbital septum and two tarsal plates.

The *orbital septum* is a thin membrane which arises from the periosteum along the entire rim of the orbit. It passes inwards into each eyelid to merge with the tarsal plates. The septum is thickest laterally. The septum is located in front of the lateral palpebral ligament but passes behind the medial palpebral ligament and lacrimal sac (but in front of the pulley of the superior oblique muscle). The palpebral ligaments are extensions of the tarsal plates (see description below) with important relationships with the orbital septum.

The orbital septum is pierced above by the levator palpebrae superioris muscle and below by the check ligament from the inferior rectus muscle. The lacrimal, supratrochlear, infratrochlear and supra-orbital nerves and vessels also pass through the septum.

The *tarsal plates* (one for each eyelid) are crescent-shaped, and about 3 cm long and 1 mm thick. The tarsal plate in the upper eyelid has a maximum height of about 1 cm, whereas the maximum height of the plate in the lower eyelid is 0.5 cm. Each plate is convex forwards, conforming to the configuration of the anterior surface of the eye. The free border is called the ciliary border as it is adjacent to the eyelashes. The ciliary border is thick and relatively straight. The attached border is termed the orbital border as it is attached to the orbital septum. The orbital border is thin and convex.

The levator palpebrae superioris muscle is attached to both the anterior surface and to the orbital border of the tarsal plate of the upper eyelid. Where it joins the orbital border, the fibres are comprised of smooth muscle. A band of smooth muscle also passes between the tarsal plate of the lower eyelid and the fascial sheath of the inferior rectus muscle.

7.14 Surface features of the right eye

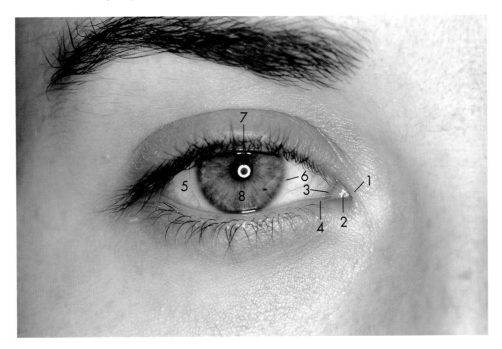

1	Medial canthus	5	Sclera
2	Lacrimal caruncle	6	Sclerocorneal junction (limbus)
3	Plica semilunaris	7	Pupil
4	Lacrimal papilla	8	Iris

7.15 Anterior view of the fibrous layer of the eyelids and the associated sensory nerves.

1 Orbital septum
2 Inferior tarsal plate
3 Lateral palpebral ligament
4 Superior tarsal plate
5 Lacrimal nerve
6 Levator palpebrae superioris muscle
7 Supra-orbital nerve
8 Supratrochlear nerve
9 Infratrochlear nerve
10 Medial palpebral ligament
11 Infra-orbital nerve

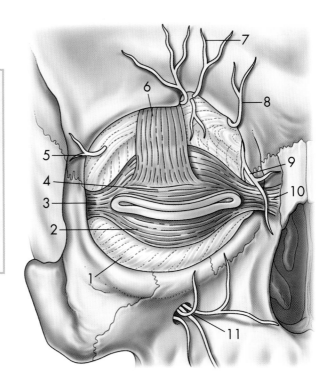

Within the tarsal plates are found tarsal glands (meibomian glands). These number about 30 in the upper eyelid and about 20 in the lower eyelid. The glands are visualised as faint yellow streaks beneath the conjunctiva. Their ducts open onto the free margin of the eyelids behind the grey line. The oily secretions of these modified sebaceous glands lubricate the lid margins and prevent the tears from overflowing onto the face. They may also retard the evaporation of the tear-film on the cornea.

The tarsal plates are connected to the margins of the orbit by the orbital septum and by medial and lateral palpebral ligaments.

The medial palpebral ligament passes from the medial ends of the two tarsal plates to the anterior lacrimal crest and the frontal process of the maxilla. It splits at its insertion into the tarsal plates to surround the lacrimal canaliculi. The medial palpebral ligament lies in front of the lacrimal sac and the orbital septum.

The lateral palpebral ligament passes from the lateral ends of the tarsal plates to a small tubercle on the zygomatic bone within the orbital margin. The ligament is relatively poorly developed. It is more deeply situated than the medial palpebral ligament, lying beneath the orbital septum and the lateral palpebral raphe of the orbicularis oculi muscle.

The *orbicularis oculi muscle* has a palpebral part, which is closely associated with the tarsal plates. It is fully described on page 104 with the muscles of facial expression. Between the muscle and overlying skin, the subcutaneous tissue is loose and easily distensible. Between the muscle and underlying tarsal plates there is a zone of loose connective tissue in which are found the main nerves to the eyelids. This region is continuous above with the subaponeurotic layer of the scalp.

The blood supply and innervation of the eyelids (7.10, 7.15)

The blood supply to the eyelids is derived mainly from vascular arcades near the lid margins. The arcades are formed by the medial and lateral palpebral arteries which are branches of the ophthalmic artery (see page 264). Additional branches supplying the eyelids come from the infra-orbital, facial, transverse facial and superficial temporal arteries. The veins are larger and more numerous than the arteries. They pass either superficially to veins on the face and forehead, or deeply to the ophthalmic veins within the orbit.

The cutaneous innervation of the eyelids comes from both the ophthalmic and maxillary divisions of the trigeminal nerve. The upper eyelid is supplied mainly by the supra-orbital branch of the frontal nerve. Additional contributions come from the lacrimal nerve, from the supratrochlear branch of the frontal nerve, and from the infratrochlear branch of the nasociliary nerve. The nerve supply to the lower eyelid is principally from the infra-orbital branch of the maxillary nerve, with small contributions from the lacrimal and infratrochlear nerves.

THE LACRIMAL APPARATUS (7.16)

This comprises the lacrimal gland, the lacrimal canaliculi, the lacrimal sac, and the nasolacrimal duct.

The lacrimal apparatus is responsible for the secretion and the drainage of tears. The tears form a thin film of fluid covering the exposed surface of the eye. This film has several functions. Firstly, it prevents drying of the cornea and the conjunctiva. Secondly, it acts as a lubricant between the eyelids and eyeballs. Thirdly, it improves the optical quality of the superficial part of the cornea. Fourthly, tears contain a bactericidal enzyme (lysozyme). Excessive production of tears results in crying. Crying is an important means of expressing emotions.

Tears are secreted mainly by the lacrimal gland which lies at the anterolateral corner of the roof of the orbit. Small, accessory lacrimal glands may also be found in both eyelids. Tears are carried from the superior fornix over the front of the eye during blinking. The fluid collects at the medial canthus of the eye where it passes through the lacrimal puncta into the lacrimal canaliculi of the eyelids. The canaliculi convey the tears into the lacrimal sac, which is located at the anteromedial corner of the floor of the orbit. A nasolacrimal canal runs from the lacrimal sac into the inferior meatus of the lateral wall of the nose. Thus, the tears eventually drain into the nose.

The lacrimal gland (7.17a)

The lacrimal gland folds around the lateral border of the tendon of the levator palpebrae superioris muscle. As a consequence it is divided into two parts, the orbital and palpebral parts. The orbital part is the larger and lies in a fossa in the frontal bone (the lacrimal fossa); the fossa is situated anterolaterally in the roof of the orbit. The palpebral part lies below the orbital part, just above the lateral aspect of the superior fornix. Thus, the palpebral part may be seen through the conjunctiva when the upper eyelid is everted.

The lacrimal gland is a compound, tubulo-alveolar gland. Its serous secretions pass into the lateral part of the superior fornix via several distinct lacrimal ducts. The ducts from the orbital part of the lacrimal gland pass through the palpebral part before draining into the fornix.

The *innervation of the lacrimal gland* is associated with the pterygopalatine parasympathetic ganglion (see page 216). Parasympathetic, secretomotor fibres arise in the superior salivatory nucleus of the brain stem and pass from the brain with the nervus intermedius of the facial nerve. These preganglionic fibres leave the facial nerve at the geniculate ganglion (without synapsing) as the greater petrosal nerve. This nerve then passes along the floor of the middle cranial fossa, beneath the trigeminal ganglion, to reach the foramen lacerum. It crosses this foramen to enter the pterygoid canal where it forms the nerve of the pterygoid canal (with the deep petrosal nerve). The greater petrosal nerve subsequently runs into the pterygopalatine fossa to relay in the pterygopalatine ganglion. Postganglionic fibres pass into the maxillary nerve and run with its zygomatic branch into the orbit. They then join the lacrimal branch of the ophthalmic nerve to reach the lacrimal gland.

Sympathetic fibres innervate the blood vessels of the lacrimal gland. These fibres originate as the deep petrosal nerve from the sympathetic plexus surrounding the internal carotid artery. The deep petrosal nerve contributes to the nerve of the pterygoid canal and passes to the pterygopalatine ganglion in the pterygopalatine fossa. The fibres do not synapse at the ganglion and pass to the lacrimal gland along the same course as the parasympathetic innervation (i.e. the zygomatic and lacrimal nerves).

Sensory fibres associated with the gland are derived from the lacrimal nerve.

There may be alternative sources of innervation for the lacrimal gland. Parasympathetic fibres may be derived from orbital branches of the pterygopalatine ganglion. Sympathetic fibres may arise directly from the sympathetic plexus surrounding the lacrimal artery.

The *vasculature of the lacrimal gland* is derived from the lacrimal branch of the ophthalmic artery. The gland may also receive blood from the transverse facial branch of the superficial temporal artery. Venous drainage is into the superior ophthalmic vein.

The lacrimal canaliculi (7.16)

The lacrimal canaliculi are fine canals, one in each eyelid, which convey tears to the lacrimal sac.

Each canaliculus opens at the margin of the eyelid, about 6 mm from the medial canthus. The canaliculus here shows a small elevation termed the lacrimal papilla. The papilla has a fine opening called the lacrimal punctum. The punctum faces backwards and is seen when the eyelid is everted. A ring of dense fibrous tissue helps to maintain the patency of the punctum.

The canaliculus in the upper eyelid initially ascends before bending to pass downwards and medially to the lacrimal sac. The canaliculus in the lower eyelid initially descends and then runs medially and slightly upwards to the lacrimal sac. The canaliculi may open either separately or together in a diverticulum near the middle of the lateral surface of the upper part of the sac.

The lacrimal sac (7.16)

The lacrimal sac is the blind-ended upper extremity of the nasolacrimal duct. It lies adjacent to the lacrimal groove in the anterior part of the medial wall of the orbit. The sac is bounded in front by the anterior lacrimal crest of the maxilla and behind by the posterior lacrimal crest of the lacrimal bone.

The sac is about 12 mm long and is surrounded by an extension of the orbital periosteum to form the lacrimal fascia. This fascia also extends along the nasolacrimal canal. The medial palpebral ligament crosses in front of the upper part of the lacrimal sac. The lacrimal part of the orbicularis oculi muscle arises behind the lacrimal sac from the posterior lacrimal crest and from the lacrimal fascia. Behind this muscle lie the orbital septum and the check ligament of the medial rectus muscle.

The nasolacrimal duct (7.16, 7.17b)

The nasolacrimal duct is the membranous canal which passes downwards from the lacrimal sac to the anterior portion of the inferior meatus on the lateral wall of the nose. The duct lies in a bony canal (the nasolacrimal canal) which is formed by the maxilla, the lacrimal bone, and the lacrimal process of the inferior nasal concha. The duct is about 15 mm long. It is directed backwards, downwards and laterally and produces a ridge in the wall of the maxillary sinus. Several folds of mucous membrane may project into the lumen of the nasolacrimal duct (the most constant projection lying at the lower end of the duct). The shape and position of the opening of the nasolacrimal duct into the inferior meatus varies considerably and may not be easy to locate.

The *innervation of the lacrimal sac and the nasolacrimal duct* is from the infratrochlear branch of the ophthalmic nerve and the anterior superior alveolar branch of the maxillary nerve.

The *vasculature of the lacrimal sac and the nasolacrimal duct* is derived from the ophthalmic (superior and inferior palpebral branches), maxillary (infra-orbital and sphenopalatine branches), and facial arteries. The venous drainage has a similar pattern to the arteries.

THE EXTRA-OCULAR MUSCLES (7.18–7.27)

Six muscles are involved in producing bodily movements of the eye — four recti and two oblique muscles. The term extra-ocular is used to differentiate these striated muscles from the intra-ocular smooth muscles inside the eye (i.e. the ciliary muscle and the dilator and sphincter pupillae muscles).

The four recti muscles are the superior, inferior, medial and lateral recti muscles. Their names indicate their positions relative to the eyeball. They all arise at the apex of the orbit from a short tendinous ring attached to the lesser wing and body of the sphenoid bone. This common tendinous ring surrounds the optic canal and the medial end of the superior orbital fissure. The recti muscles run forwards as a cone of muscles and pierce the fascia bulbi to insert into the sclera over the anterior half of the eye.

The oblique muscles are the superior and inferior oblique muscles. The superior oblique muscle arises from the apex of the orbit and runs above the eye. The inferior oblique muscle is the only muscle which arises from the front of the orbit. It runs below the eye. As indicated by the names, both muscles have an oblique course. They pierce the fascia bulbi to insert into the sclera over the posterior half of the eye.

The extra-ocular muscles exhibit a number of specialised features which probably relate to the need for very fine control of eye movements. Among these features are: the small size of the muscle fibres, the high ratio of nerve to muscle fibres, the high firing rate of the motor units.

7.16 The lacrimal apparatus

1 Tendon of levator palpebrae superioris muscle
2 Orbital part – lacrimal gland
3 Palpebral part – lacrimal gland
4 Lacrimal punctum on lacrimal papilla
5 Superior canaliculus
6 Ethmoidal air cells
7 Lacrimal sac
8 Inferior canaliculus
9 Nasolacrimal duct
10 Inferior concha
11 Inferior meatus

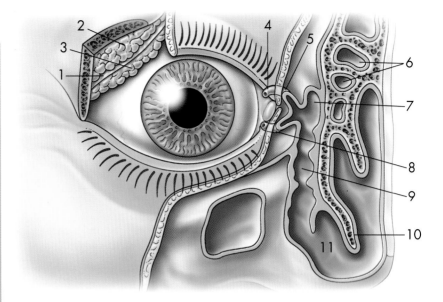

7.17a Lateral wall of orbit showing lacrimal gland and the disposition of some muscles

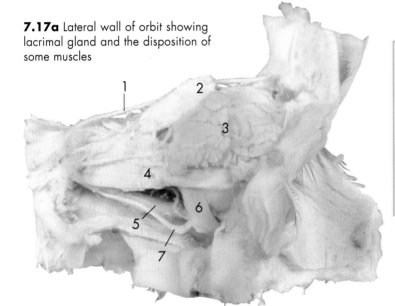

1 Frontal nerve
2 Levator palpebrae superioris
3 Lacrimal gland folded around tendon of levator palpebrae superioris
4 Lateral rectus muscle
5 Inferior rectus muscle
6 Inferior oblique muscle
7 Oculomotor nerve (inferior division)

7.17b Lateral wall of nose with bristle through opening of nasolacrimal duct in inferior meatus

1 Middle ethimoidal sinus
2 Bulla ethmoidalis
3 Hiatus semilunaris
4 Opening of maxillary sinus
5 Middle meatus
6 Inferior concha (cut)
7 Inferior meatus
8 Bristle in nasolacrimal duct opening
9 Greater palatine nerve
10 Pterygopalatine ganglion
11 Nerve of pterygoid canal
12 Maxillary nerve

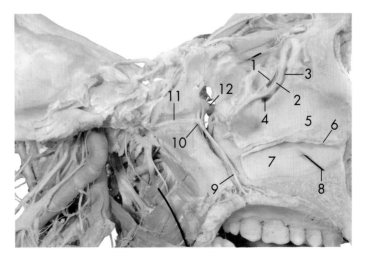

The descriptions of the extra-ocular muscles that follow include actions that assume the eye is in the primary position (i.e. the gaze is directed straight ahead). However, the muscles can have quite different actions if the eye is already displaced from the primary position. For example, the superior and inferior recti muscles act as elevators or depressors alone only when the eye is in abduction.

The superior rectus muscle (7.19, 7.21, 7.24–7.27)

Attachments: The superior rectus muscle is slightly larger than the other recti muscles. It arises from the upper part of the common tendinous ring, above and lateral to the optic foramen. Some fibres also arise from the dural sheath of the optic nerve. The fibres pass forwards and laterally (at an angle of about 25° to the median plane of the eye in the primary position) to insert into the upper part of the sclera about 8 mm from the limbus. The insertion of the superior rectus muscle is slightly oblique, the medial margin being more anterior than the lateral margin.

Innervation: The muscle is supplied by the superior division of the oculomotor nerve. This nerve enters the inferior surface of the muscle.

Vasculature: The arterial supply is derived both directly from the ophthalmic artery and indirectly from its supra-orbital branch.

Actions: Superior rectus moves the eye so that the cornea is directed upwards (elevation) and medially (adduction). To obtain upward movement alone, the muscle must function with the inferior oblique muscle. The superior rectus muscle also causes intorsion of the eye (i.e. medial rotation). Because a check ligament extends from the muscle to the levator palpebrae superioris muscle, elevation of the cornea also results in elevation of the upper eyelid.

The inferior rectus muscle (7.19, 7.20a, 7.24–7.27)

Attachments: This muscle arises from the common tendinous ring, below the optic canal. It runs along the orbital floor in a similar direction to superior rectus (i.e. forwards and laterally). The muscle inserts obliquely into the sclera below the cornea, 6 mm from the limbus.

Innervation: The inferior rectus muscle is innervated by a branch of the inferior division of the oculomotor nerve. This branch enters the superior surface of the muscle.

Vasculature: The arterial supply is derived from the ophthalmic artery and from the infra-orbital branch of the maxillary artery.

Actions: The principal activity of the muscle is to move the eye so that the cornea is directed downwards (depression). The muscle also causes the cornea to deviate medially. To obtain downward movement alone, the muscle must function with the superior oblique muscle. The inferior rectus muscle is responsible for extorsion of the eye (i.e. lateral rotation). A check ligament passes from the inferior rectus muscle to the inferior tarsal plate of the eyelid. This causes the lower eyelid to be slightly depressed when the inferior rectus muscle contracts.

7.18 Orbit viewed from above showing disposition of muscles

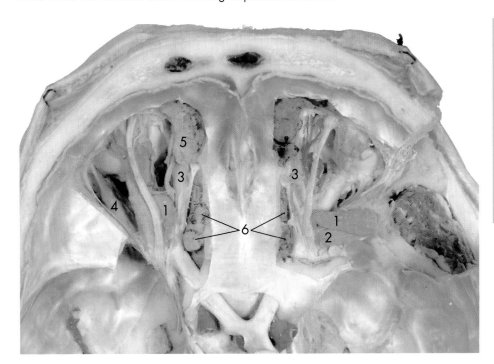

1	Levator palpebrae superioris muscles
2	Superior rectus muscle
3	Superior oblique muscles
4	Lateral rectus muscle
5	Lacrimal gland
6	Ethmoidal air sinuses

7.19 Lateral view of orbit showing disposition of muscles

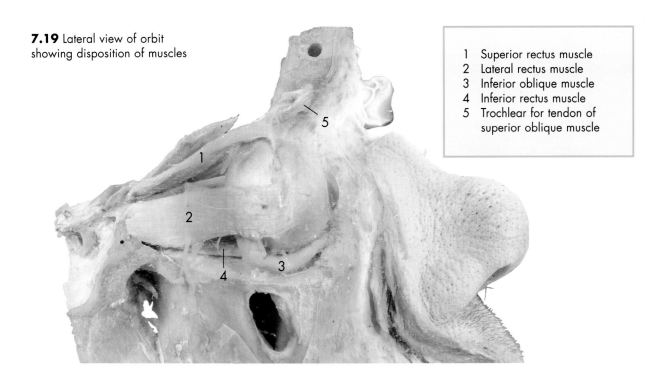

1	Superior rectus muscle
2	Lateral rectus muscle
3	Inferior oblique muscle
4	Inferior rectus muscle
5	Trochlear for tendon of superior oblique muscle

The medial rectus muscle (7.20a, 7.24–7.27)

Attachments: The medial rectus muscle is slightly shorter than the other recti muscles, but is said to be the strongest. It arises from the medial part of the common tendinous ring. In addition, some fibres arise from the dural sheath of the optic nerve. It passes horizontally forwards along the medial wall of the orbit, below the superior oblique muscle. It inserts into the medial surface of the sclera, approximately 5.5 mm from the limbus and slightly anterior to the other recti muscles.

Innervation: The muscle is supplied by a branch from the inferior division of the oculomotor nerve. This branch enters the lateral surface of the muscle.

Vasculature: The arterial supply is derived from the ophthalmic artery.

Actions: The medial rectus muscle moves the eye so that the cornea is directed medially (adducted). The two medial recti muscles acting together are responsible for convergence.

The lateral rectus muscle (7.21, 7.24–7.27)

Attachments: This muscle arises from the lateral part of the common tendinous ring. It bridges the superior orbital fissure. Some fibres also arise from a spine on the greater wing of the sphenoid. The fibres pass horizontally forward along the lateral wall of the orbit to insert into the lateral surface of the sclera, about 7 mm from the limbus.

Innervation: Lateral rectus receives its nerve supply from the abducent nerve. This nerve enters the medial surface of the muscle.

Vasculature: The artery to this muscle arises from the ophthalmic artery directly and/or from its lacrimal branch.

Actions: Contraction of the lateral rectus muscle moves the eye so that the cornea is directed laterally (abducted).

The superior oblique muscle (7.20, 7.22, 7.24–7.27)

Attachments: This muscle arises from the body of the sphenoid bone, above and medial to the common tendinous ring. It runs forwards, above the medial rectus muscle, in the angle between the roof and medial wall of the orbit. The superior oblique muscle becomes narrower and tendinous as it approaches the orbital margin. The tendon passes through a fibrocartilaginous pulley (the trochlea) on the medial wall of the orbit to re-emerge at a completely different angle, being now directed backwards, outwards and downwards. The reflected tendon approaches the eye in the primary position at an angle of about 50°, passing beneath the superior rectus muscle to fan out into a broad insertion over the posterolateral aspect of the sclera.

Innervation: The superior oblique muscle is supplied by the trochlear nerve. This nerve enters the superior surface of the muscle.

Vasculature: The muscle is supplied both directly from the ophthalmic artery and indirectly from its supra-orbital branch.

Actions: Because of its insertion into the posterior part of the eye, contraction of the superior oblique muscle will elevate the back of the eye, thus resulting in depression of the cornea (particularly with the eye in the adducted position). The superior oblique muscle moves the eye laterally and also causes intorsion.

7.20a Medial wall of orbit showing disposition of muscles

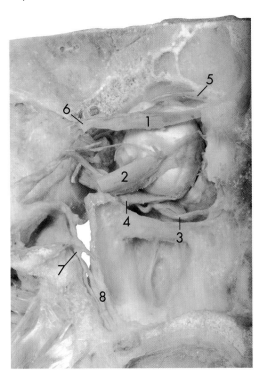

7.20b Orbit viewed from above showing superior oblique muscle

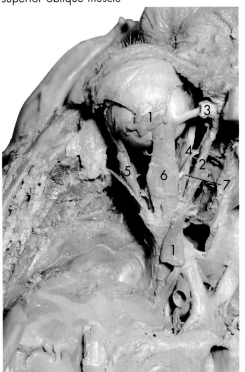

1	Superior oblique muscle
2	Medial rectus muscle
3	Inferior oblique muscle
4	Inferior rectus muscle
5	Trochlear for tendon of superior oblique muscle
6	Trochlear nerve
7	Pterygopalatine ganglion
8	Greater and lesser palatine nerves

1	Cut ends of levator palpebrae superioris muscle
2	Superior oblique muscle
3	Trochlea of superior oblique muscle
4	Medial rectus muscle
5	Lateral rectus muscle
6	Superior rectus muscle
7	Nasociliary nerve

7.21 Lateral view of orbit showing disposition of muscles

1	Superior rectus muscle
2	Lateral rectus muscle
3	Inferior rectus muscle
4	Inferior oblique muscle
5	Maxillary artery (third part)
6	Maxillary sinus

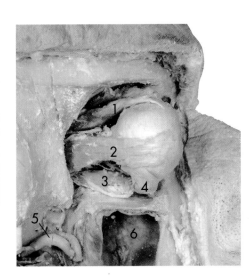

The inferior oblique muscle (7.20a, 7.21, 7.24–7.27)

Attachments: Unlike the other extra-ocular muscles, the inferior oblique muscle arises anteriorly from the floor of the orbit. Its origin is from the maxilla, immediately lateral to the lacrimal groove. The muscle passes backwards, outwards and upwards along the floor of the orbit and below the inferior rectus muscle. The direction of the inferior oblique muscle parallels that of the tendon of the superior oblique muscle. The inferior oblique muscle passes beneath the lateral rectus muscle to insert into the postero-inferior aspect of the sclera.

Innervation: The muscle receives its nerve supply from a branch of the inferior division of the oculomotor nerve. This branch enters the superior surface of the muscle.

Vasculature: The arteries supplying the muscle are derived from the ophthalmic artery and from the infra-orbital branch of the maxillary artery.

Actions: Because of its insertion into the posterior part of the eye, contraction of the inferior oblique muscle depresses the back of the eye, resulting in elevation of the cornea (particularly in the adducted position). The muscle moves the eye laterally and also causes extorsion.

The levator palpebrae superioris muscle (7.13, 7.15, 7.18)

Although this muscle is not responsible for movements of the eye, it is considered here because of its close anatomical association with the extra-ocular muscles and because of its functional relationship with the superior rectus muscle.

Attachments: The levator palpebrae superioris muscle arises from the lesser wing of the sphenoid bone, above the superior rectus muscle and lateral to the superior oblique muscle. Levator palpebrae superioris runs horizontally forwards between superior rectus and the roof of the orbit. Near the superior fornix of the conjunctival sac, the muscle fans out into a wide aponeurosis which passes into the skin and tarsal plate of the upper eyelid. The attachment to the tarsal plate is to the anterior surface and to the orbital border. At the orbital border, the fibres are comprised primarily of smooth muscle. There is also an attachment to the superior fornix, via the fascial sheath of the muscle.

Innervation: The muscle is supplied by a branch of the superior division of the oculomotor nerve. This branch enters the inferior surface of the muscle. Sympathetic fibres to the smooth muscle component of levator palpebrae superioris are derived from the plexus surrounding the internal carotid artery. These nerve fibres join the oculomotor nerve in the cavernous sinus.

Vasculature: The arterial supply is derived both directly from the ophthalmic artery and indirectly from its supra-orbital branch.

Actions: As its name suggests, the levator palpebrae superioris muscle elevates the upper eyelid. (This action is opposed by the palpebral part of the orbicularis oculi muscle.) The muscle is linked to the superior rectus muscle by a check ligament, thus there is elevation of the upper eyelid when the gaze of the eye is directed upwards.

Although for descriptive convenience the actions of the extra-ocular muscles have been described for each individual muscle, it is important to appreciate that all eye movements usually require the co-ordinated activity of several muscles. Muscles which aid each other in a particular movement are termed synergists; muscles which oppose each other are termed antagonists. Muscles which are synergistic for one type of movement may be antagonistic for another type of movement. These concepts are further complicated in the case of the eye where co-ordinated movements of both eyes are required in order that corresponding points of each retina will fixate on the same object. For example, when looking to the left, contraction of the left lateral rectus muscle and the right medial rectus muscle occurs together with relaxation of the left medial rectus muscle and the right lateral rectus muscle. Left and right pairs of synergistic eye muscles are called yoke muscles.

7.22 Frontal view of orbit showing oblique muscles

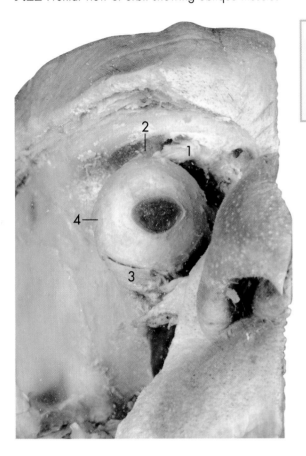

1	Superior oblique muscle
2	Tendon of superior rectus muscle
3	Inferior oblique muscle
4	Tendon of lateral rectus muscle

7.23 Orbit viewed from above showing the levator palpebrae superioris muscle

1	Levator palpebrae superioris muscle
2	Frontal nerve
3	Trochlear nerve on superior oblique muscle
4	Nasociliary nerve dividing into anterior ethmoidal and infratrochlear nerves
5	Ophthalmic artery
6	Mandibular nerve
7	Maxillary nerve
8	Oculomotor nerve
9	Optic nerve
10	Trochlear nerve
11	Middle meningeal artery

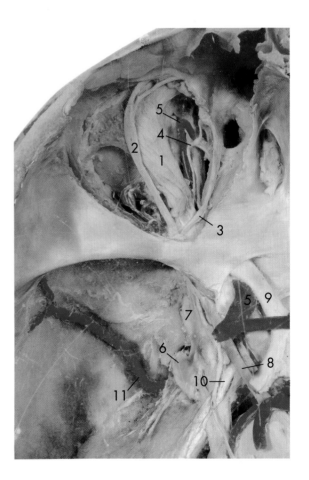

7.24 The extra-ocular muscles viewed from above. A portion of the superior rectus muscle has been removed to display the optic nerve and inferior rectus muscle

1 Ethmoidal air cells
2 Medical rectus muscle
3 Superior oblique muscle
4 Pulley (trochlea)
5 Lateral check ligament
6 Insertion of inferior oblique muscle
7 Superior rectus muscle
8 Lateral rectus muscle
9 Inferior rectus muscle
10 Optic nerve

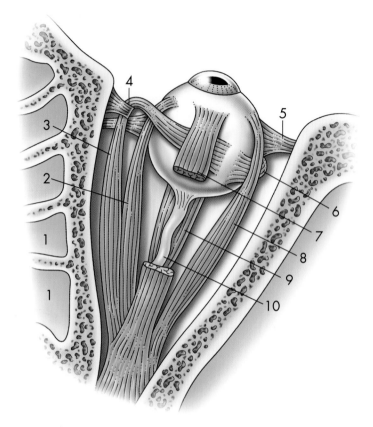

7.25 The extra-ocular muscles viewed from below. A portion of the inferior rectus muscle has been removed to display the optic nerve and superior rectus muscle

1 Lateral rectus muscle
2 Optic nerve
3 Lateral check ligament
4 Inferior oblique muscle
5 Inferior rectus muscle
6 Superior rectus muscle
7 Medial rectus muscle

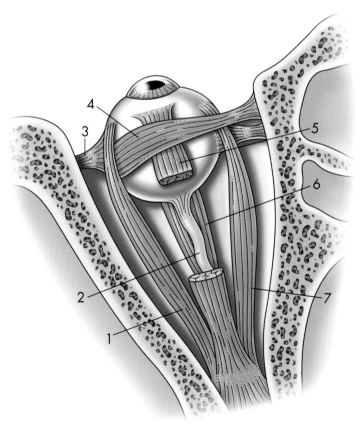

7.26 The extra-ocular muscles viewed from the lateral side. A portion of the lateral rectus muscle has been removed to display the optic nerve and medial rectus muscle

1 Medial rectus muscle
2 Inferior rectus muscle
3 Optic nerve
4 Superior rectus muscle
5 Levator palpebrae superioris muscle
6 Superior oblique muscle
7 Pulley (trochlea)
8 Lateral rectus muscle
9 Inferior oblique muscle

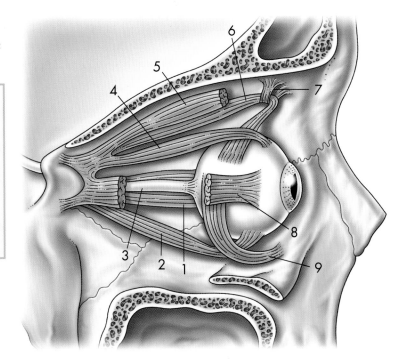

7.27 The surfaces of the eye showing the sties of attachment of the extra-ocular muscles

I Lateral surface
II Superior surface
III Medial surface
IV Inferior surface

1 Superior rectus
2 Inferior rectus
3 Medial rectus
4 Lateral rectus
5 Superior oblique
6 Inferior oblique

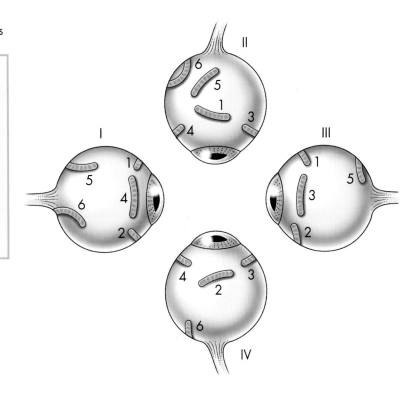

SMOOTH MUSCLE IN THE ORBIT

As well as the main striated extra-ocular muscles, several aggregations of nonstriated, smooth muscle are found within the orbit:

- The levator palpebrae superioris muscle has a smooth muscle component near its insertion onto the orbital border of the tarsal plate in the upper eyelid.

- The orbitalis muscle is a thin layer of smooth muscle located in the periosteum covering the floor of the orbit. It crosses the inferior orbital fissure and extends as far backwards as the cavernous sinus.

- Other groups of smooth muscle lie in the fascia bulbi, where they almost encircle the eye (being deficient laterally). There is also a band of smooth muscle which passes between the levator palpebrae superioris muscle and the tarsal plate in the upper eyelid. Another band runs between the inferior rectus muscle and the tarsal plate in the lower eyelid.

The functional significance of smooth muscle in the orbit is not fully understood. The muscle is innervated by sympathetic nerves.

THE NERVES WITHIN THE ORBIT (7.28–7.33)

Both motor and sensory nerves are found in the orbit. The motor nerves are the oculomotor, trochlear and abducent nerves. They supply the extra-ocular muscles. There are also motor nerves derived from the autonomic nervous system. Parasympathetic fibres from the oculomotor nerve (via the ciliary ganglion) supply the sphincter pupillae and ciliary muscles. Parasympathetic fibres from the facial nerve (via the pterygopalatine ganglion) supply the lacrimal gland. Sympathetic fibres supply the dilator pupillae muscle. The sensory nerves within the orbit are the optic, ophthalmic and maxillary nerves. The ophthalmic and maxillary nerves are essentially only passing through the orbit to supply the face and jaws.

The oculomotor nerve (7.28)

This is the third cranial nerve. It is the main source of innervation of the extra-ocular muscles. The oculomotor nerve also contains parasympathetic fibres which relay in the ciliary ganglion.

The oculomotor nerve emerges at the midbrain, on the medial side of the crus of the cerebral peduncle. It passes along the lateral dural wall of the cavernous sinus. The oculomotor nerve then divides into superior and inferior divisions and runs beneath the trochlear and ophthalmic nerves. The two divisions of the oculomotor nerve enter the orbit through the superior orbital fissure, within the common tendinous ring of the recti muscles. Here, the nasociliary branch of the ophthalmic nerve lies between the divisions of the oculomotor nerve.

The superior division of the oculomotor nerve passes above the optic nerve to enter the inferior surface of the superior rectus muscle. It supplies this muscle and provides a branch which runs to the levator palpebrae superioris muscle.

The inferior division of the oculomotor nerve divides into three branches, medial, central and lateral. The medial branch passes beneath the optic nerve to enter the lateral surface of the medial rectus muscle. The central branch runs downwards and forwards to enter the superior surface of the inferior rectus muscle. The lateral branch travels forwards on the lateral side of the inferior rectus muscle to enter the superior surface of the inferior oblique muscle. The lateral branch also communicates with the ciliary ganglion to distribute parasympathetic fibres to the sphincter pupillae and ciliary muscles.

7.28 Lateral view of orbit showing the abducent nerve, the inferior division of oculomotor nerve and the ciliary ganglion

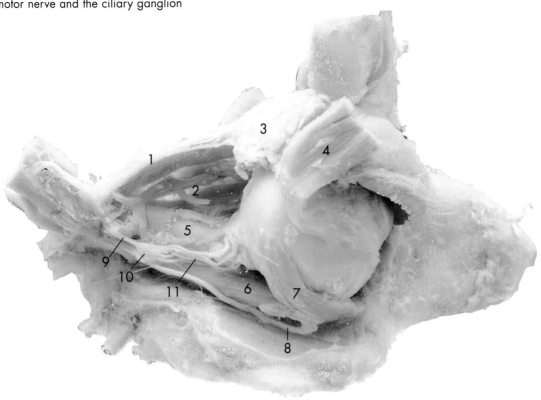

1	Superior rectus muscle
2	Ophthalmic artery
3	Lacrimal gland
4	Lateral rectus muscle (reflected)
5	Optic nerve
6	Inferior rectus muscle
7	Inferior oblique muscle
8	Inferior division of oculomotor nerve
9	Ganglionic branch from nasociliary nerve
10	Ciliary ganglion
11	Short ciliary nerves

The trochlear nerve (7.29, 7.30)

This is the fourth cranial nerve. It is the only cranial nerve which emerges from the dorsal surface of the brain. The trochlear nerve passes from the midbrain onto the lateral surface of the crus of the cerebral peduncle. It runs through the lateral dural wall of the cavernous sinus. The nerve then crosses the oculomotor nerve and enters the orbit through the superior orbital fissure, above the common tendinous ring of the recti muscles. Here, it lies above the levator palpebrae superioris muscle and medial to the frontal and lacrimal nerves. The trochlear nerve travels but a short distance to enter the superior surface of the superior oblique muscle. Indeed, the innervation of the superior oblique muscle is the sole function of the trochlear nerve.

The abducent nerve (7.3, 7.33)

The abducent nerve is the sixth cranial nerve. It emerges from the brain stem, between the pons and the medulla oblongata. The abducent nerve is related to the cavernous sinus but, unlike the oculomotor, trochlear, ophthalmic and maxillary nerves which merely invaginate the lateral dural wall, it passes through the sinus itself. The abducent nerve enters the orbit through the superior orbital fissure. It is here situated within the common tendinous ring of the recti muscles, first below and then between the two divisions of the oculomotor nerve and lateral to the nasociliary nerve. The abducent nerve passes forwards to enter the medial surface of the lateral rectus muscle. The innervation of this muscle is the sole function of the abducent nerve.

The ophthalmic nerve and its branches (7.29–7.33)

The ophthalmic nerve is a division of the trigeminal nerve (the fifth cranial nerve) and is a sensory nerve that travels through the orbit to supply primarily the upper part of the face. Developmentally, it is the nerve of the frontonasal process.

The trigeminal ganglion in the floor of the middle cranial fossa is the site where the ophthalmic nerve arises. The nerve passes along the lateral dural wall of the cavernous sinus and gives off three main branches just before the superior orbital fissure.

Branches of the ophthalmic nerve:

- Lacrimal nerve

- Frontal nerve:
  Supra-orbital nerve
  Supratrochlear nerve

- Nasociliary nerve:
  Sensory branches to the ciliary ganglion
  Long ciliary nerves
  Posterior ethmoidal nerve
  Anterior ethmoidal nerve
  (and external nasal nerve)
  Infratrochlear nerve

The *lacrimal nerve* enters the orbit through the superior orbital fissure, above the common tendinous ring of the recti muscles. Here, it is situated lateral to the frontal and trochlear nerves. The lacrimal nerve passes forwards along the lateral wall of the orbit on the superior border of the lateral rectus muscle. It passes through the lacrimal gland and the orbital septum to supply conjunctiva and skin covering the lateral part of the upper eyelid (see page 116). The lacrimal nerve communicates with the zygomatic branch of the maxillary nerve. By this means, para-sympathetic fibres associated with the pterygopalatine ganglion are conveyed to the lacrimal gland.

7.29 Orbit viewed from above showing distribution of nerves

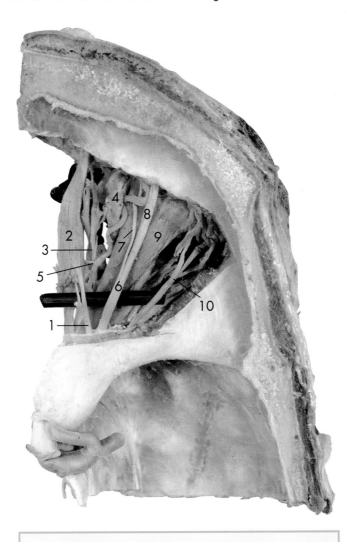

1	Trochlear nerve
2	Superior oblique muscle
3	Nasociliary nerve
4	Superior ophthalmic vein
5	Ophthalmic artery
6	Frontal nerve
7	Supratrochlear nerve
8	Supra-orbital nerve
9	Levator palpebrae superioris
10	Lacrimal nerve and artery

The *frontal nerve* is the largest branch of the ophthalmic nerve. It enters the orbit through the superior orbital fissure, above the common tendinous ring of the recti muscles, and lies between the lacrimal nerve laterally and the trochlear nerve medially. The frontal nerve passes forwards on the levator palpebrae superioris muscle, towards the rim of the orbit. About halfway along this course, it divides into the supra-orbital and supratrochlear nerves.

The supra-orbital nerve is the larger of the terminal branches of the frontal nerve. It continues forwards along the levator palpebrae superioris muscle and leaves the orbit through the supra-orbital notch (or foramen) to emerge onto the forehead. The supra-orbital nerve supplies mucous membrane lining the frontal sinus, skin and conjunctiva covering the upper eyelid, and skin over the forehead and scalp (see page 116).

The supratrochlear nerve runs medially above the pulley for the superior oblique muscle. It gives a descending branch to the infratrochlear nerve and ascends onto the forehead through the frontal notch. It supplies skin and conjunctiva covering the upper eyelid, and skin over the forehead (see page 116).

The *nasociliary nerve* passes into the orbit through the superior orbital fissure, within the common tendinous ring of the recti muscles. Initially, the nerve lies lateral to the optic nerve. It then runs forwards and medially across the optic nerve and, coursing between the superior oblique and medial rectus muscles, comes to lie close to the medial wall of the orbit. Near the anterior ethmoidal foramen, the nasociliary nerve divides into its terminal branches: the anterior ethmoidal and infratrochlear nerves.

The first branches of the nasociliary nerve are sensory branches to the ciliary ganglion. They leave the ganglion in the short ciliary nerves, running to the eyeball to supply the cornea, the ciliary body and the iris.

Two or three long ciliary branches arise from the nasociliary nerve as it crosses the optic nerve. These ciliary nerves pierce the sclera at the back of the eye and pass forwards to provide sensory innervation to the cornea and iris. They also distribute sympathetic fibres to the dilator pupillae muscle. The sympathetic fibres originate from the superior cervical ganglion. They are postganglionic fibres which travel in the plexus surrounding the internal carotid artery. They join the ophthalmic nerve in the cavernous sinus.

The posterior ethmoidal nerve passes beneath the superior oblique muscle and leaves the orbit through the posterior ethmoidal foramen to enter the nose. It supplies the sphenoidal sinus and the posterior ethmoidal air cells.

The anterior ethmoidal nerve exits the orbit through the anterior ethmoidal foramen. It enters the anterior cranial fossa where the cribriform plate of the ethmoid bone meets the orbital part of the frontal bone. It then runs into the roof of the nose through a small foramen at the side of the crista galli. The anterior ethmoidal nerve supplies the anterior and middle ethmoidal air cells and some of the mucosa covering the nasal septum and the lateral wall of the nose (see page 200). It terminates on the face as the external nasal nerve (see page 116).

7.30 Orbit viewed from above showing distribution of nerves

1   Superior oblique muscle
2   Trochlear nerve
3   Frontal nerve dividing into supra-orbital and supratrochlear nerves
4   Lacrimal nerve
5   Ophthalmic artery
6   Nasociliary nerve
7   Superior ophthalmic vein
8   Optic nerve

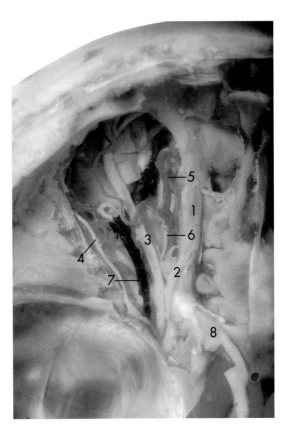

7.31 View of medial wall of orbit showing distribution of nerves

1   Frontal nerve
2   Supra-orbital nerve
3   Supratrochlear nerve
4   Nasociliary nerve
5   Ciliary ganglion
6   Short ciliary nerves
7   Anterior ethmoidal nerve
8   Infratrochlear nerve
9   Infra-orbital nerve
10 External nasal nerve
11 Zygomaticofacial nerve

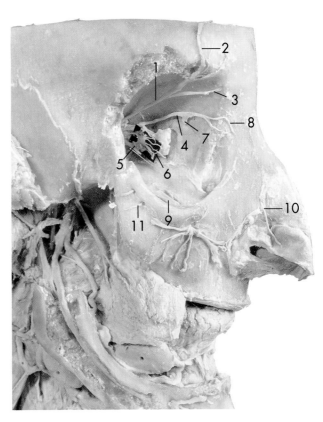

The infratrochlear nerve passes forwards along the medial wall of the orbit below the pulley of the superior oblique muscle. It passes above the medial palpebral ligament to reach the side of the nose. It supplies the lacrimal sac, the caruncle, the conjunctiva at the medial canthus, and the skin on the medial aspect of the upper eyelid (see pages 116).

The maxillary nerve and its branches (7.31, 7.33)

The maxillary nerve is a sensory division of the trigeminal nerve (fifth cranial nerve). Most of the branches from the maxillary nerve arise in the pterygopalatine fossa (see page 216). The maxillary nerve gives rise directly to two nerves that pass into the orbit — the zygomatic and infra-orbital nerves — and indirectly to an orbital branch from the pterygopalatine ganglion. All three nerves enter the orbit through the inferior orbital fissure.

The *zygomatic nerve* in the orbit is located close to the base of the lateral wall. It soon divides into two branches, the zygomaticotemporal and the zygomaticofacial nerves. These nerves run only for a short distance in the orbit before passing onto the face through the lateral wall of the orbit. They may either enter separate canals within the zygomatic bone or the zygomatic nerve itself may enter the bone before dividing.

The zygomaticotemporal nerve exits the zygomatic bone at its temporal (medial) surface. It pierces the temporal fascia to supply skin over the temple (see page 116). The zygomaticotemporal nerve also gives a branch to the lacrimal nerve which carries parasympathetic fibres to the lacrimal gland (see page 241).

The zygomaticofacial nerve leaves the zygomatic bone on its lateral surface to supply skin overlying the prominence of the cheek (see page 116).

The *infra-orbital nerve* initially lies in a groove (the infra-orbital groove) on the floor of the orbit. As it approaches the rim of the orbit, it runs into a canal (the infra-orbital canal) and passes onto the face at the infra-orbital foramen. The infra-orbital nerve supplies the conjunctiva and skin of the lower eyelid. It also innervates the skin over the upper jaw (see page 116) and provides the middle and anterior superior alveolar nerves (see page 176).

The orbital branch from the pterygopalatine ganglion supplies the orbitalis muscle and some periosteum. It may connect with the ciliary ganglion. The orbital branch may also leave the orbit through the posterior ethmoidal foramen to supply the posterior ethmoidal air cells and the sphenoidal air sinus.

The optic nerve (7.28, 7.33)

The optic nerve is the second cranial nerve. It arises from the optic chiasma on the floor of the diencephalon. It enters the orbit through the optic canal, accompanied by the ophthalmic artery. The shape of the optic nerve changes from being flattened at the chiasma to being rounded as it passes through the optic canal. The optic nerve in the orbit passes forwards, laterally and downwards. It pierces the sclera at the lamina cribrosa, slightly medial to the posterior pole. The optic nerve has a slightly wavy course which allows for movements of the eye.

Within the orbit, the optic nerve is surrounded by extensions of the three meninges. This reflects the fact that the nerve is really an 'outgrowth' of the brain.

The optic nerve has important relationships with other orbital structures. As the nerve leaves the optic canal, it lies superomedial to the ophthalmic artery. The oculomotor, nasociliary and abducent nerves (and sometimes the ophthalmic veins) are situated between the optic nerve and the lateral rectus muscle. The optic nerve is also closely related to the origins of the four recti muscles. More anteriorly, however, the muscles diverge and the nerve becomes separated from them by a substantial amount of orbital fat. Just beyond the optic canal, the ophthalmic artery and the nasociliary nerve cross the optic nerve to reach the medial wall of the orbit. The central artery of the retina enters the substance of the optic nerve about halfway along its length. Near the back of the eye, the optic nerve becomes surrounded by long and short ciliary nerves and vessels.

7.32 Frontal view of orbit showing course of maxillary nerve

1   Lacrimal nerve
2   Frontal nerve
3   Nasociliary nerve
4   Infra-orbital nerve
5   Zygomatic nerve
6   Zygomaticofacial branch
7   Zygomaticotemporal branch

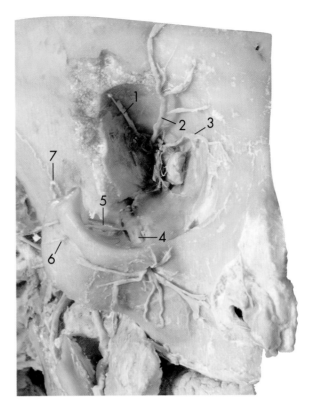

7.33 Lateral view of orbit showing maxillary and optic nerves

1   Oculomotor nerve
2   Trochlear nerve
3   Abducent nerve
4   Internal carotid artery
5   Maxillary nerve
6   Posterior superior
    alveolar nerve
7   Zygomatic nerve
8   Zygomaticofacial nerve
9   Zygomaticotemporal
    nerve
10 Ciliary ganglion
11 Short ciliary nerve
12 Optic nerve
13 Inferior division of
    oculomotor nerve
14 Inferior rectus muscle
15 Inferior oblique muscle
16 Lacrimal nerve
17 Infraorbital nerve

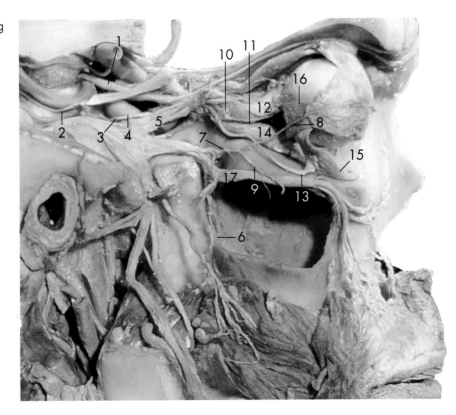

THE CILIARY GANGLION (7.28, 7.33, 7.34, 7.35)

The ciliary ganglion is a parasympathetic ganglion which is located near the apex of the orbit. It lies in front of the optic canal, between the lateral rectus muscle and the optic nerve, and close to the ophthalmic artery. The ganglion appears as a small swelling connected to the nasociliary nerve. Short ciliary nerves pass from the ganglion to the eyeball. Functionally, the ciliary ganglion is related to the eye, in particular the motor supply of intra-ocular muscles.

The parasympathetic fibres to the ciliary ganglion arise from the Edinger–Westphal nucleus of the oculomotor nerve. The preganglionic fibres run with the oculomotor nerve into the orbit, leaving in the branch to the inferior oblique muscle. The fibres then pass to the ciliary ganglion where they synapse. Postganglionic fibres travel to the back of the eye in the short ciliary nerves.

The sympathetic fibres to the ciliary ganglion arise from the plexus around the internal carotid artery within the cavernous sinus. These postganglionic fibres form a fine branch which enters the orbit through the superior orbital fissure, inside the common tendinous ring of the recti muscles. This branch then travels through the ganglion without synapsing and into the short ciliary nerves.

The sensory fibres to the ciliary ganglion are derived from the nasociliary nerve. They also pass through the ganglion to the short ciliary nerves without synapsing.

The *short ciliary nerves* convey parasympathetic, sympathetic and sensory fibres between the eyeball and the ciliary ganglion. The nerves pierce the sclera at the back of the eye and run forwards between the sclera and the choroid. The parasympathetic fibres are distributed to the sphincter pupillae and ciliary muscles. Contraction of the ciliary muscles is associated with the accommodation reflex. The sympathetic fibres supply arteries within the eye. (The sympathetic fibres supplying the dilator pupillae muscle are thought to run in the long ciliary nerves.) The sensory fibres carry sensation from the cornea, the ciliary body and the iris.

THE ARTERIES WITHIN THE ORBIT (7.36, 7.37)

The main vessel supplying orbital structures is the ophthalmic artery. Its terminal branches anastomose on the face and scalp with those of the facial, maxillary and superficial temporal arteries, thus establishing connections between the external and internal carotid arteries. In addition to the ophthalmic artery, the infra-orbital branch of the maxillary artery supplies orbital structures.

The ophthalmic artery

The ophthalmic artery arises from the internal carotid artery as it emerges from the roof of the cavernous sinus. It traverses the optic canal below the optic nerve and within the dural sheath.

Within the orbit, the ophthalmic artery winds across the optic nerve, passing from the lateral side to the medial side of the orbit. In this position, the artery lies immediately beneath the superior rectus muscle. It then runs a tortuous course with the nasociliary nerve and, passing between the superior oblique and medial rectus muscles, terminates near the medial canthus of the eye by dividing into the dorsal nasal and supratrochlear arteries.

7.34 The ciliary parsympathetic ganglion

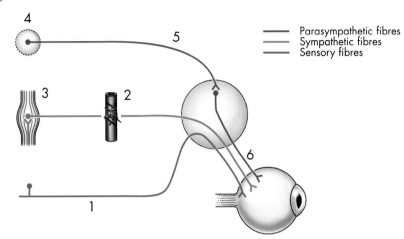

1 Nasociliary nerve
2 Internal carotid artery
3 Superior cervical ganglion
4 Edinger–Westphal nucleus
   in midbrain
5 Oculomotor nerve
6 Short ciliary nerve

Parasympathetic fibres
Sympathetic fibres
Sensory fibres

7.35 Lateral view of orbit to show the ciliary ganglion

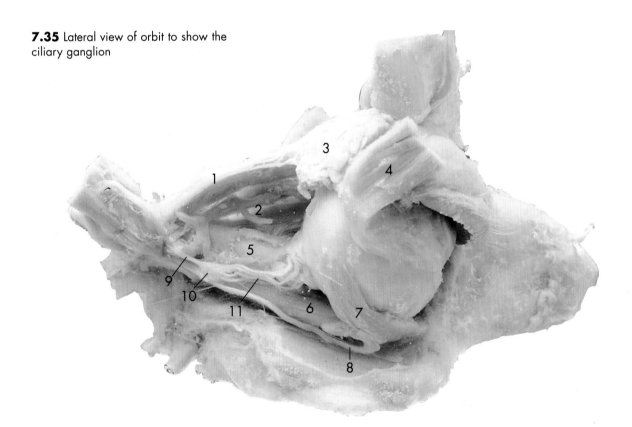

1 Superior rectus muscle	7 Inferior oblique muscle
2 Ophthalmic artery	8 Inferior division of oculomotor nerve
3 Lacrimal gland	9 Ganglionic branch from nasociliary nerve
4 Lateral rectus muscle (reflected)	10 Ciliary ganglion
5 Optic nerve	11 Short ciliary nerves
6 Inferior rectus muscle	

The branches of the ophthalmic artery include:

- Central artery of the retina

- Lacrimal artery

- Muscular branches

- Ciliary arteries

- Supra-orbital artery

- Posterior ethmoidal artery

- Anterior ethmoidal artery

- Meningeal branch

- Medial palpebral arteries

- Supratrochlear artery

- Dorsal nasal artery

Many of the branches of the ophthalmic artery accompany sensory nerves of the same name and have a similar distribution: i.e. the lacrimal, supra-orbital, posterior ethmoidal, anterior ethmoidal, and supratrochlear arteries.

The *central artery of the retina* is the first branch of the ophthalmic artery and is given off close to the optic canal. It initially runs beneath the optic nerve and then within the accompanying dural sheath. Before reaching the back of the eye, the artery enters the substance of the optic nerve itself (through the inferomedial surface). It then runs forwards (accompanied by the central retinal vein) in the central part of the nerve to the retina. Passing through the lamina cribrosa of the sclera, the artery divides into superior and inferior branches. Each branch then divides into nasal and temporal branches, usually in the region of the margin of the optic disc. These vessels supply the inner, neural part of the retina. (The photoreceptors, including the fovea centralis, are supplied by the choriocapillaris of the choroid.) The central artery of the retina is an end artery (its capillaries not anastomosing with those of any other blood vessel); therefore damage or blockage will result in varying degrees of blindness.

The ophthalmic artery gives off two main *muscular branches* (within the common tendinous ring of the recti muscles) to supply all the extra-ocular muscles. A lateral muscular branch supplies the levator palpebrae superioris, superior oblique, and lateral and superior recti muscles. A medial muscular branch supplies the inferior oblique, and inferior and medial recti muscles.

Three branches of the ophthalmic artery supply the eye: the central artery of the retina (see above) and the *ciliary arteries*.

Anterior ciliary arteries arise from the muscular branches of the ophthalmic artery. They accompany the tendons of the four recti muscles (usually in pairs, although only one artery with the lateral rectus muscle). After supplying the conjunctiva and sclera, the anterior ciliary arteries pierce the sclera (close to the attachments of the tendons of the recti muscles) to enter the ciliary body. Here, they anastomose with the long posterior ciliary arteries to form the major arterial circle of the iris.

Posterior ciliary arteries (usually two) arise from the ophthalmic artery as it runs below the optic nerve. From these arteries arise a series of short and long posterior ciliary branches. There are usually between 10 and 20 short posterior ciliary arteries. They closely surround the optic nerve and, accompanied by the short ciliary nerves, pierce the sclera close to the optic nerve. The short posterior ciliary arteries run in the choroid and supply the greater part of this layer. There are two long posterior ciliary arteries; one lies medial and one lies lateral to the optic nerve. These vessels pierce the sclera close to the attachments of the medial and lateral recti muscles. The long posterior ciliary arteries run forwards in the choroid to the ciliary body. They supply the anterior part of the choroid and the ciliary body. They anastomose with the anterior ciliary arteries at the ciliary body to form the major arterial circle of the iris.

7.36 The ophthalmic artery (left) and the nasociliary nerve (right)

1 Optic chiasma
2 Middle meningeal artery
3 Internal carotid artery
4 Meningeal branch
5 Lacrimal artery
6 Muscular branch
7 Zygomatic branch
8 Posterior ciliary artery
9 Supra-orbital artery
10 Supratrochlear artery
11 Anterior ethmoidal artery
12 Anterior ethmoidal nerve
13 Infratrochlear nerve
14 Long ciliary nerve
15 Short ciliary nerve
16 Ciliary ganglion
17 Ophthalmic division of trigeminal nerve
18 Posterior ethmoidal nerve

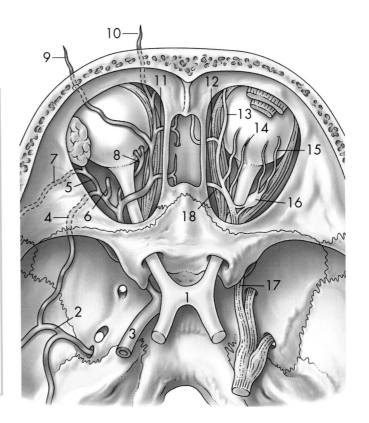

7.37 Orbit viewed from above showing the ophthalmic artery

1 Optic nerve
2 Internal carotid artery
3 Ophthalmic artery
4 Nasociliary nerve
5 Superior oblique muscle
6 Frontal nerve
7 Lacrimal nerve
8 Superior ophthalmic vein

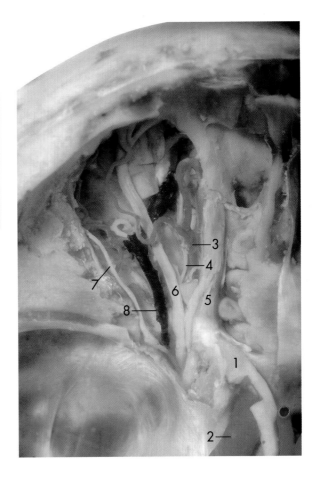

The ophthalmic artery also provides a *meningeal branch,* either directly, or as a branch of the lacrimal artery. The meningeal branch runs back through the superior orbital fissure to anastomose with the middle meningeal artery.

The eyelids derive their blood supply from two sources. Two *medial palpebral arteries* (superior and inferior) arise directly from the ophthalmic artery near the medial canthus. Two *lateral palpebral arteries* (superior and inferior) arise as branches of the lacrimal artery. The superior arteries supply the upper eyelid, the inferior arteries the lower eyelid.

The *dorsal nasal artery* is a terminal branch of the ophthalmic artery. It pierces the orbital septum above the medial palpebral ligament to supply the lacrimal sac and adjacent skin on the nose. It anastomoses with adjacent branches of the facial artery.

The *infra-orbital branch of the maxillary artery* enters the orbit through the posterior part of the inferior orbital fissure. It passes along the infra-orbital groove of the maxillary bone in the floor of the orbit before entering the infra-orbital canal. Eventually, it comes out onto the face through the infra-orbital foramen. As the infra-orbital artery traverses the infra-orbital canal, it provides branches which supply the inferior rectus and inferior oblique muscles and the lacrimal sac.

THE VEINS WITHIN THE ORBIT (7.37, 7.38)

The veins draining the orbit are the superior and inferior ophthalmic veins and the infra-orbital vein. The veins of the eyeball mainly drain into the vortex veins (see page 230).

The *superior ophthalmic vein* originates just above the medial palpebral ligament, where it communicates with the supra-orbital vein and with the first part of the facial vein (the angular vein). The superior ophthalmic vein passes backwards alongside the ophthalmic artery, lying between the optic nerve and the superior rectus muscle. It leaves the orbit through the superior orbital fissure to drain into the anterior part of the cavernous sinus. The superior ophthalmic vein usually passes through the superior orbital fissure above the common tendinous ring of the recti muscles. Occasionally, it can pass within or below the common tendinous ring.

The superior ophthalmic vein receives tributaries which accompany branches from the ophthalmic artery (i.e. lacrimal, muscular, anterior and posterior ethmoidal, anterior ciliary veins). It also receives the two superior vortex veins of the eyeball, and the central vein of the retina. Alternatively, the central vein of the retina drains directly into the cavernous sinus (although still having a communicating branch to the superior ophthalmic vein). The superior ophthalmic vein may also receive the inferior ophthalmic vein.

The *inferior ophthalmic vein* originates as a plexus in the anterior part of the floor of the orbit. It runs backwards on the inferior rectus muscle and across the inferior orbital fissure. It then either joins the superior ophthalmic vein or passes through the superior orbital fissure (within or below the common tendinous ring of the recti muscles) to drain directly into the cavernous sinus.

The inferior ophthalmic vein receives tributaries from the inferior rectus and inferior oblique muscles, and from the lacrimal sac and the eyelids. It also receives the two inferior vortex veins of the eyeball. The inferior ophthalmic vein communicates with the pterygoid venous plexus by a branch passing through the inferior orbital fissure. It may also communicate with the facial vein across the inferior margin of the orbit.

The *infra-orbital vein* runs with the infra-orbital nerve and artery in the floor of the orbit. It passes backwards through the inferior orbital fissure into the pterygoid venous plexus. It drains structures in the floor of the orbit and communicates with the inferior ophthalmic vein. On the face, the infra-orbital vein may communicate with the facial vein.

It is evident that the veins of the orbit link the cavernous sinus with veins on the face and in the infratemporal fossa (see page 147). All of these veins lack valves. A pathway therefore exists for the intracranial spread of infection.

7.38 Veins associated with the orbit

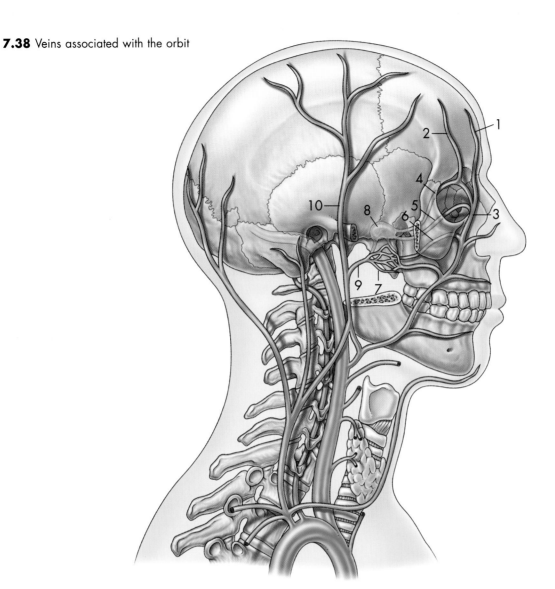

1	Supratrochlear vein
2	Supra-orbital vein
3	Facial vein
4	Superior ophthalmic vein
5	Inferior ophthalmic vein
6	Infra-orbital vein
7	Pterygoid venous plexus
8	Cavernous sinus
9	Maxillary vein
10	Superficial temporal vein

chapter 8

THE CRANIAL
CAVITY

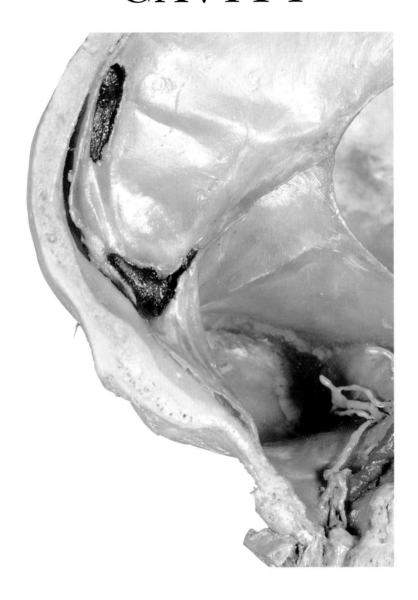

Chapter 8 THE CRANIAL CAVITY

The cranial cavity is the interior of the skull that accommodates the brain and associated structures. Many of the contents are located near the floor of the cranial cavity, and this region can be divided into three distinct fossae: the anterior, middle and posterior cranial fossae. The fossae have a marked step-like appearance, such that the floor of the anterior cranial fossa is at the highest level and the floor of the posterior cranial fossa is lowest (see pages 28–31 for a detailed description of the osteology).

The anterior cranial fossa is formed by the orbital part of the frontal bone, the cribriform plates of the ethmoid bone with the crista galli, and the lesser wings and jugum of the sphenoid bone. It is occupied mainly by the frontal lobes of the cerebral hemispheres of the brain.

The middle cranial fossa consists of a central part formed by the body of the sphenoid bone, and right and left lateral parts each formed by the greater wing of the sphenoid bone and the squamous and petrous parts of the temporal bone. The central part is occupied mainly by the pituitary gland. The lateral parts contain the temporal lobes of the cerebral hemispheres of the brain.

The posterior cranial fossa is formed by the basilar, lateral and lower squamous parts of the occipital bone, the petrous and mastoid parts of the temporal bones, a small part of the mastoid angles of the parietal bones, and the dorsum sellae and posterior part of the body of the sphenoid bone. Unlike the other cranial fossae, the posterior cranial fossa has a well-defined roof. This roof is formed by a fold or septum of dura mater called the tentorium cerebelli. The posterior cranial fossa contains the lowest part of the midbrain and the pons, cerebellum and medulla oblongata. The region of the cranial cavity immediately above the tentorium cerebelli contains the occipital lobes of the cerebral hemispheres of the brain.

Intervening between the brain and the bones of the cranial cavity are three layers called the meninges.

THE MENINGES (4.1, 8.2–8.5)

The whole of the brain and spinal cord are enveloped by three membranes or meninges: dura mater, arachnoid mater and pia mater. The meninges line the cranial cavity and the vertebral canal, providing support and protection for the neural tissue within.

The dura mater is sometimes called the pachymeninx (pachy meaning thick). The arachnoid and pia mater together constitute the leptomeninges (lepto meaning thin).

THE DURA MATER (8.2–8.5)

The dura mater is the outermost and thickest meninx. It is inelastic with a high content of collagen fibres.

The dura mater in the cranial cavity is fused for much of its extent with the internal periosteum of the skull bones. The dura is a combined membrane comprising outer and inner layers. The outer layer is called the endosteal layer; the inner layer is called the meningeal layer. These layers are not easily separable, except where venous sinuses occur between them.

The dura is particularly adherent to the bones of the cranium at the base of the skull and along the sutures (most notably in childhood and old age). The attachment is mediated by fibrous tissue and the connective tissue of blood vessels. The endosteal layer of the dura is continuous with the pericranium through sutures and foramina, and also with the periosteal lining of the orbital cavity via the superior orbital fissure.

8.1 The osteology of the cranial cavity

1 Anterior cranial fossa
2 Orbital plate of frontal bone
3 Cribriform plate of ethmoid bone
4 Crista galli
5 Lesser wing of sphenoid bone
6 Jugum of the sphenoid bone
7 Middle cranial fossa
8 Optic canal
9 Body of sphenoid bone with
  sella tursica (pituitary fossa)
10 Greater wing of sphenoid bone
11 Superior orbital fissure
12 Foramen rotundum
13 Foramen ovale
14 Foramen spinosum
15 Squamous part of temporal bone
16 Petrous process of temporal bone
17 Foramen lacerum and opening of
  the carotid canal
18 Grooves for meningeal vessels
19 Groove for petrosal nerve
20 Posterior cranial fossa
21 Basilar part of occipital bone
22 Dorsum sellae
23 Foramen magnum
24 Squamous part of occipital bone
25 Hypoglossal canal
26 Groove for transverse dural
  venous sinus
27 Groove for sigmoid dural
  venous sinus
28 Jugular foramen
29 Internal acoustic meatus

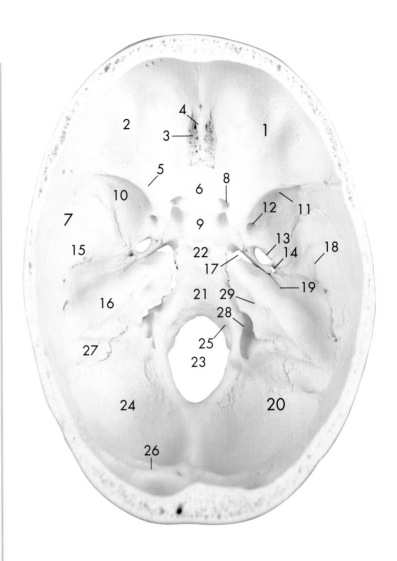

8.2 Coronal section through the superior sagittal sinus showing the arrangement of the meninges

1 Cerebral cortex
2 White matter
3 Falx cerebri
4 Pia mater
5 Trabeculae of arachnoid
6 Cranial vault
7 Arachnoid granulation
8 Superior sagittal sinus
9 Outer (endosteal) layer of dura mater
10 Venous lacuna
11 Superficial cerebral vein
12 Inner (meningeal) layer of dura mater
13 Arachnoid mater
14 Subarachnoid space

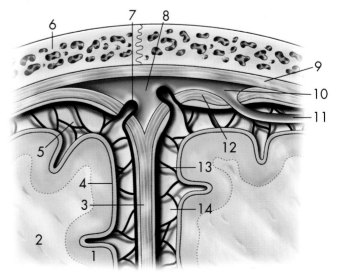

The dura forms sleeves around the cranial nerves, being continuous with their epineuria. The dura surrounds the whole of the optic nerve, becoming continuous with the sclera of the eyeball.

The inner surface of the dura is smooth. It has a ubiquitous lining of arachnoid mater from which it is separated by only a thin film of serous fluid.

Folds of the meningeal layer of the dura form four fibrous partitions or septa that broadly divide the cranial cavity. These are the large falx cerebri and tentorium cerebelli, and the smaller falx cerebelli and diaphragma sellae.

The *falx cerebri* is a sickle-shaped fold of dura that lies along the median sagittal plane in the longitudinal fissure between the two cerebral hemispheres (i.e. above the corpus callosum). Anteriorly, it is attached to the crista galli. Its attachment to the skull continues superiorly and posteriorly along the margins of the superior sagittal venous sinus to the internal occipital protuberance. At its posterior and inferior limit, the falx cerebri is continuous with the tentorium cerebelli. The inferior sagittal venous sinus runs in its free inferior border, and the straight sinus along its junction with the tentorium cerebelli.

The *tentorium cerebelli* lies between the cerebellum and the occipital lobes of the cerebral hemispheres. It forms the crescent-shaped roof to the posterior cranial fossa. The tentorium cerebelli is notched anteriorly so that the roof of the posterior cranial fossa is incomplete behind the dorsum sellae of the sphenoid bone. This notch is called the tentorial incisure, its margin being named the free border of the tentorium. The midbrain lies in this incisure,

together with part of the adjacent cerebellar vermis. Closely related to the free border of the tentorium are the great cerebral vein (of Galen) and medial regions of the temporal lobes of the cerebral hemispheres (the parahippocampal gyri). The tentorium cerebelli is attached at its periphery to the margins of the transverse and superior petrosal venous sinuses, and to the posterior clinoid processes of the dorsum sellae. However, the free border of the tentorium continues anteriorly to gain attachment to the anterior clinoid processes. A cavernous venous sinus is located on each side of the sella turcica between two layers of dura mater (i.e. the layer lining the sella turcica and the layer extending from the free border of the tentorium).

A recess is present in the tentorium cerebelli near its attachment to the apex of the petrous part of the temporal bone and beneath the superior petrosal sinus. This recess is called the trigeminal cave and is occupied by the roots of the trigeminal nerve connecting with the pons, and by part of the trigeminal ganglion.

The *falx cerebelli* is a small median fold at the back of the cranial cavity, which extends from the inferior surface of the tentorium cerebelli. It passes into the cerebellar notch between the cerebellar hemispheres. Posteriorly, the falx cerebelli is attached to the internal occipital crest and to the margins of the occipital sinus.

The *diaphragma sellae* roofs the sella turcica. The pituitary gland (hypophysis) lies beneath it, with the pituitary stalk (infundibulum) passing through a central aperture. Within the sella turcica, the dura (together with the arachnoid and pia mater) blends with the capsule of the pituitary gland.

8.3 The appearance of the falx cerebri, seen in a sagittal section of the head

1 Falx cerebri
2 Attachment of falx to crista galli
3 Superior sagittal dural venous sinus
4 Inferior sagittal dural venous sinus
5 Straight dural venous sinus where falx cerebri meets tentorium cerebelli
6 Confluence of sinuses
7 Falx cerebelli

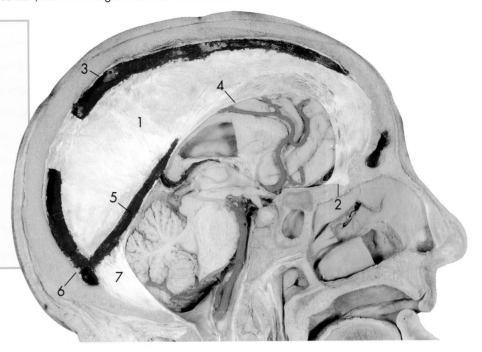

8.4 The appearance of the tentorium cerebelli and the falx cerebri, seen in a coronal section of the back of the head

1 Falx cerebri
2 Tentorium cerebelli

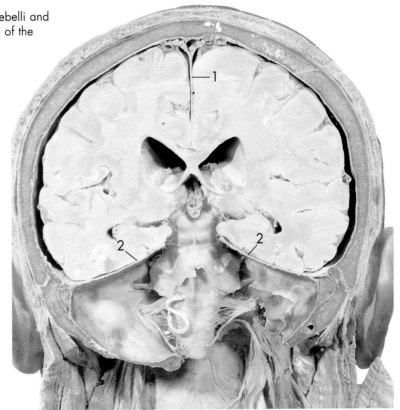

THE ARACHNOID MATER (4.1, 8.2)

The arachnoid mater closely lines the dura mater, being separated from it by a potential space called the subdural space. This space contains a thin film of serous fluid and is probably in continuity with the lymph spaces of the cranial and spinal nerves. The arachnoid mater does not follow the sulci and fissures of the brain (except where these are occupied by the septa of the dura mater). In this respect, it resembles the dura mater but not the pia mater.

Between the arachnoid and pia mater is a variable space called the subarachnoid space. This is filled with cerebrospinal fluid and it contains the major arteries and veins supplying the central nervous system. The arachnoid in the cranial cavity is connected to the pia mater by a close meshwork of fine trabeculae. Indeed, it lies so close to the pia mater that virtually a single membrane is formed (the 'pia-arachnoid'). In some regions, however, named cisternae containing cerebrospinal fluid occur where separation of the pia and arachnoid is greater. The subarachnoid space is in communication with the brain ventricles via the three apertures of the fourth ventricle, and with the venous system via arachnoid villi and granulations. The space also continues into the roof of the nasal cavity along the olfactory nerves.

THE PIA MATER (8.2)

The pia mater is a vascularised, areolar membrane. The pia mater covers almost the whole external surface of the brain. Indeed, the pia is in intimate contact with the brain, extending into every sulcus and fissure.

The pia mater forms the tela choroidea of the third ventricle (roof) and of the fourth ventricle (inferior part) and the choroid plexuses of all the ventricles of the brain. It ensheaths precapillary blood vessels entering the nervous tissue, forming perivascular cuffs (with the arachnoid mater). The ensheathment is particularly marked for the minute blood vessels that pass perpendicularly into the cerebral cortex. The interface between the pia and the nervous tissue is provided by a basement membrane in contact with the end-feet of astrocytic glial cells. Breaches in the pia roofing the fourth ventricle allow passage of cerebrospinal fluid into the subarachnoid space via a median aperture (foramen of Magendie) and two lateral apertures (foramina of Luschka).

THE DURAL VENOUS SINUSES (8.3, 8.6–8.9)

Between the meningeal and endosteal layers of the dura mater are found a series of venous sinuses. (The inferior sagittal and straight sinuses are exceptional in being located between two layers of meningeal dura.) The venous sinuses drain blood from the brain and from the bones of the cranium. Many of the sinuses can be easily located on the dry skull because they lie in prominent grooves along the cranium. The sinuses may be subdivided into two groups, depending upon location. There is an antero-inferior group at the base of the cranium and a posterosuperior group.

Antero-inferior sinuses

- Cavernous (paired)
- Intercavernous
- Basilar plexus
- Sphenoparietal (paired)
- Superior petrosal (paired)
- Inferior petrosal (paired)
- Middle meningeal (paired)

Posterosuperior sinuses

- Superior sagittal
- Inferior sagittal
- Straight
- Transverse (paired)
- Sigmoid (paired)
- Occipital

(The unpaired sinuses are situated in the midline.)

8.5 Cranial nerve roots in the floor of the cranial cavity, seen in relationship to the falx cerebri and tentorium cerebelli

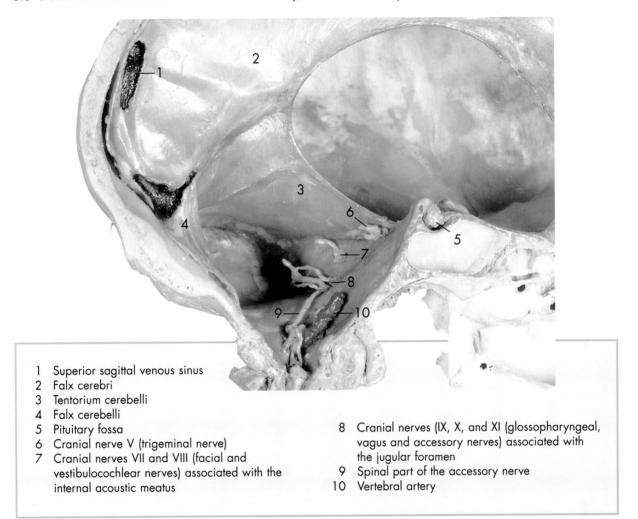

1   Superior sagittal venous sinus
2   Falx cerebri
3   Tentorium cerebelli
4   Falx cerebelli
5   Pituitary fossa
6   Cranial nerve V (trigeminal nerve)
7   Cranial nerves VII and VIII (facial and vestibulocochlear nerves) associated with the internal acoustic meatus

8   Cranial nerves (IX, X, and XI (glossopharyngeal, vagus and accessory nerves) associated with the jugular foramen
9   Spinal part of the accessory nerve
10 Vertebral artery

8.6 The dural venous sinuses and the main cerebral veins

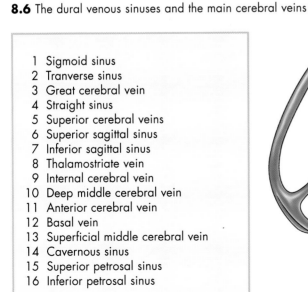

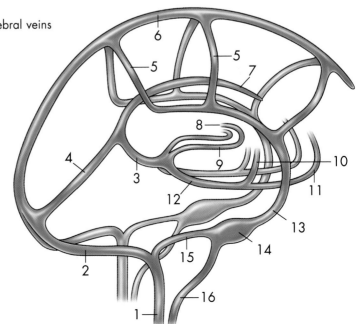

1   Sigmoid sinus
2   Tranverse sinus
3   Great cerebral vein
4   Straight sinus
5   Superior cerebral veins
6   Superior sagittal sinus
7   Inferior sagittal sinus
8   Thalamostriate vein
9   Internal cerebral vein
10 Deep middle cerebral vein
11 Anterior cerebral vein
12 Basal vein
13 Superficial middle cerebral vein
14 Cavernous sinus
15 Superior petrosal sinus
16 Inferior petrosal sinus

The *cavernous sinus* lies adjacent to the body of the sphenoid bone. Although most of the dural venous sinuses are open channels, the cavernous sinus is crossed by many trabeculae.

Communication between the two cavernous sinuses occurs in front of and behind the pituitary gland. These are called the anterior and posterior inter-cavernous sinuses. The two cavernous sinuses and the intercavernous sinuses together are sometimes referred to as the circular sinus.

The tributaries of the cavernous sinus are: the sphenoparietal sinus, the superficial middle cerebral vein, the inferior cerebral veins, veins from the orbit (superior and inferior ophthalmic veins, and sometimes the central vein of the retina).

The cavernous sinus drains via the superior petrosal sinus into the transverse sinus close to its junction with the sigmoid sinus. It also drains into the internal jugular vein via the inferior petrosal sinus.

Emissary veins link the cavernous sinuses with the pterygoid venous plexuses in the infratemporal fossa, passing through the foramen lacerum, foramen ovale and the emissary sphenoidal foramen.

Several important structures lie within the walls of the cavernous sinus. The oculomotor and trochlear nerves, and the ophthalmic and maxillary divisions of the trigeminal nerve invaginate the lateral dural wall of the sinus. The internal carotid artery (with its sympathetic plexus) and the abducent nerve lie inside the cavernous sinus.

The *basilar venous plexus* is located in the dura covering the clivus of the posterior cranial fossa. It connects with a number of other venous sinuses, including the superior and inferior petrosal sinuses and the cavernous sinus. Further connections are with the marginal sinuses of the occipital sinus (around the foramen magnum) and with the internal vertebral plexus (within the vertebral canal).

The *sphenoparietal sinus* arises from meningeal veins, particularly the middle meningeal vein. It is located near the posterior rim of the lesser wing of the sphenoid bone and empties into the cavernous sinus. It usually receives anterior temporal diploic veins and often the superficial middle cerebral vein.

The *superior petrosal sinus*, as its name suggests, occupies a groove on the upper border of the petrous part of the temporal bone. It is situated in the anterior part of the attached margin of the tentorium cerebelli. The superior petrosal sinus passes backwards and outwards from the cavernous sinus to the transverse sinus at the junction with the sigmoid sinus. It may pass above, below or even surround the trigeminal cave. Tributaries of the superior petrosal sinus include superior cerebellar and inferior cerebral veins, and veins from the brain stem.

The *inferior petrosal sinus* lies at the lower border of the petrous bone, occupying a groove in the region of the petro-occipital suture. It passes from the back of the cavernous sinus to terminate at the jugular foramen in the superior bulb of the internal jugular vein. The inferior petrosal sinus receives veins from the internal ear, the brain stem and the lower surface of the cerebellum.

8.7a The dural venus sinuses seen in the floor of the cranial cavity

1 Cribriform plate of ethmoid bone in anterior cranial fossa
2 Optic nerve
3 Oculomotor nerve
4 Diaphragma sella overlying pituitary fossa
5 Sectioned midbrain
6 Tentorium cerebelli
7 Site of a cavemous sinus
8 Superior sagittal sinus draining into the confluence of sinuses
9 Transverse sinus
10 Superior petrosal sinus
11 Sigmoid sinus
12 Middle meningeal artery

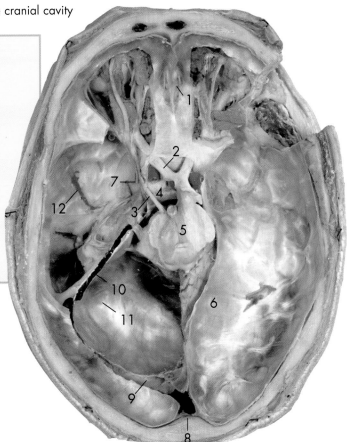

8.7b Floor of posterior and middle cranial fossa showing inferior petrosal, sigmoid and transverse vendus sinuses

1 Internal carotid artery
2 Trigeminal nerve
3 Inferior petrosal sinus
4 Sigmoid sinus
5 Transverse sinus

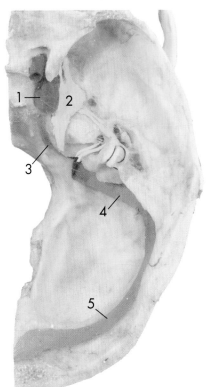

The *middle meningeal veins*, despite their name, are two small venous sinuses that run with the middle meningeal artery. These sinuses may be designated the frontal and parietal branches. They lie in meningeal grooves on the parietal bone, and pass backwards to drain into the pterygoid venous plexus (via the foramen spinosum and/or the foramen ovale). The middle meningeal veins may have a direct connection with the cavernous sinus or an indirect one through the sphenoparietal sinus. In addition to draining the meninges, they may receive as tributaries some diploic veins and the superficial cerebral and inferior cerebral veins.

The *superior sagittal sinus* runs along the median sagittal plane of the calvaria. It is situated in the attached margin of the falx cerebri. Small at its origin near the crista galli of the ethmoid bone, the sinus enlarges as it passes posteriorly. At its termination in the region of the internal occipital protuberance, the superior sagittal sinus becomes dilated to form the confluence of sinuses. Here, the superior sagittal sinus is usually displaced to the right side to join the right transverse sinus.

The superior sagittal sinus drains the superior cerebral veins. These veins pass into the sinus at an oblique angle. Along the sides of the sinus are situated the openings of some irregularly shaped dilations called venous lacunae. There are usually three lacunae on each side, and they connect with the meningeal and diploic veins. The lacunae contain arachnoid villi and are therefore thought to be a site at which cerebrospinal fluid passes into the bloodstream.

The superior sagittal sinus is connected to the veins of the face and the scalp through emissary veins. Rarely, an emissary vein passes through the foramen caecum lying immediately in front of the crista galli, linking the anterior extremity of the sinus with nasal veins. Emissary veins may also join the facial veins. Parietal emissary veins pass through the parietal foramina to link the superior sagittal sinus with the superficial temporal and occipital veins.

The *inferior sagittal sinus* is considerably smaller than the superior sagittal sinus. It lies in the free edge of the falx cerebri, above the corpus callosum. The inferior sagittal sinus drains the falx cerebri and receives some small veins from the medial surface of the cerebral hemispheres. At the anterior end of the junction between the falx cerebri and the tentorium cerebelli, the inferior sagittal sinus unites with the great cerebral vein to form the straight sinus.

The *straight sinus* is found at the site of attachment between the falx cerebri and the tentorium cerebelli. It is formed by the union of the inferior sagittal sinus and the great cerebral vein. The straight sinus passes downwards and backwards to enter the confluence of sinuses. It continues as the transverse sinus opposite to that receiving blood from the superior sagittal sinus (i.e. usually the left transverse sinus). The straight sinus receives some superior cerebellar veins.

The *transverse sinuses* begin at the confluence of sinuses. They are large sinuses, the right being generally larger. The right sinus is usually a continuation of the superior sagittal sinus, the left usually a continuation of the straight sinus. The transverse sinus passes laterally across the occipital bone in the attached margin of the tentorium cerebelli. It drains into the sigmoid sinus. The transverse sinus receives inferior cerebellar and inferior cerebral veins, and posterior temporal and occipital diploic veins. It also receives the superior petrosal sinus where it continues into the sigmoid sinus (at the postero-inferior corner of the parietal bone).

8.8 The dural venous sinuses associated with the falx cerebri

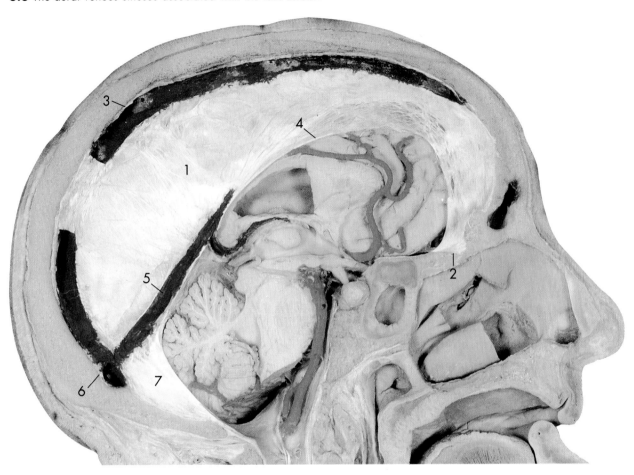

1 Falx cerebri
2 Attachment of falx to crista galli
3 Superior sagittal dural venous sinus
4 Inferior sagittal dural venous sinus
5 Straight dural venous sinus where falx
   cerebri meets tentorium cerebelli
6 Confluence of sinuses
7 Falx cerebelli

The *sigmoid sinus* is the main site of drainage for the dural venous sinus system. The sinus runs from the transverse sinus into the internal jugular vein at the jugular foramen. It has an S-shaped course, grooving the temporal and occipital bones. The sigmoid sinus communicates with the occipital veins extracranially via mastoid and condylar emissary veins. The mastoid emissary vein passes through the mastoid foramen near the posterior border of the mastoid part of the temporal bone. The condylar emissary vein passes through the condylar canal (posterior condylar canal) of the occipital bone. Emissary veins through this canal may also link with vertebral veins.

The *occipital sinus* has two parts. First, there are two marginal sinuses that pass around the margins of the foramen magnum. Second, there is a single sinus that links the marginal sinuses with the confluence of sinuses. This part of the occipital sinus runs upwards from the foramen magnum in the attached margin of the falx cerebelli. The marginal sinuses communicate with the internal vertebral venous plexus (see page 94). There are also communications with the terminal part of the sigmoid sinus and with the basilar venous plexus.

The dural venous sinuses eventually drain into the extracranial venous system via the sigmoid sinuses and the internal jugular veins. Additional communications exist through the diploic veins of the skull and the emissary veins.

The *diploic vessels* run in the diploe of the cranial vault. The diploic arteries are small and numerous, and arise from the arteries of the scalp and/or of the dura mater. The diploic veins show considerable anastomoses and eventually drain into the meningeal veins, the dural venous sinuses, and the pericranial veins. Although the anastomotic pattern is complex, five main diploic veins can usually be recognised on each side: the frontal, anterior temporal (two), posterior temporal, and occipital diploic veins.

The frontal diploic vein is found at the front of the cranium. It drains extracranially into the supra-orbital vein of the forehead, and intracranially into the superior sagittal sinus. The anterior temporal diploic veins run either side of the coronal suture. They drain extracranially into the superficial temporal vein and/or intracranially into the sphenoparietal sinus. The posterior temporal vein runs in the parietal bone. It drains intracranially into the transverse sinus. The occipital diploic vein either drains extracranially into the occipital vein (at the suboccipital region of the neck) or intracranially into the transverse sinus (near the confluence of sinuses). It may also drain into the occipital emissary vein.

Emissary veins are veins that pass through foramina in the cranium to link the dural venous sinuses intracranially with veins extracranially. They show considerable variability. Emissary veins may be found associated with both the vault of the skull and the cranial base.

For the cranial vault, there are three named emissary veins: the parietal, mastoid and occipital emissary veins. The parietal emissary vein passes through the parietal foramen to link the superior sagittal sinus with veins on the scalp. The mastoid emissary vein passes through the mastoid foramen to connect the sigmoid sinus and the posterior auricular or occipital veins. The occipital emissary vein passes through the region of the occipital protuberances to link the confluence of sinuses and the occipital vein. It may receive the occipital diploic vein.

8.9a The dural venous sinuses seen in the posterior cranial fossa viewed from behind

1	Superior sagittal sinus
2	Right transverse sinus
3	Sigmoid sinus
4	Internal jugular vein

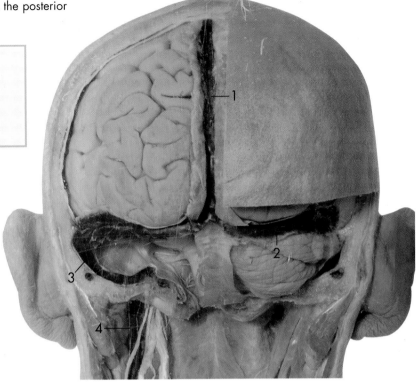

8.9b Lateral view of face showing course of middle meningeal artery

1	Dura mater
2	Middle meningeal artery entering skull
3	Temporal lobe of cerebrum
4	Anterior branch of middle meningeal artery
5	Internal carotid artery

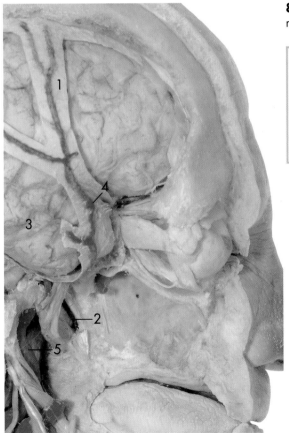

The emissary veins at the cranial base are particularly variable and are often not named. Several emissary veins link the cavernous sinus and the pterygoid venous plexus. These may pass through the foramen ovale, the foramen lacerum and/or the emissary sphenoidal foramen. An unnamed emissary vein passes through the carotid canal to connect the cavernous sinus with the internal jugular vein. Another unnamed emissary vein traverses the hypoglossal canal to link the basilar plexus or sigmoid sinus with the internal jugular vein. A condylar emissary vein runs through the condylar canal to join the sigmoid sinus and the occipital vein. An unnamed emissary vein may pass through the squamous part of the temporal bone to link the transverse sinus to the external jugular vein via a petrosquamous sinus.

An emissary vein may traverse the foramen caecum in the region of the crista galli of the ethmoid bone to join the superior sagittal sinus to veins in the nose.

The ophthalmic veins are not usually categorised as emissary veins, but they link the veins on the face extracranially with the cavernous sinus intracranially.

THE VASCULATURE OF THE MENINGES (8.9b, 8.13)

The meningeal arteries are numerous and are derived from several sources: the ascending pharyngeal, occipital and maxillary branches of the external carotid artery, the internal carotid artery and its ophthalmic branch, and the vertebral branch of the subclavian artery. Despite being called meningeal vessels, they principally supply the bones of the skull. Indeed, the cranial dura mater is relatively avascular. Furthermore, the arachnoid mater does not appear to have a direct blood supply and the pia mater receives numerous vessels derived from arteries supplying the brain.

The largest and principal meningeal artery is the middle meningeal artery. This is a branch of the first part of the maxillary artery (i.e. before the lateral pterygoid muscle in the infratemporal fossa; see page 144). It enters the middle cranial fossa of the skull through the foramen spinosum of the greater wing of the sphenoid bone. Passing up the squamous part of the temporal bone, the middle meningeal artery divides into frontal (anterior) and parietal (posterior) branches which ramify over the anterior and middle cranial fossa (with some small branches to the posterior cranial fossa). The frontal branch passes close to the pterion, where it frequently lies in a small canal in the greater wing of the sphenoid bone. A branch of the middle meningeal artery passes through the superior orbital fissure to anastomose with the lacrimal artery. Although mainly supplying the cranial bones, the middle meningeal artery also provides branches to the trigeminal ganglion and to the tympanic cavity (including a branch to the tensor tympani muscle). In addition to its intracranial branches, the middle meningeal artery gives off small branches that pass through the greater wing of the sphenoid bone to anastomose with the deep temporal branches of the maxillary artery in the temporal fossa.

Other arteries supplying the middle cranial fossa include the accessory meningeal artery and small branches from the internal carotid. The accessory meningeal artery arises from the first part of the maxillary artery and enters the middle cranial fossa through the foramen ovale. A meningeal branch from the ophthalmic branch of the internal carotid artery enters the middle cranial fossa through the superior orbital fissure.

Other arteries supplying the anterior cranial fossa are derived from the anterior and posterior ethmoidal branches of the ophthalmic artery. These enter the anterior cranial fossa from the orbit via the anterior and posterior ethmoidal foramina.

The posterior cranial fossa is provided with meningeal arteries which arise from the occipital artery, the vertebral artery, and the ascending pharyngeal artery. The meningeal branches from the occipital artery enter through the jugular and mastoid foramina, and the condylar canal. There is also an occasional branch of the occipital artery which passes through the parietal foramen. The meningeal branches from the ascending pharyngeal artery enter through the foramen lacerum and the hypoglossal canal.

The meningeal veins accompany the meningeal arteries and should be more correctly considered as small venous sinuses. They connect with some of the large venous sinuses and with the diploic veins. The most prominent are the middle meningeal veins accompanying the middle meningeal artery and these are described with the venous sinuses on page 276.

THE INNERVATION OF THE MENINGES

The dura mater is supplied by branches derived mainly from the trigeminal cranial nerve and from the upper cervical spinal nerves. The leptomeninges do not appear to have a sensory nerve supply.

The meningeal nerves of the anterior cranial fossa are derived chiefly from the anterior and posterior ethmoidal branches of the ophthalmic division of the trigeminal nerve. The ethmoidal nerves enter the anterior cranial fossa through the anterior and posterior ethmoidal foramina of the orbit. Their meningeal branches also innervate the anterior part of the falx cerebri. The meningeal branch of the mandibular nerve also contributes to the supply of the anterior cranial fossa.

The middle cranial fossa is innervated by the meningeal branch (nervus spinosus) of the mandibular division of the trigeminal nerve. This enters the cranial cavity through the foramen spinosum. An additional supply is derived via the meningeal branch of the maxillary nerve, and some twigs arise directly from the trigeminal ganglion.

The posterior cranial fossa is supplied by ascending meningeal branches derived from the upper three cervical spinal nerves. Branches from the second and third cervical nerves pass through the foramen magnum. Those of the first and second cervical nerves pass through the hypoglossal canal (perhaps as the meningeal branch of the hypoglossal nerve) and through the jugular foramen (perhaps as the meningeal branch of the vagus nerve). The tentorium cerebelli and the posterior part of the falx cerebri are innervated by the recurrent tentorial branch of the ophthalmic division of the trigeminal. The supratentorial dura is supplied by branches from all three divisions of the trigeminal nerve and also directly from its ganglion.

Sensory and sympathetic fibres pass to the cranial meninges with branches of the internal carotid and vertebral arteries. Meningeal blood vessels, including vessels in the pia mater, are also innervated by sympathetic fibres that arise directly from the superior cervical ganglion as lateral branches.

THE CONTENTS OF THE ANTERIOR CRANIAL FOSSA (8.10)

This fossa contains mainly the frontal lobes of the cerebral hemispheres. Located in the floor of the fossa are the olfactory nerves and the anterior ethmoidal nerves and vessels.

The *olfactory nerve* is the first cranial nerve. Approximately 15 to 20 delicate olfactory nerves pass on each side from the roof of the nasal fossa through the cribriform plate of the ethmoid bone to the olfactory bulb. These nerves are accompanied by minute sheaths of the meningeal layer of the dura mater and of the leptomeninges. From the olfactory bulbs, olfactory tracts can be seen passing along the base of the frontal lobes of the brain. Running with the olfactory system on each side is a small nerve called the nervus terminalis. It passes from the nose and alongside the olfactory bulb. However, its functional significance is unknown.

The *anterior ethmoidal nerve and vessels* pass across the cribriform plate and enter the nasal cavity through a fissure situated close to the crista galli. The anterior ethmoidal nerve is derived from the nasociliary branch of the ophthalmic division of the trigeminal nerve (6.3).

There are few venous sinuses in the anterior cranial fossa. The superior and inferior sagittal sinuses commence in this region.

THE CONTENTS OF THE MIDDLE CRANIAL FOSSA

Laterally, the middle cranial fossa supports the temporal lobes of the cerebral hemispheres. Centrally, the pituitary gland is retained in the sella turcica by the overlying diaphragma sellae.

The *pituitary gland* or hypophysis cerebri is an endocrine gland connected to the hypothalamus of the brain by a pituitary stalk or infundibulum. This stalk passes through a central aperture in the diaphragma sellae. The gland is surrounded by a capsule that merges with the meninges accompanying the stalk through the central aperture. The gland can be subdivided into an anterior lobe and a posterior lobe. This subdivision indicates different embryological and functional characteristics. The anterior lobe develops from Rathke's pouch, whereas the posterior lobe develops as a downgrowth of the brain. The anterior lobe can also be referred to as the adenohypophysis. Although some endocrinologists regard the terms posterior lobe and neurohypophysis as being synonymous, strictly speaking the neurohypophysis includes the posterior lobe, the pituitary stalk, and the median eminence of the tuber cincereum at the base of the brain.

The hormones of the anterior lobe of the pituitary gland are controlled by hormone-releasing factors from the hypothalamus which pass to the gland by means of a hypophyseoportal venous system. The hormones of the posterior lobe are transported in precursor form directly from the hypothalamus by axons within the pituitary stalk. These axons arise from cells of the supra-optic and paraventricular nuclei in the hypothalamus. Accessory or ectopic pituitary tissue can be found between the pituitary fossa and the nasopharynx. This reflects the embryonic path of Rathke's pouch.

The pituitary gland has a number of important relationships. Below are the sphenoidal air sinuses in the body of the sphenoid bone. The optic chiasma is situated above the pituitary gland and in front of the pituitary stalk. However, in only a small percentage of individuals does the chiasma lie in the chiasmatic groove between the optic canals. Lying lateral to the pituitary gland are the cavernous sinuses and their contents. Indeed, the internal carotid arteries within the sinuses often lie immediately adjacent to the pituitary gland (8.11).

8.10 The contents of the anterior cranial fossa

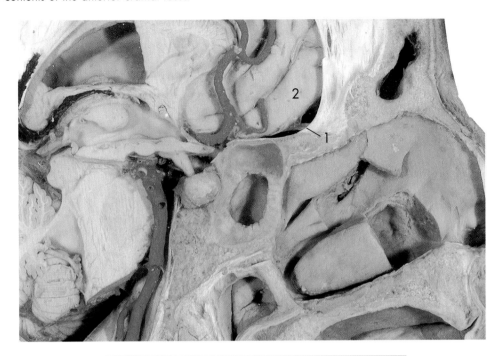

1	Olfactory tract
2	Frontal lobe of a cerebral hemisphere

8.11 Relationships of the pituitary gland

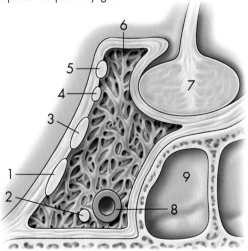

1	Maxillary nerve
2	Abducent nerve
3	Ophthalmic nerve
4	Trochlear nerve
5	Oculomotor nerve
6	Cavernous sinus
7	Pituitary gland
8	Internal carotid artery
9	Sphenoidal sinus

The blood supply of the pituitary gland is derived from inferior and superior hypophyseal arteries which originate from the internal carotid arteries. The inferior hypophyseal artery comes from the internal carotid as it passes through the cavernous sinus. The superior hypophyseal artery may arise as a series of arteries that appear either directly from the internal carotid artery as it emerges from the cavernous sinus or from the anterior and posterior cerebral arteries. The inferior hypophyseal artery divides into lateral and medial branches. These anastomose with their fellows of the opposite side to form a complete arterial ring around the posterior lobe of the pituitary gland. The superior hypophyseal arteries are arranged into anterior and posterior branches which pass to the region of the pituitary stalk. Trabecular arteries are branches of the superior hypophyseal arteries which pass down to the posterior lobe. Thus, the posterior lobe and the pituitary stalk receive their blood supply directly from the hypophyseal arteries. However, the anterior lobe of the pituitary gland has no arterial branches supplying it and receives its blood from a hypophyseoportal system of veins. The portal system begins around the pituitary stalk as a series of long and short portal vessels. These veins pass into vascular sinusoids between clumps of secretory cells in the anterior lobe. A region of the pituitary gland between the anterior and posterior lobes called the pars intermedia appears to be avascular. From the hypophyseoportal system, blood drains into inferior hypophyseal veins. These veins drain into the dural venous sinuses. The venous drainage of the posterior lobe is by three routes: directly into superior hypophyseal veins, indirectly via the hypophyseoportal system, and into veins in the hypothalamic region. The hypophyseoportal system is important functionally because it is the route by which hormone-releasing factors pass from the hypothalamus to the anterior lobe of the pituitary gland.

The innervation of the pituitary gland can be subdivided into a constituent intrinsic innervation and a vasomotor innervation. The constituent innervation is composed of the numerous nerve fibres that pass from the hypothalamus, down the pituitary stalk to the posterior lobe. The vasomotor supply is derived from the sympathetic plexus associated with the internal carotid artery.

The cranial nerves found in the floor of the middle cranial fossa are the optic, oculomotor, trochlear, trigeminal and abducent nerves. Other nerves passing across the floor of this fossa are the greater and lesser petrosal nerves, meningeal branches of the trigeminal nerve and sympathetic nerves.

The *optic nerve* is the second cranial nerve. It is seen just above the internal carotid artery, entering the optic canal. The nerve is connected to the optic chiasma in the central part of the middle cranial fossa. On entering the cranial cavity, the meningeal sheaths of the optic nerve become continuous with the cranial meninges. Although it is usually stated that the optic chiasma lies within the chiasmatic groove of the sphenoid bone, this appears to occur in very few cases. Furthermore, in most instances the chiasma lies above the diaphragma sellae, which roofs the central part of the fossa. At the optic chiasma, the nerve fibres are so arranged that those associated with the nasal parts of the retinae of the eyeballs decussate. From the optic chiasma two optic tracts appear, but soon merge into the substance of the base of the brain.

The *oculomotor, trochlear and abducent nerves* pass through the cavernous sinus towards the superior orbital fissure. The oculomotor nerve is the third cranial nerve. It enters the cavernous sinus in the area where the free and attached margins of the tentorium cerebelli cross over. Immediately behind the oculomotor nerve lies the very fine root of the trochlear nerve. This is the fourth cranial nerve. The oculomotor and trochlear nerves emerge from the midbrain. The abducent nerve is the sixth cranial nerve. It has a long course, arising from the brain stem in the posterior cranial fossa (see below) and then in the cavernous sinus in the middle cranial fossa. The abducent nerve is situated inside the cavernous sinus with the internal carotid artery.

8.12 Blood supply of the pituitary gland

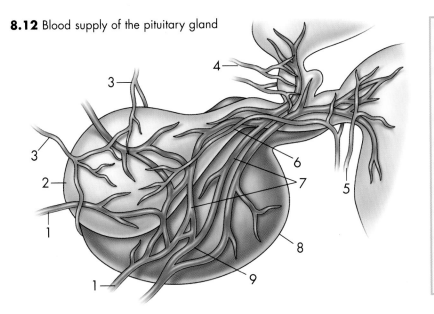

1	Inferior hypophyseal vein
2	Posterior lobe
3	Branches of inferior hypophyseal artery
4	Posterior branches of superior hypophyseal artery
5	Anterior branches of superior hypophyseal artery
6	Trabecular artery
7	Long and short portal veins
8	Anterior lobe
9	Hypophyseal system of veins

8.13 The contents of the middle cranial fossa

1	Internal carotid artery
2	Middle cerebral artery
3	Anterior cerebral artery
4	Optic nerve
5	Oculomotor nerve
6	Trochlear nerve
7	Trigeminal nerve
8	Mandibular nerve
9	Maxillary nerve
10	Ophthalmic nerve
11	Middle meningeal artery
12	Greater petrosal nerve
13	Posterior communicating artery

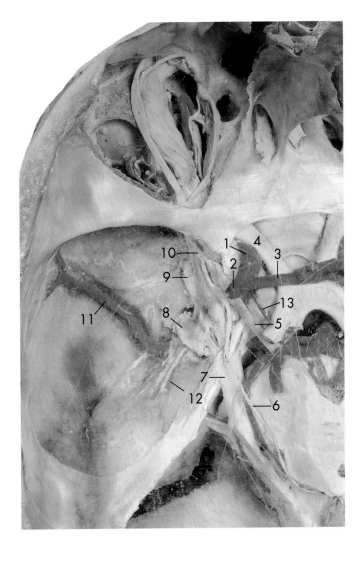

The *trigeminal nerve* is the fifth cranial nerve. It appears on the floor of the middle cranial fossa, first as nerve roots crossing the petrous ridge of the temporal bone, then as a trigeminal ganglion, and finally as three major divisions (the ophthalmic, maxillary and mandibular divisions). The trigeminal ganglion is situated in a recess of the dura (the trigeminal cave) close to the apex of the petrous part of the temporal bone. When the dura is removed, the ophthalmic, maxillary and mandibular nerves may be identified. The ophthalmic and maxillary nerves pass through the lateral wall of the cavernous sinus. The mandibular nerve passes directly to the foramen ovale, through which it leaves the skull to reach the infratemporal fossa. The ophthalmic nerve passes into the orbit through the superior orbital fissure, but before doing so divides into lacrimal, frontal and nasociliary branches in the middle cranial fossa. The maxillary nerve leaves the middle cranial fossa through the foramen rotundum and eventually emerges into the pterygopalatine fossa. All three divisions of the trigeminal nerve (and the ganglion itself) have meningeal branches. The branches associated with the ophthalmic and maxillary nerves arise within the middle cranial fossa. The meningeal branch from the mandibular nerve is given off in the infratemporal fossa and enters the cranium through the foramen spinosum.

The *greater petrosal nerve* is a branch of the facial nerve and carries parasympathetic fibres to the pterygopalatine fossa. It emerges from the region of the middle ear on to the floor of the middle cranial fossa at a hiatus, and then grooves the bone as it passes forwards to the foramen.

The *lesser petrosal nerve* is a branch of the glossopharyngeal nerve and carries parasympathetic fibres to the otic ganglion. Like the greater petrosal nerve, the lesser petrosal nerve arises in the middle ear and passes on to the floor of the middle cranial fossa through a hiatus in the petrous part of the temporal bone. The nerve lies in a groove located lateral to that of the greater petrosal nerve and runs towards the foramen ovale.

The venous sinuses within the middle cranial fossa are the cavernous, intercavernous, sphenoparietal and superior petrosal. The internal carotid artery is seen by the side of the body of the sphenoid bone, associated with the cavernous sinus. Just behind the optic canal, it gives off the ophthalmic artery. The meningeal arteries are the middle meningeal and the accessory meningeal branches from the maxillary artery, and branches from the ascending pharyngeal, ophthalmic and lacrimal arteries.

THE CONTENTS OF THE POSTERIOR CRANIAL FOSSA (8.15)

This fossa contains the lowest part of the midbrain and the pons, cerebellum and medulla oblongata. Located in its floor are the roots of the trigeminal nerve and the abducent, facial, vestibulocochlear, glossopharyngeal, vagus, accessory (both cranial and spinal parts) and hypoglossal nerves. Also found are the meningeal branches of the upper cervical spinal nerves.

The *roots of the trigeminal nerve* are seen passing between the trigeminal cave at the back of the middle cranial fossa and the lateral side of the pons. They cross the petrous part of the temporal bone close to the apex.

The *root of the abducent nerve* is seen lying medial to and slightly below the roots of the trigeminal nerve, on the clivus of the posterior cranial fossa. It penetrates the dura mater between the apex of the petrous part of the temporal bone and the dorsum sellae to reach the cavernous sinus.

Both the trigeminal and abducent nerves run much of their intracranial course in the medial cranial fossa and have already been described.

8.14 Cranial nerves associated with the petrous ridge dividing the middle and posterior cranial fossae

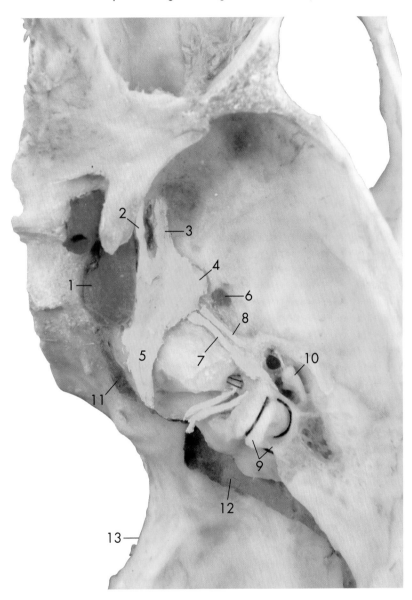

 1 Internal carotid artery
 2 Ophthalmic nerve
 3 Maxillary nerve
 4 Mandibular nerve
 5 Trigeminal nerve
 6 Middle meningeal artery (cut end)
 7 Greater petrosal nerve
 8 Lesser petrosal nerve
 9 Semicircular canals of internal ear
10 Incus of middle ear
11 Inferior petrosal sinus
12 Sigmoid sinus
13 Margin of foramen magnum

The *facial and vestibulocochlear nerves* are respectively the seventh and eighth cranial nerves. They both pass into the opening of the internal acoustic meatus, lying below and lateral to the roots of the trigeminal nerve.

The *glossopharyngeal, vagus and accessory nerves* are the ninth, tenth and eleventh cranial nerves. All pass into the jugular foramen which lies just below the internal acoustic meatus. The spinal accessory nerve is seen passing up from the cervical region of the spinal cord, through the foramen magnum, to join the cranial part of the accessory nerve shortly before the jugular foramen.

The *hypoglossal nerve* is the twelfth cranial nerve and is situated below the jugular foramen and behind the vertebral artery. It leaves the posterior cranial fossa through the hypoglossal canal.

The *meningeal branches from the upper three cervical nerves* pass through the foramen magnum to supply dura in the posterior cranial fossa.

The dural venous sinuses in the posterior cranial fossa: the sigmoid, inferior petrosal, basilar, occipital and straight sinuses, with the transverse and superior petrosal sinuses in the attached margins of the tentorium cerebelli. The vertebral arteries pass up through the foramen magnum and unite to form the basilar artery on the clivus. Meningeal branches from the ascending pharyngeal and occipital arteries are also present.

8.15 Contents of the posterior cranial fossa

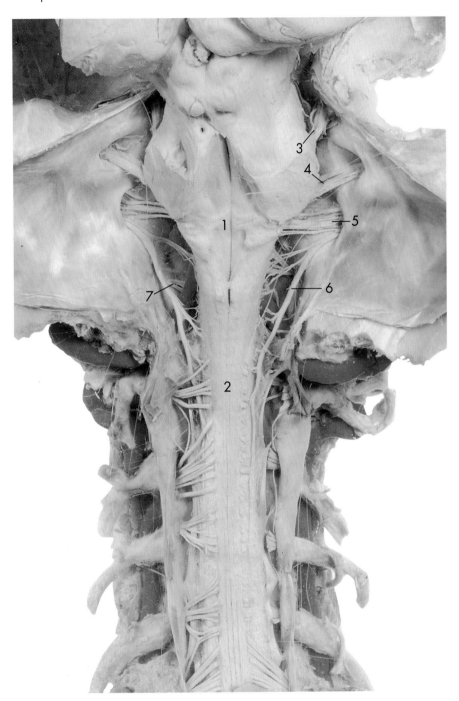

1   Floor of fourth ventricle
2   Spinal cord
3   Trigeminal nerve
4   Facial and vestibulocochlear nerves
5   Glossopharyngeal and vagus nerves
6   Spinal part of accessory nerve
7   Hypoglossal nerve

chapter 9
THE EAR

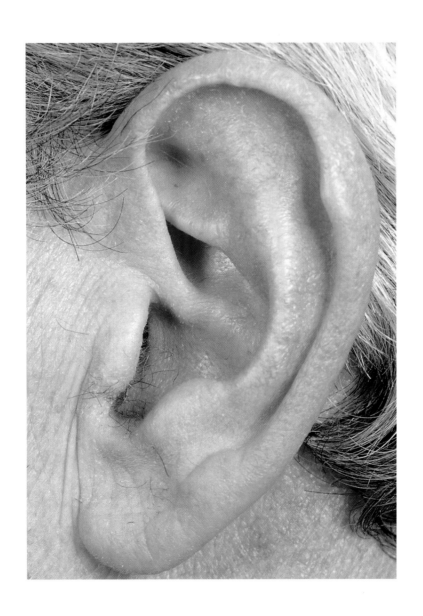

Chapter 9 THE EAR

The ear is the sense organ concerned with hearing and balance. It can be subdivided into three parts: the external, middle and internal ear. All parts are associated with, or lie within, the temporal bone on the lateral aspect of the skull.

The external ear consists of the auricle, external acoustic meatus and tympanic membrane. It is the part which funnels air vibrations towards the middle ear.

The middle ear is a cavity within the temporal bone (the tympanic cavity) which contains the ear ossicles. These small bones conduct vibrations from the tympanic membrane, across the tympanic cavity, to the internal ear.

The internal ear consists essentially of a convoluted tube (the membranous labyrinth) in which lie the receptors for hearing and balance. The membranous labyrinth itself is housed in a bony chamber termed the osseous labyrinth. Movements of fluids within the internal ear (perilymph and endolymph) are responsible for stimulating the various receptors. The vestibulocochlear nerve reaches the internal ear through the internal acoustic meatus.

THE EXTERNAL EAR

THE AURICLE (9.1–9.4)

The auricle is composed of a thin, elastic, fibro-cartilaginous plate covered by adherent, hairy skin.

Laterally, the auricle appears irregular in shape, showing a number of more or less consistent folds and depressions. The curved rim of the auricle is know as the helix. The anterior end of the helix is termed the crus of the helix. A small tubercle (the auricular tubercle of Darwin) may be seen where the curve turns postero-inferiorly. Running within and alongside the helix is the antihelix. The antihelix divides anteriorly into two crura, between which is situated a depression called the triangular fossa. The depression between the helix and the antihelix is termed the scaphoid fossa. The antihelix circumscribes the concha of the auricle, a prominent depression which leads into the external acoustic meatus. Projecting into the concha are two folds of tissue, the tragus and the antitragus. The tragus lies anteriorly and projects from the face. The antitragus lies inferiorly and above the lobule of the auricle. The tragus and the antitragus are separated by an intertragic notch. Unlike other parts of the auricle, the lobule is composed of soft tissues and does not have a cartilaginous skeleton.

The *cartilage of the auricle* has a shape which conforms closely with the folds and depressions described above. The part of the cartilage corresponding to the helix shows a small process anteriorly, which is called the spine of the helix. Separating the tail of the helix posteriorly from the antitragus is a fissure (the antitragohelicine notch). The cranial or medial surface of the cartilage shows an eminence that corresponds to the depression of the concha. This conchal eminence is crossed by an oblique ridge (the ponticulus) which marks the site of attachment of the posterior auricular muscle. The cartilage of the auricle is continuous with the cartilaginous part of the external acoustic meatus.

The *muscles of the auricle* can be subdivided into extrinsic and intrinsic sets of muscles. The extrinsic muscles are the posterior, superior and anterior auricular muscles, which belong to the muscles of facial expression (see page 107). The intrinsic muscles are rudimentary. The muscles are innervated by the facial nerve.

9.1 The auricle

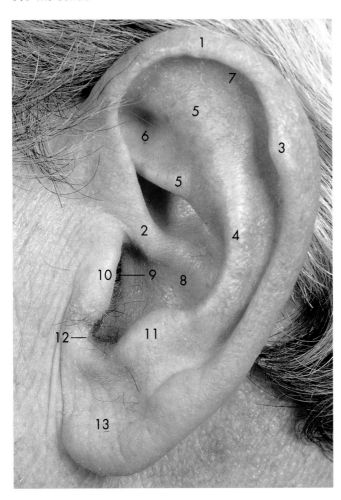

9.2 Diagram to show sensory supply of surface of external ear

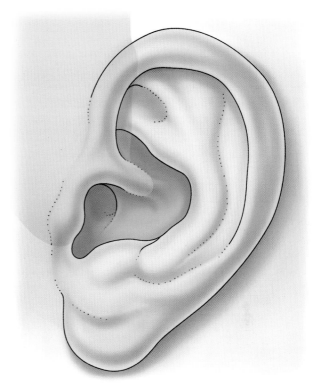

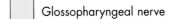

Auriculotemporal nerve

Glossopharyngeal nerve

Vagus nerve

1	Helix
2	Crus of the helix
3	Auricular tubercle
4	Antihelix
5	Crura of antihelix
6	Triangular fossa
7	Scaphoid fossa
8	Concha of auricle
9	External acoustic meatus
10	Tragus
11	Antitragus
12	Intertragic notch
13	Lobule of auricle

The *cutaneous innervation of the auricle* is complex and is not fully determined. This is perhaps because the external ear represents an area where skin originally derived from the branchial region meets skin from the postbranchial region. Most of the skin is innervated by the great auricular nerve from the cervical plexus (second and third cervical nerves). The lesser occipital nerve from the cervical plexus (the second and sometimes the third cervical nerves) may supply the upper part of the cranial surface of the auricle. The auriculotemporal branch of the mandibular division of the trigeminal innervates skin around the tragus and the crus of the helix. The concavity of the concha and a small area of the cranial surface near the mastoid is supplied by the auricular branch of the vagus and by the facial nerve.

The great auricular nerve, the lesser occipital nerve and the auriculotemporal nerve are described on pages 140 and 320 respectively. The auricular branch of the vagus nerve arises from the superior ganglion below the jugular foramen. It then enters the temporal bone through the mastoid canaliculus near the base of the styloid process. After passing through the temporal bone, the auricular branch exits through the tympanomastoid fissure on the posterior aspect of the opening of the external acoustic meatus. It now divides into two branches, one supplying the skin of the auricle and the other joining the posterior auricular branch of the facial nerve. Fibres from the facial nerve supplying the auricle may be derived from either its posterior auricular branch or from fibres joining the auricular branch of the vagus during its passage through the temporal bone.

The *vasculature of the auricle* is rich and there are many arteriovenous anastomoses. The vessels are derived mainly from the posterior auricular and the superficial temporal branches of the external carotid artery. The occipital artery may also contribute. The venous drainage is via the posterior auricular and superficial temporal veins. The lymphatics of the auricle empty into parotid, retro-auricular, and superficial cervical nodes.

THE EXTERNAL ACOUSTIC MEATUS (9.4, 9.5, 9.9)

The external acoustic meatus is a tunnel into the temporal bone that extends medially from the concha of the auricle to the tympanic membrane. It does not run a straight course, but is S-shaped. In front of the meatus lies the temporomandibular joint and a portion of the parotid salivary gland. Behind lie the mastoid air cells.

The external acoustic meatus can be subdivided into two parts. The outer third of the meatus is cartilaginous; the inner two-thirds is osseous. The cartilaginous portion is continuous with the cartilage of the auricle. It is fixed by fibrous tissue to the circumference of the osseous portion. The osseous portion is formed chiefly by the C-shaped tympanic part of the temporal bone. The wall is completed above by the squamous and petrous parts of the temporal bone. The osseous portion is narrower than the cartilaginous portion.

Both the cartilaginous and osseous portions of the external acoustic meatus are covered by firmly adherent skin. The skin over the cartilaginous portion possesses numerous hairs and sebaceous glands and the wax-secreting ceruminous glands.

The *innervation of the skin of the meatus* has a dual origin. The auriculotemporal branch of the mandibular division of the trigeminal nerve supplies the anterior and superior walls. The auricular branch of the vagus nerve supplies the posterior and inferior walls. The facial nerve may also contribute via its communication with the vagus nerve.

The *blood supply of the meatus* is derived from the posterior auricular artery, the superficial temporal artery and, near the tympanic membrane, the deep auricular branch of the maxillary artery. The veins drain into the external jugular and maxillary veins and into the pterygoid venous plexus. The lymphatics of the external acoustic meatus drain into the parotid, retro-auricular and superficial cervical nodes.

9.3 The subdivisions of the ear

I   Internal ear
II Middle ear
III External ear

1 Auditory tube
2 Cochlea
3 Vestibulocochlear nerve
4 Semicircular canals
5 Stapes – ear ossicle
6 Incus – ear ossicle
7 Malleus – ear ossicle
8 Auricle
9 External acoustic meatus
10 Tympanic membrane

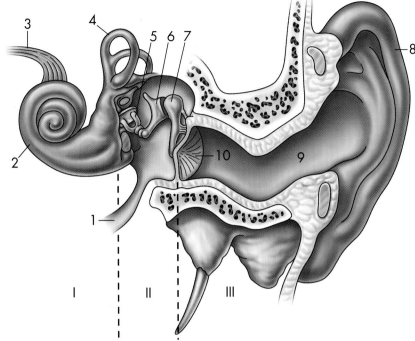

9.4 The external acoustic meatus

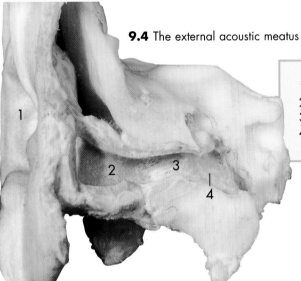

1 Auricle
2 Outer third of external acoustic meatus (cartilaginous)
3 Inner two-thirds of external acoustic meatus (bony)
4 Tympanic membrane

9.5 The external acoustic meatus seen in a transverse section of the head

1 External acoustic meatus
2 Auricle
3 Tympanic membrane
4 Tympanic cavity (middle ear)
5 Temporomandibular joint
6 Mastoid air cells

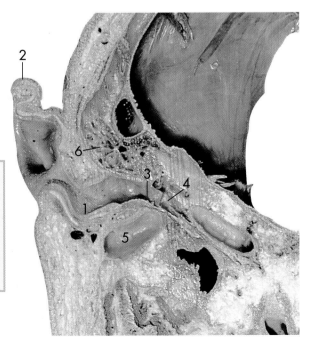

THE TYMPANIC MEMBRANE (9.6–9.8, 9.11)

The tympanic membrane is commonly known as the ear drum. It is a thin, semi-transparent membrane that lies at the medial end of the external acoustic meatus, separating the external ear from the middle ear.

The tympanic membrane consists of three layers. The outer layer is derived from the skin overlying the external acoustic meatus and consists of a stratified squamous epithelium. The inner layer is part of the mucous membrane lining the middle ear and consists of a ciliated columnar epithelium. The intermediate layer is fibrous. The fibres are attached to the handle of the malleus ear ossicle and radiate to the periphery. At the periphery, many circular fibres are also found. The margin of the tympanic membrane is thickened and forms a fibrocartilaginous ring.

The tympanic membrane lies obliquely at the end of the external acoustic meatus such that it slopes downwards and forwards as well as laterally. The fibrocartilaginous ring slots into a groove (the tympanic sulcus) in the tympanic plate of the temporal bone. The groove is, however, deficient superiorly where two bands called the anterior and posterior malleolar folds pass across the membrane to the lateral process of the malleus. The membrane is lax above these folds. The terms pars flaccida and pars tensa are employed to distinguish the lax and tense parts of the tympanic membrane. The membrane is tensed by the activity of the tensor tympani muscle within the middle ear (see page 305).

When viewed with an auriscope, the tympanic membrane appears as a concave, pearly-grey disc. In the depth of the concavity, a reddish-yellow streak indicates the site of the handle of the malleus. This is referred to as the umbo. A bright cone of light is seen in the antero-inferior quadrant of the membrane when it is illuminated for inspection. Above the umbo and close to the roof of the external acoustic meatus lies a white spot which represents the lateral process of the malleus. The anterior and posterior malleolar folds and the pars flaccida can also be observed in this region. The long process of the incus ear ossicle may be discerned as a whitish streak lying posterior and parallel to the upper part of the handle of the malleus.

The *innervation of the tympanic membrane* differs for outer and inner surfaces. The outer surface of the membrane is supplied by the auriculotemporal branch of the mandibular nerve and the vagus nerve. The facial nerve may also contribute. The tympanic branch of the glossopharyngeal nerve supplies the inner surface of the tympanic membrane.

The *arterial supply of the tympanic membrane* is derived from the deep auricular and anterior tympanic arteries and from the stylomastoid artery. The deep auricular artery arises from the maxillary artery before the lateral pterygoid muscle in the infratemporal fossa and pierces the wall of the external acoustic meatus. The anterior tympanic artery also arises from the maxillary artery before the lateral pterygoid. It enters the tympanic cavity through the petrotympanic fissure. The stylomastoid artery is a branch of the posterior auricular artery. It passes through the stylomastoid foramen. The deep auricular artery supplies the outer surface of the tympanic membrane, the others supply the inner surface. For both surfaces, a vascular ring is found around the margin of the membrane. However, although numerous small branches enter the membrane around the margins, significant branches also descend across the pars flaccida and the umbo.

The *venous drainage of the tympanic membrane* is complex. The veins from its outer surface drain into the external jugular vein, whereas those from the deep surface drain into the transverse sinus, the dural veins and the venous plexus of the auditory tube.

9.6 Right tympanic membrane (external surface)

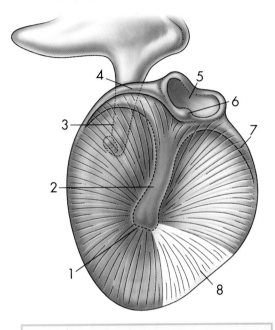

1 Position of umbo
2 Outline of handle of malleus
3 Long process of incus
4 Posterior malleolar fold
5 Pars flaccida
6 Lateral process of malleus
7 Anterior malleolar fold
8 Cone of light

9.7 Sensory innervation of the external and middle ears. Horizontal section

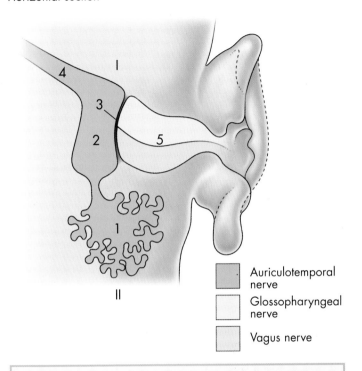

Auriculotemporal nerve

Glossopharyngeal nerve

Vagus nerve

I Anterior
II Posterior

1 Mastoid air cells

2 Tympanic cavity
3 Tympanic membrane
4 Auditory tube
5 External acoustic meatus

9.8 The tympanic membrane, seen through an auriscope

1 Umbo (handle of malleus)
2 Cone of light
3 Position of lateral process of malleus
4 Anterior malleolar fold
5 Posterior malleolar fold
6 Pars flaccida

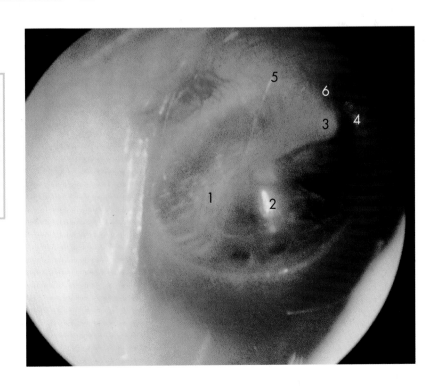

THE MIDDLE EAR

THE TYMPANIC CAVITY (9.9–9.12)

The tympanic cavity lies mainly within the petrous part of the temporal bone. It can be thought of as a diverticulum of the pharynx as it is connected to the nasopharynx by the auditory tube and is derived embryologically from the first (and possibly second) pharyngeal pouch.

The tympanic cavity is irregular in shape but resembles a biconcave lens. It is compressed laterally, the antero-posterior diameter (~15 mm) being about four times greater than the transverse diameter (~4 mm). It is narrowest opposite the centre of the tympanic membrane (~2 mm). The cavity can be subdivided into the tympanic cavity proper opposite the tympanic membrane, and the epitympanic recess above the membrane.

The roof of the tympanic cavity

This is formed by a thin plate of bone called the tegmen tympani. This plate projects anteriorly to form the roof of the canal for the tensor tympani muscle, posteriorly into the mastoid antrum and laterally into the epitympanic recess. The tegmen tympani separates the middle ear from the middle cranial fossa and the temporal lobe of the brain.

The floor of the tympanic cavity

A thin plate of bone separates the floor of the tympanic cavity from the internal jugular vein. Where the vein is small, the bone is thick and may contain accessory mastoid cells. In places, however, the bone may be deficient such that only a thin membrane separates the vein from the tympanic cavity. A small aperture lies near the medial wall of the tympanic cavity, the (inferior) tympanic canaliculus for the tympanic branch of the glossopharyngeal nerve.

The lateral wall of the tympanic cavity

This wall is largely occupied by the tympanic membrane with the attached handle of the malleus. In the angle between the lateral and posterior walls lies a small aperture called the posterior canaliculus for the chorda tympani nerve. From this canaliculus, the chorda tympani branch of the facial nerve and the posterior tympanic branch of the stylomastoid artery enter the tympanic cavity. The chorda tympani then passes across the upper part of the tympanic membrane beneath the mucous layer and over the neck of the malleus. It leaves the tympanic cavity through the anterior canaliculus for the chorda tympani nerve. The anterior canaliculus demarcates the medial end of the petrotympanic fissure through which the chorda tympani emerges into the infratemporal fossa. The fissure also allows the passage of the anterior tympanic branch of the maxillary artery into the tympanic cavity.

The *epitympanic recess* is a small portion of the tympanic cavity that extends upwards and beyond the lateral wall. It can be likened to the peak of a cap extending laterally from the middle ear above the external acoustic meatus. It contains the head of the malleus and the body and short process of the incus.

9.9 Diagram to show the shape of the middle ear and its position within the temporal bone

1 Vestibulocochlear nerve
2 Internal ear
3 Tympanic cavity
4 External acoustic meatus
5 Auditory tube

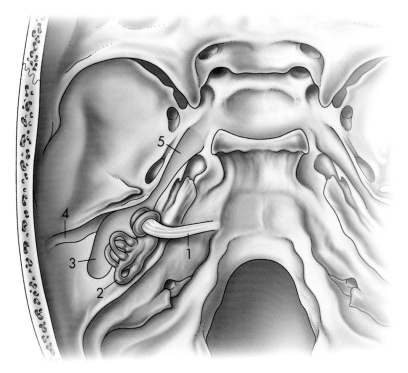

9.10 Diagram representing the walls of the tympanic cavity to show the contents of the middle ear. Note that the lateral wall is displaced to display the remaining parts of the tympanic cavity

1 Tympanic branch of glossopharyngeal nerve
2 Fenestra cochleae with secondary tympanic membrane
3 Tympanic plexus on promontory
4 Auditory tube
5 Lesser petrosal nerve
6 Tendon of tensor tympani muscle at processus cochleariformis
7 Stapes in fenestra vestibuli
8 Facial canal with facial nerve
9 Lateral semicircular canal
10 Epitympanic recess
11 Malleus
12 Incus
13 Mastoid antrum
14 Tympanic membrane
15 Stapedius muscle with nerve supply from facial nerve
16 Chorda tympani of facial nerve
17 Pyramid
18 Tendon of tensor tympani muscle
19 Articulation of incus with stapes

I Roof
II Anterior wall
III Medial wall
IV Posterior wall
V Lateral wall
VI Floor

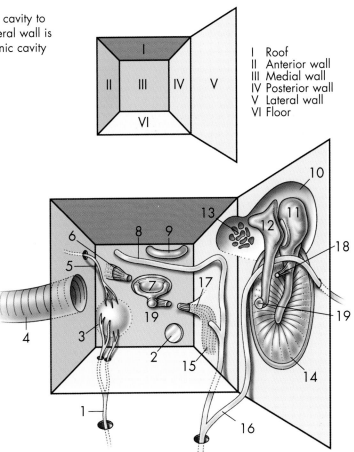

The anterior wall of the tympanic cavity

This wall is occupied mainly by the opening of the auditory tube. This tube communicates with the nasopharynx and has a dual purpose. First, it allows pressures on either side of the tympanic membrane to be equalised. Second, it allows drainage of the secretions from the middle ear, including the mastoid air cells. The auditory tube is fully described on pages 398–400. Above the auditory tube lies a canal which contains the tensor tympani muscle. The canal runs on to the medial wall of the tympanic cavity where the tendon of the muscle emerges. Below the auditory tube, the anterior wall is often thin where it forms the posterior wall of the carotid canal. This part is perforated by the caroticotympanic nerves from the sympathetic plexus on the internal carotid artery and by tympanic branches of the internal carotid artery.

The posterior wall of the tympanic cavity

Running vertically from the roof to the floor is the facial canal, containing the facial nerve. This canal is a continuation of the canal found in the medial wall and terminates as the stylomastoid foramen. Close to the roof of the posterior wall of the tympanic cavity lies the opening or aditus of the mastoid antrum. Below the aditus is a small depression (the fossa incudis) where the short process of the incus is attached by ligamentous fibres. Below the fossa incudis projects a hollow cone called the pyramid, through which emerges the tendon of the stapedius muscle. A canal for the muscle runs down within the posterior wall in front of the facial canal. Behind the posterior wall of the tympanic cavity is the posterior cranial fossa and the sigmoid sinus.

The *mastoid antrum* can be regarded as the air sinus of the petrous part of the temporal bone. Unlike the other cranial air sinuses, the mastoid antrum is almost adult size at birth. It communicates with the middle ear through the aditus. This aperture leads forwards from the posterior wall of the tympanic cavity into the epitympanic recess.

In view of the surgical importance of the mastoid antrum (viz mastoidotomy, mastoidectomy), its topographical relationships are of significance. The anterior wall of the antrum shows the aditus in its upper part. Here, it is closely related to the lateral semicircular canal of the internal ear. Antero-inferiorly lies the descending part of the facial canal. The posterior wall of the antrum has the sigmoid sinus and the cerebellum behind it. The medial wall of the antrum is related to the posterior semicircular canal of the internal ear. The lateral wall of the antrum relates to the suprameatal triangle on the outer surface of the temporal bone. The roof of the antrum is part of the tegmen tympani and is related to the middle cranial fossa and the temporal lobe of the brain. The floor of the antrum is the site for communication with the mastoid air cells.

The *mastoid air cells* lie mainly, but not exclusively, within the mastoid process of the temporal bone. At birth, the air cells are only just beginning to appear.

The mastoid air cells generally comprise a series of intercommunicating chains of thin-walled cavities. However, there is considerable variation in both number and arrangement. Indeed, three types of mastoid process can be identified: sclerotic (where there are few air cells), pneumatic (where there are many air cells), and mixed (where there are some regions with air cells and others with bone marrow). The air cells within the mastoid process are sometimes separated into two distinct groups by a plate of bone (the false bottom). This reflects the fact that the mastoid arises from both the squamous and petrous parts of the temporal bone divided by an extension of the petrosquamous fissure.

9.11 Diagram of the lateral wall of the tympanic cavity (internal surface) illustrating the shapes and positions of the malleus and incus ear ossicles

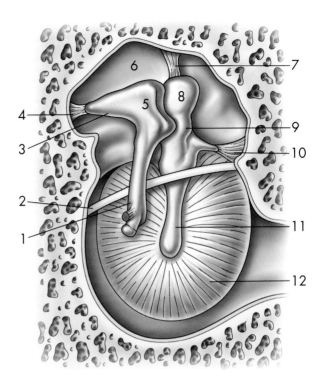

1 Long limb of incus
2 Chorda tympani nerve
3 Short limb of incus
4 Posterior ligament of incus
5 Body of incus
6 Epitympanic recess
7 Superior malleolar ligament
8 Head of malleus
9 Neck of malleus
10 Anterior malleolar ligament extending from anterior process
11 Handle (manubrium) of malleus
12 Tympanic membrane

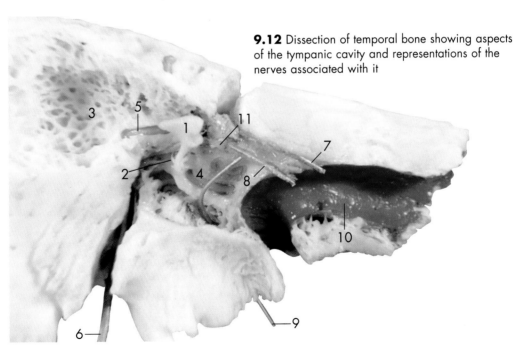

9.12 Dissection of temporal bone showing aspects of the tympanic cavity and representations of the nerves associated with it

1 Incus ear ossicle in tympanic cavity
2 Stapes ear ossicle
3 Mastoid antrum
4 Turn of the cochlea of inner ear
5 Lateral semicircular canal of inner ear
6 Representation of facial nerve exiting at stylomastoid foramen
7 Representation of greater petrosal nerve
8 Representation of lesser petrosal nerve
9 Representation of tympanic branch of glossopharyngeal nerve
10 Representation of internal carotid artery in carotid canal
11 Representation of the genu of the facial nerve

The medial wall of the tympanic cavity (9.13)
This separates the cavities of the middle and internal ears.

The most prominent feature of the medial wall is a bulge (called the promontory) formed by the cochlea of the internal ear. Above the promontory and close to the roof of the middle ear is a ridge related to the lateral semicircular canal of the internal ear. Between this ridge and the promontory lie the horizontal part of the facial canal, the fenestra vestibuli and the processus cochleariformis.

The horizontal part of the facial canal transports the facial nerve towards the posterior wall of the tympanic cavity. The fenestra vestibuli is one of the two sites of communication between the middle and internal ears (the other being the fenestra cochleae). The fenestra vestibuli lies above and behind the promontory and just below the facial canal. It is an oval opening that houses the footplate of the stapes ear ossicle. The processus cochleariformis is situated anterior to the fenestra vestibuli. It is a hollow bony process around which the tendon of the tensor tympani muscle bends. Although present on the medial wall, the processus cochleariformis is derived from the partition between the auditory tube and the canal for the tensor tympani on the anterior wall of the tympanic cavity.

The fenestra cochleae lies below and behind the promontory. It is a round opening covered by a membrane, the secondary tympanic membrane. Also behind the promontory is a depression called the sinus tympani. The sinus is a site which is susceptible to harbouring infections.

THE BONES OF THE MIDDLE EAR (9.14)

The tympanic cavity is bridged by a chain of three ossicles (the malleus, incus and stapes) which passes from the lateral to the medial wall.

The malleus
This is the largest ossicle. It is situated most laterally, alongside the tympanic membrane.

The name is derived from its shape, being like a hammer or mallet in appearance. Five parts can be identified: the head, neck, handle and anterior and lateral processes.

The head of the malleus extends above the tympanic membrane into the epitympanic recess. It is the part which articulates with the incus. The articulation is demarcated by a facet on the posterior surface.

The narrow neck of the malleus lies adjacent to the pars flaccida of the tympanic membrane. The chorda tympani nerve crosses it medially.

The handle of the malleus may also be referred to as the manubrium. It is attached to the tympanic membrane.

The lateral process of the malleus projects from the upper end of the handle. Anterior and posterior malleolar folds pass from the process to connect with the tympanic sulcus.

The anterior process of the malleus also projects from the upper end of the handle. In the fetus, it is continuous with the cartilage of the first branchial arch. It is much less distinct in the adult and it connects with the petrotympanic fissure by some ligamentous fibres.

9.13 The tympanic cavity dissected from the petrous ridge of the temporal bone

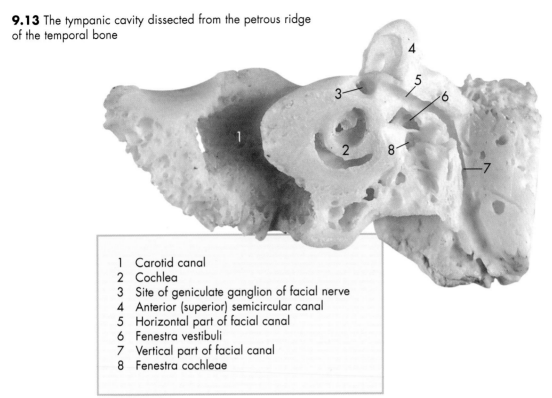

1 Carotid canal
2 Cochlea
3 Site of geniculate ganglion of facial nerve
4 Anterior (superior) semicircular canal
5 Horizontal part of facial canal
6 Fenestra vestibuli
7 Vertical part of facial canal
8 Fenestra cochleae

9.14 The ear ossicles

A Malleus
1 Head
2 Neck
3 Handle
4 Anterior process
5 Lateral process

B Incus
6 Body
7 Short limb
8 Long limb

C Stapes
9 Head
10 Neck
11 Limb
12 Base (footplate)

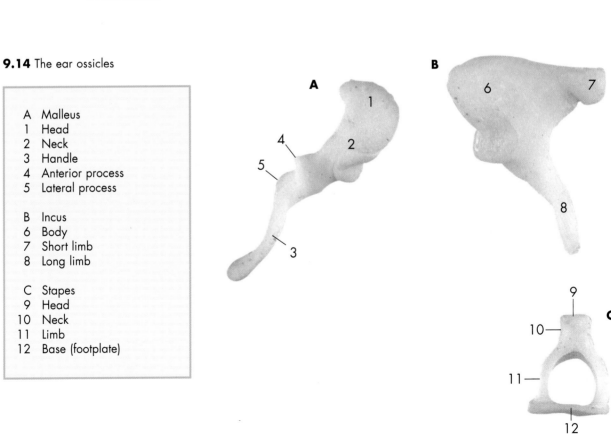

The incus

The incus is situated in the epitympanic recess and articulates with both the malleus and stapes. It resembles an anvil or a bicuspid tooth. It shows a body and two slender, root-like processes (the long and short limbs of the incus).

The body of the incus articulates with the malleus. The long limb of the incus projects nearly vertically downwards into the tympanic cavity. It terminates as the lenticular process, which articulates with the head of the stapes. The short limb of the incus passes posteriorly and is attached by ligamentous fibres to the fossa incudis on the posterior wall of the tympanic cavity.

The stapes

This is the smallest ear ossicle. It takes its name from its resemblance to a stirrup.

The head of the stapes articulates with the incus. At the neck of the stapes lies the attachment for the stapedius muscle. Anterior and posterior limbs connect the neck to the base (footplate) of the stapes. The footplate fits into the fenestra vestibuli on the medial wall of the tympanic cavity. A ring of ligamentous fibres (annular ligament) attaches the margins of the footplate and the fenestra.

The *joints between the ear ossicles* are synovial. Their articular capsules possess much elastic tissue. The following ligaments attach the ossicles to the walls of the tympanic cavity:

- The anterior ligament of the malleus connects the malleus to the petrotympanic fissure and then passes to the spine of the sphenoid where it is continuous with the sphenomandibular ligament.

- The lateral ligament of the malleus passes from the head of the malleus to the posterior part of the tympanic notch.

- The superior ligament of the malleus joins the head to the roof of the epitympanic recess.

- The superior ligament of the incus attaches the body of the incus to the roof of the epitympanic recess.

- The posterior ligament of the incus passes from the short process of the incus to the fossa incudis.

- The annular ligament of the stapes attaches the baseplate to the margin of the fenestra vestibuli.

THE MUSCLES OF THE MIDDLE EAR (9.10)

Two muscles are found in the tympanic cavity, the tensor tympani and the stapedius muscles.

The tensor tympani muscle

Attachments: This muscle lies within a bony canal situated above the auditory tube in the anterior wall of the tympanic cavity. It originates from this canal, from the cartilaginous part of the auditory tube and from an adjacent area of the greater wing of the sphenoid. It emerges into the tympanic cavity as a slender, tendinous structure. This turns sharply around the processus cochleariformis and crosses the tympanic cavity to insert into the upper part of the handle of the malleus.

Innervation: The nerve to the tensor tympani muscle is derived from the mandibular division of the trigeminal nerve. It initially forms part of the nerve to the medial pterygoid muscle but then passes through the otic ganglion to enter the muscle. The glossopharyngeal nerve (via the tympanic plexus) may also contribute to the motor innervation of the muscle.

Vasculature: The arterial supply is derived from the superior tympanic branch of the middle meningeal artery.

Actions: By drawing the handle of the malleus medially, the muscle tenses the tympanic membrane and helps to damp sound vibrations.

The stapedius muscle

Attachments: The muscle arises from within the hollow pyramid on the posterior wall of the tympanic cavity. It emerges at the apex of the pyramid as a tendinous structure and then inserts into the neck of the stapes.

Innervation: It is supplied by a branch of the facial nerve that is given off in the facial canal.

Vasculature: The muscle receives its blood supply from branches of the posterior auricular, anterior tympanic and middle meningeal arteries.

Actions: It helps to damp excessive sound vibrations and functions when sound is too loud.

THE MUCOSA OF THE MIDDLE EAR

The mucosa covers not only the walls of the tympanic cavity but also the structures contained within it, including the ossicles and their musculature. It is a ciliated columnar epithelium, except for regions posteriorly and within the mastoid antrum and air cells, where it is non-ciliated. Goblet cells are limited to an area around the orifice of the auditory tube. The sensory innervation of the mucosa is derived from the tympanic branch of the glossopharyngeal nerve via the tympanic plexus.

THE NERVES OF THE MIDDLE EAR (5.30, 9.10, 9.12, 9.15, 9.16)

The tympanic plexus

This plexus lies on the promontory of the medial wall of the tympanic cavity. It receives contributions from two main sources:

- Sensory fibres from the tympanic branch of the glossopharyngeal nerve (with possible contributions from the facial nerve).

- Vasomotor, sympathetic fibres from the internal carotid plexus.

The tympanic branch of the glossopharyngeal nerve passes into the temporal bone through the ridge between the carotid canal and the jugular foramen.

The following branches emanate from the plexus:

- Branches supplying the mucosa of the tympanic cavity and the auditory tube. The mucosa of the mastoid air cells is innervated from both the tympanic plexus and the nervus spinosus (meningeal branch) of the mandibular nerve.

- The lesser petrosal nerve destined to supply the parotid gland (5.30, and see page 126).

- Communicating branches to the greater petrosal nerve.

The facial nerve within the temporal bone

The facial nerve enters the temporal bone through the internal acoustic meatus (accompanied by the vestibulo-cochlear nerve). Initially, there are two separate components: the motor root supplying the muscles of the face, and the nervus intermedius which contains sensory fibres concerned with the perception of taste and parasympathetic (secreto-motor) fibres to various glands. The two components merge within the meatus. At the end of the meatus, the facial nerve enters its own canal, the facial canal, which runs across the medial wall and down the posterior wall of the tympanic cavity to the stylo-mastoid foramen. As the nerve enters the facial canal, there is a bend in which lies the geniculate ganglion. The branches which arise from the facial nerve within the temporal bone can be subdivided into those which come from the geniculate ganglion and those which arise within the facial canal.

The main branch from the geniculate ganglion is the greater (superficial) petrosal nerve, a branch of the nervus intermedius. The nerve passes anteriorly to exit the petrous bone and enter the middle cranial fossa. It contains parasympathetic fibres going to the pterygopalatine ganglion, and taste fibres from the palate (see page 216). The geniculate ganglion also communicates with the lesser petrosal nerve.

Within the facial canal, close to the pyramid, arises the nerve to the stapedius muscle. The chorda tympani is given off just before the stylomastoid foramen. This is the second, and last, branch from the nervus intermedius. It contains parasympathetic fibres going to the submandibular ganglion and taste fibres from the anterior two-thirds of the tongue. The nerve initially runs within its own canal before entering the tympanic cavity to cross the malleus. It then enters another canal before leaving the temporal bone through the petrotympanic fissure (see page 142 for the subsequent course). Another branch of the facial nerve is the branch communicating with the auricular branch of the vagus.

9.15 The tympanic plexus and the course of the facial nerve within the temporal bone

1 Glossopharyngeal nerve
2 Tympanic branch of glossopharyngeal nerve
3 Sympathetic plexus on internal carotid artery giving caroticotympanic nerves to tympanic plexus
4 Tympanic plexus
5 Lesser petrosal nerve
6 Greater petrosal nerve
7 Facial nerve in internal acoustic meatus
8 Geniculate ganglion
9 Facial nerve in facial canal
10 Stapedial nerve
11 Chorda tympani nerve
12 Facial nerve emerging through stylomastoid foramen

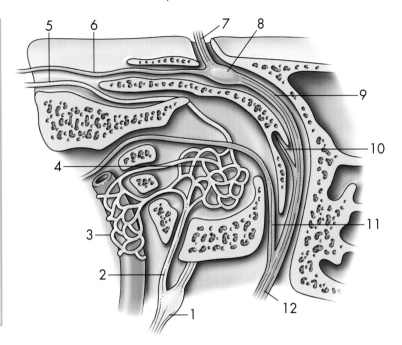

9.16 The course and branches of the facial nerve around the middle ear

1 Internal carotid artery
2 Ophthalmic nerve
3 Maxillary nerve
4 Mandibular nerve
5 Middle menigeal artery (cut end)
6 Lesser petrosal nerve
7 Greater pertrosal nerve
8 Anterior (superior) semicircular canal
9 Lateral semicircular canal
10 Incus in middle ear cavity
11 Facial and vestibulocochlear nerves
12 Trigeminal nerve

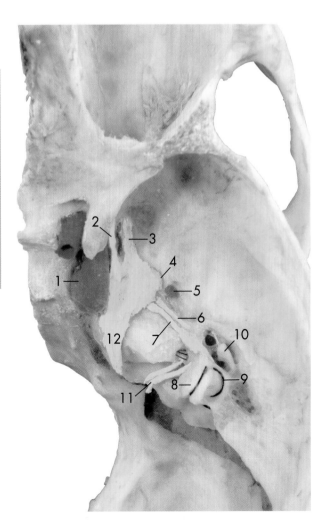

THE BLOOD SUPPLY OF THE MIDDLE EAR

The inner surface of the tympanic membrane and the anterior part of the tympanic cavity are supplied chiefly by the anterior tympanic branch of the maxillary artery. The posterior part, including the mastoid air cells, is supplied by the stylomastoid branch of the posterior auricular (or of the occipital) artery. The anterior tympanic artery enters the tympanic bone through the petrotympanic fissure, and the stylomastoid artery enters via the stylomastoid foramen. Additional sources of supply come from the inferior tympanic branch of the ascending pharyngeal artery, the middle meningeal artery, the caroticotympanic branches from the internal carotid, and branches from the artery of the pterygoid canal.

The veins of the tympanic cavity drain either externally into the pterygoid venous plexus or internally into the superior petrosal sinus. The lymphatics drain into the upper deep cervical or parotid nodes and the retropharyngeal nodes.

THE INTERNAL EAR

THE OSSEOUS LABYRINTH (9.17–9.19)

The osseous labyrinth consists of a series of chambers within the petrous part of the temporal bone. It contains the membranous labyrinth and some clear fluid called perilymph, and is lined with a thin layer of internal periosteum. The osseous labyrinth communicates with the middle ear by means of the fenestra vestibuli and the fenestra cochleae. It opens into the posterior cranial fossa via the aqueducts of the vestibule and the cochlea. The osseous labyrinth can be subdivided into three parts — the vestibule, the cochlea, and the semicircular canals — although it is crossed by a sponge-like arrangement of bony trabeculae.

The *vestibule* is the central portion of the osseous labyrinth. It contains the saccule and utricle of the membranous labyrinth. Indeed, the medial wall of the vestibule shows two distinct depressions for these structures. Anteriorly lies a spherical recess for the saccule. Posterosuperiorly lies an elliptical recess for the utricle. At the lower margin of the elliptical recess is the opening of the aqueduct of the vestibule. In this aqueduct lies the ductus endolymphaticus of the membranous labyrinth. On the lateral wall of the vestibule is found the fenestra vestibuli which is occupied by the base of the stapes. On the medial wall and the floor of the vestibule are minute foramina for the passage of branches of the vestibular nerve.

The *cochlea* is situated anterior to the vestibule and contains the cochlear duct of the membranous labyrinth. It is the part of the internal ear concerned with sound perception. In appearance, the cochlea resembles the shell of a snail. It presents as a hollowed canal of two and three-quarter turns, which diminishes in size from its base to its apex (the cupola). The cochlea spirals around a bony central pillar called the modiolus. A shelf of bone (the spiral lamina) projects from the modiolus in a manner likened to the thread of a screw. The lamina thus partially divides the canal of the cochlea. The division is completed by the cochlear duct. The cochlear duct occupies only the central portion of the canal, two passageways being seen on either side — the scala vestibuli and the scala tympani. The scala vestibuli is functionally the ascending spiral and the scala tympani the descending spiral. The scalae are continuous at the cupola around the apical extremity of the membranous cochlear duct. This region is termed the helicotrema. The cochlear nerve passes centrally through the modiolus. Branches from the nerve run out along the spiral lamina to reach the sound receptors in the cochlear duct. Three openings lie near the base of the cochlea:

- The fenestra vestibuli leads into the scala vestibuli.

- The fenestra cochleae marks the termination of the scala tympani and is closed in life by the secondary tympanic membrane. This membrane allows for the dissipation of pressure from the internal ear into the tympanic cavity.

- The aqueduct of the cochlea also lies at the end of the scala tympani. It passes through the petrous bone as the cochlear canaliculus to open below the internal acoustic meatus where, because the arachnoid mater is attached to the margins of the opening, it allows the drainage of perilymph into the cerebrospinal fluid in the subarachnoid space.

9.17 View of the medial wall of middle ear showing features associated with internal ear

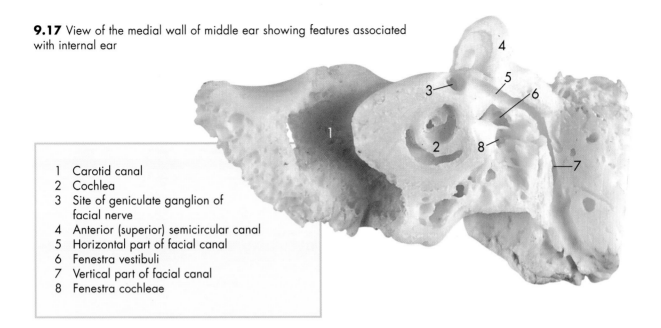

1 Carotid canal
2 Cochlea
3 Site of geniculate ganglion of facial nerve
4 Anterior (superior) semicircular canal
5 Horizontal part of facial canal
6 Fenestra vestibuli
7 Vertical part of facial canal
8 Fenestra cochleae

9.18 The osseus labyrinth within the petrous part of the temporal bone

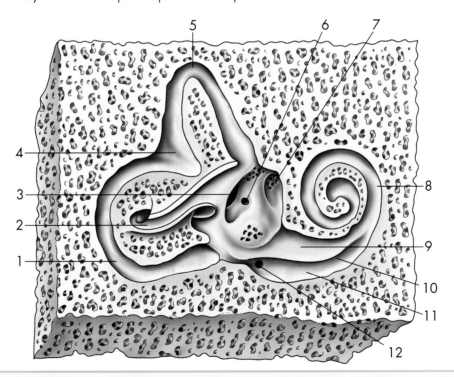

1 Posterior semicircular canal
2 Lateral semicircular canal
3 Opening of common crus into vestibule
4 Common crus
5 Anterior semicircular canal
6 Opening of aqueduct of vestibule below elliptical recess
7 Spherical recess
8 Cochlea
9 Scala vestibuli
10 Spiral lamina
11 Scala tympani
12 Opening of aqueduct of cochlea

The *semicircular canals* are concerned with balance, particularly by maintaining a stable retinal image with head movement. They lie posterosuperiorly to the vestibule and are three in number: anterior (superior), posterior and lateral. Each canal occupies about two-thirds of a circle and thus opens into the vestibule at two ends. However, as the posterior end of the anterior canal and the anterosuperior end of the posterior canal join to form a common crus, there are in total five orifices for the semicircular canals into the vestibule. One end of each canal is dilated to form a structure called the ampulla.

The anterior semicircular canal lies in a vertical plane across the long axis of the petrous bone. Its ends are posterior (at the common crus) and anterolateral (the ampullated end). The canal may be responsible for the ridge known as the arcuate eminence on the floor of the middle cranial fossa. However, the ridge may correspond to the occipitotemporal sulcus of the temporal lobe of the brain.

The posterior semicircular canal also lies in a vertical plane but along the long axis of the petrous bone. Thus, it lies approximately at right angles to the anterior canal. Its ends are anterosuperior (at the common crus) and inferior (the ampullated end).

The lateral semicircular canal is 30° off the horizontal plane. Its ends are posterior and anterior (the ampullated end). Its ampulla produces a bulge in the middle ear, on the medial wall of the aditus and epitympanic recess above the facial canal.

The relationship between the semicircular canals is such that, whereas the lateral canals lie in the same plane, the posterior canal of one side lies nearly parallel with the anterior canal of the opposite side.

THE MEMBRANOUS LABYRINTH (9.20–9.24)

The shape of the membranous labyrinth gives form to the osseous labyrinth. Essentially, the membranous labyrinth consists of a convoluted tube containing a fluid called endolymph. It is subdivided into four parts: the cochlear duct, the saccule, the utricle, the semicircular ducts.

The *cochlear duct* is the spirally-arranged tube that comprises the anterior part of the membranous labyrinth. It lies within the cochlea of the osseous labyrinth and is attached to the outer wall and the spiral lamina. The duct commences at a blind extremity below the cupola and spirals downwards to end by joining the saccule through a minute canal (the ductus reuniens).

The cochlear duct appears triangular in cross-section. The base of the triangle is the endosteum lining the bony canal. The endosteum is greatly thickened to form the spiral ligament of the cochlea. A specialised zone, the stria vascularis, lies on the outer wall of the cochlear duct. It is a stratified epithelium carrying a rich plexus of intra-epithelial capillaries. The floor of the cochlear duct is formed by the spiral lamina from the modiolus and by a fibrous band called the basilar membrane. This membrane runs from the lamina to the spiral ligament of the cochlea. It supports the spiral organ of Corti which contains the sound receptors. The roof of the cochlear duct is formed by a delicate membrane called the vestibular membrane.

The *saccule* is a small sac of the membranous labyrinth which lies in the spherical recess of the vestibule of the osseous labyrinth. It is connected anteriorly with the cochlear duct by the ductus reuniens and posteriorly with the utricle by the ductus endolymphaticus and the utriculosaccular duct. The anterior wall of the saccule shows a discrete, oval thickening called the macula of the saccule. This contains sensory nerve endings concerned with balance.

9.19 Posterior view to show orientation of the three semicircular canals of the internal ear

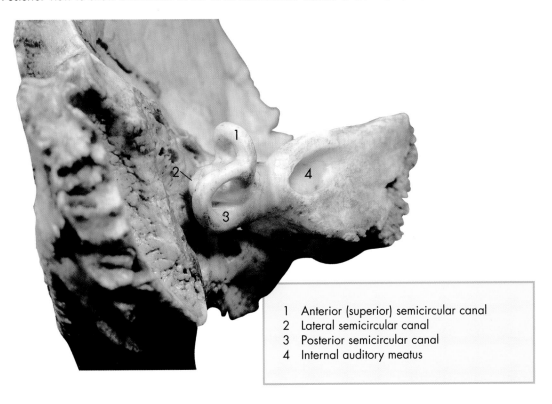

1	Anterior (superior) semicircular canal
2	Lateral semicircular canal
3	Posterior semicircular canal
4	Internal auditory meatus

9.20 The membranous labyrinth

1	Lateral semicircular canal
2	Posterior semicircular canal
3	Anterior semicircular canal
4	Utricle
5	Saccule
6	Cochlear duct
7	Ductus reuniens
8	Endolymphatic sac
9	Utriculosaccular duct

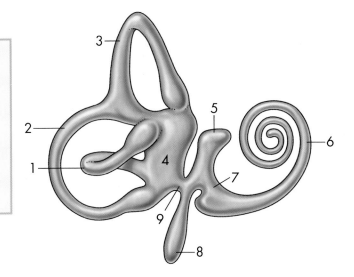

The *utricle* is a fibrous sac that is larger and less round than the saccule. It lies within the elliptical recess of the osseous labyrinth. Within the floor of the utricle is a thickening called the macula of the utricle. This is in a plane approximately at right angles to the macula of the saccule. It also contains sensory endings concerned with balance. The five openings of the semicircular ducts appear posteriorly. Anteromedially, the utriculosaccular duct passes towards the saccule and ductus endolymphaticus.

The *ductus endolymphaticus* arises between the saccule and the utricle. It passes along the aqueduct of the vestibule of the osseous labyrinth and, on emerging through an aperture close to the internal acoustic meatus, ends in the endolymphatic sac beneath the dura on the posterior surface of the petrous bone.

The *semicircular ducts* are three in number (anterior, posterior, lateral), corresponding to the semicircular canals of the osseous labyrinth. The ducts are only one-quarter of the width of the bony canals but are similar in form. At the ampullae, they almost fill the canals. Each duct lies against the outer surface of the lining periosteum of its canal. The ducts open into five orifices in the posterior part of the utricle. The sensory receptors are concerned with balance and are situated in the ampulla at a transverse crest called the crista.

PERILYMPH AND ENDOLYMPH

Perilymph is a fluid that occupies the perilymphatic spaces between the osseous and the membranous labyrinths. In composition, perilymph resembles cerebrospinal fluid or extracellular tissue fluid. The source of the fluid and its precise mode of drainage is uncertain, though the connection between the perilymphatic space and the subarachnoid space through the cochlear canaliculus has been implicated.

Endolymph is the fluid within the membranous labyrinth. It closely resembles intracellular fluid, being rich in potassium. The source of the fluid is unknown, but it is thought to drain via a vascular plexus associated with the endolymphatic sac.

The perilymph and endolymph have important roles in both auditory and vestibular functions. When the stapes moves within the fenestra vestibuli, there is movement of perilymph within the scala tympani. This stimulates the auditory receptors in the spiral organ of Corti. The fluid movements continue down the scala tympani and pressure is dissipated by displacement of the secondary tympanic membrane which overlies the fenestra cochleae. Concerning the vestibular apparatus, the semicircular canals give information about movements, the saccule and utricle about the position of the head. Movement of the head results in movement of the endolymph in the semicircular canals. This stimulates receptors in the ampullae. The receptors in the maculae of the saccule and utricle are essentially stretch receptors. The saccule is affected when there has been lateral tilting of the head, while the utricle is affected following anterior or posterior flexion.

9.21 Section through the cochlea of the internal eye

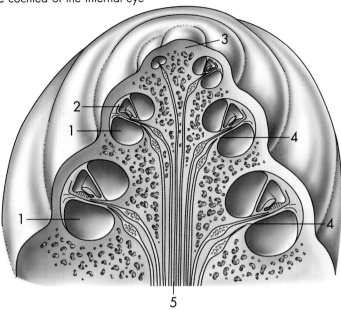

1 Cochlear canal
2 Cochlear duct
3 Cupola of cochlea
4 Spiral lamina
5 Cochlear nerve passing through modiolus

9.22 Diagram to show the appearance of a single turn of cochlea

1 Modiolus with cochlear nerve
2 Spiral ganglion
3 Spiral lamina with branch
  of cochlear nerve
4 Scala vestibuli
5 Cochlear duct
6 Spiral ligament
7 Basilar membrane and
  spiral organ
8 Scala tympani

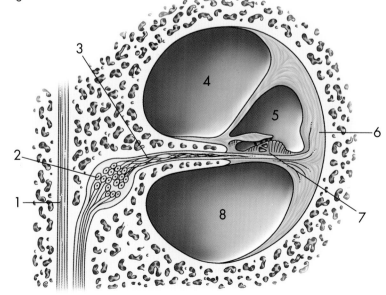

THE INNERVATION OF THE INTERNAL EAR (9.16, 9.21, 9.22)

The nerve to the internal ear is the vestibulocochlear nerve (eighth cranial nerve). It arises alongside the facial nerve on the lateral side of the brain between the pons and the medulla oblongata. It passes into the petrous part of the temporal bone through the internal acoustic meatus. Within the meatus, the nerve divides into two vestibular branches (superior and inferior) and a cochlear branch.

The vestibular nerves arise from a ganglion (Scarpa's ganglion). The superior vestibular nerve supplies the maculae of both the saccule and utricle, and the ampullae of the anterior and lateral semicircular ducts. The inferior vestibular nerve supplies the ampulla of the posterior semicircular duct and the macula of the saccule. A small branch of the nerve communicates with the cochlear nerve.

The cochlear nerve is associated with a ganglion (the spiral ganglion), which is situated within the modiolus along the spiral lamina. Fibres pass through the lamina to end in the spiral organ of Corti. A branch of the cochlear nerve may also contribute to the innervation of the macula of the saccule.

THE BLOOD SUPPLY OF THE INTERNAL EAR

The arteries of the internal ear are derived from two sources: the labyrinthine artery and the stylomastoid artery.

The labyrinthine artery arises from the anterior inferior cerebellar artery, or directly from the basilar artery. It passes through the internal acoustic meatus and divides into vestibular and cochlear branches.

A labyrinthine vein accompanies the artery and drains into the superior petrosal sinus or the transverse sinus. In addition, a small vein from the cochlea passes through the cochlear canaliculus to drain into the internal jugular vein.

9.23 Section through the cochlear duct

1 Basilar membrane
2 Osseous spiral lamina
3 Vestibular membrane
4 Stria vascularis
5 Spiral ligament
6 Spiral organ of Corti

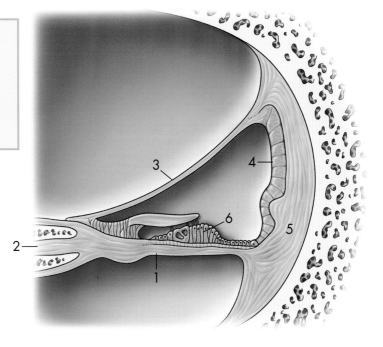

9.24 The distribution of the vestibulocochlear nerve to the membranous labyrinth of the internal ear

1 Cochlear duct
2 Macula of saccule
3 Posterior semicircular duct
4 Lateral semicircular duct
5 Anterior semicircular duct
6 Macula of utricle
7 Superior branch of vestibular nerve
8 Inferior branch of vestibular nerve
9 Cochlear nerve

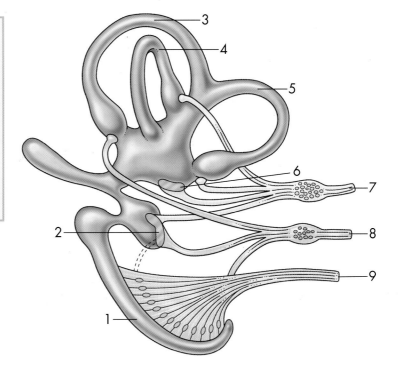

chapter 10
THE NECK

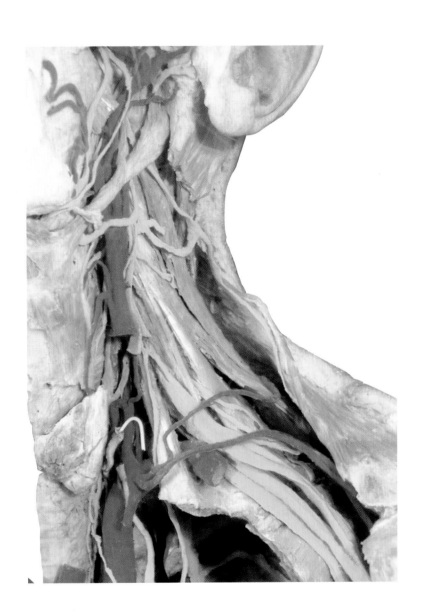

Chapter 10 THE NECK

THE GENERAL ARRANGEMENT OF STRUCTURES IN THE NECK (10.13)

The neck extends from the base of the cranium and the inferior border of the mandible to the thoracic inlet.

Superficially, the neck is surrounded by a sleeve of fascia known as the investing layer of deep cervical fascia. The fascia encloses the trapezius and sternocleidomastoid muscles. At the front of the neck, the platysma muscles lie between the fascia and the skin; the infrahyoid muscles (strap muscles) lie behind the fascia.

Posteriorly, there is a musculoskeletal compartment which consists of the vertebral column and the muscles immediately surrounding it. This is enclosed by a sleeve of fascia which is prominent in front of the vertebral bodies and is therefore called the prevertebral fascia.

There is also a visceral compartment in the neck which, depending on the level, contains the pharynx, the oesophagus, the larynx and the trachea. This compartment is enclosed by fascia which, because it is prominent in front of the trachea, is called the pretracheal fascia. The thyroid gland lies on the trachea at the root of the neck.

On each side of the neck, beneath the sternocleidomastoid muscle, lies a neurovascular compartment — the carotid sheath. Within the sheath lies the common carotid and internal carotid arteries, the internal jugular vein, and the vagus nerve. Detailed information concerning the fascia of the neck is given on pages 332–338.

SURFACE MARKINGS OF THE NECK (10.1)

Superiorly, ridges indicating the mastoid process and the mandible (the angle and inferior border) can be clearly seen. At the back of the head in the midline lies a prominence termed the external occipital protuberance. Below and in front of the mastoid process, the tip of the transverse process of the atlas can be palpated using deep pressure. Behind the angle of the mandible lies a point indicating the lowest part of the parotid gland. The submandibular gland is situated below the inferior border of the mandible and above the hyoid bone.

Inferiorly are ridges indicating the manubrium of the sternum, the clavicle and the scapula. A depression immediately above the superior border of the manubrium (the jugular notch) is termed the suprasternal fossa. It is bounded on each side by prominent ridges produced by the sternal heads of the sternocleidomastoid muscles. A supraclavicular fossa lies above the middle third of the clavicle. It is bounded medially by the clavicular head of the sternocleidomastoid muscle and behind and laterally by the lateral margin of the trapezius muscle. If the shoulders are shrugged, the margin produced by the trapezius becomes prominent. Within the supraclavicular fossa are landmarks indicating the inferior belly of the omohyoid muscle and the upper trunk of the brachial plexus. Between the sternal and clavicular heads of the sternocleidomastoid muscle lies a depression which is sometimes referred to as the lesser supraclavicular fossa. This fossa marks the site of the sternoclavicular joint and the union between the internal jugular and subclavian veins to form the brachiocephalic vein.

Anteriorly, the thyroid cartilage of the larynx presents a laryngeal prominence ('Adam's apple') which is most conspicuous in the adult male. The upper border of the thyroid cartilage is at the level of the lower part of the fourth cervical vertebra in males, but is slightly higher in females and in children. This is the level at which the common carotid artery bifurcates. The arch of the cricoid cartilage of the larynx can be palpated at the level of the sixth cervical vertebra. At about this level, the recurrent laryngeal nerve enters the larynx, the vertebral artery enters the foramen transversarium of the sixth cervical vertebra, the cervical sympathetic trunk presents the middle cervical ganglion, the pharynx becomes the oesophagus, and the larynx leads into the trachea. The trachea passes down from the cricoid cartilage and enters the thorax behind the jugular notch of the manubrium. The thyroid gland is

10.1 Surface markings of the neck

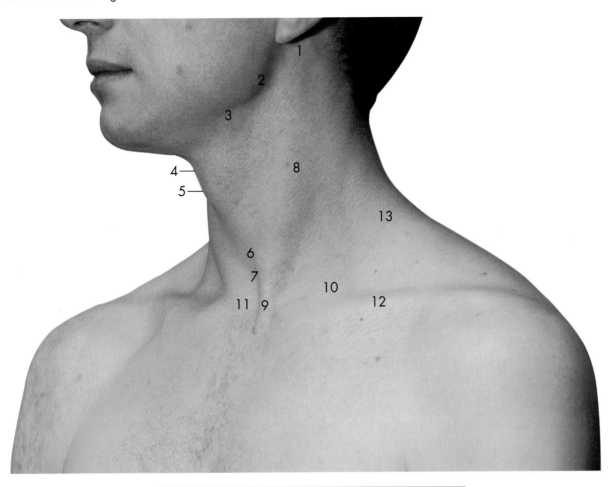

1 Mastoid process
2 Angle of the mandible
3 Submandibular gland
4 Hyoid bone
5 Laryngeal prominence
6 Arch of the cricoid cartilage
7 Isthmus of the thyroid gland
8 Sternocleidomastoid muscle
9 Sternal head of the sternocleidomastoid muscle
10 Clavicular head of sternocleidomastoid muscle
11 Jugular notch
12 Clavicle
13 Trapezius muscle

closely related to the trachea in the root of the neck, the isthmus joining the two lobes of the thyroid lying 1.5 cm below the cricoid cartilage. The hyoid bone is situated above the thyroid cartilage of the larynx and below the inferior border of the mandible, at the level of the upper part of the fourth cervical vertebra. Its horseshoe shape is easily discerned, the body lying in the midline and the two greater horns extending laterally towards the anterior borders of the sternocleidomastoid muscles below the angle of the mandible. At about this level the lingual and occipital arteries arise from the external carotid artery.

Laterally, the sternocleidomastoid muscle can be seen running from the manubrium sterni and the clavicle up to the mastoid process. It is particularly prominent when it is activated by turning the head to the opposite side against resistance. The muscle is crossed superficially by the external jugular vein. The course of the vein is indicated by a line running from a point 3.0 cm below and behind the angle of the mandible to a point on the clavicle lateral to the attachment of the sternocleidomastoid muscle. The carotid pulse can be felt below the angle of the mandible and in front of the anterior border of the sternocleidomastoid muscle.

Posteriorly, the spines of the upper thoracic vertebrae and the seventh cervical vertebra are prominent. The remaining cervical vertebrae are indistinct, the spines being covered by the ligamentum nuchae which separates the postvertebral musculature on both sides. A groove runs down the midline of the neck. This is particularly marked in the young. The upper limit of the neck muscles is indicated by the external occipital protuberance and the superior nuchal lines on the back of the skull.

THE CUTANEOUS INNERVATION OF THE NECK (10.2, 10.3)

The skin of the neck is innervated by branches of cervical spinal nerves, via both dorsal and ventral rami. The dorsal rami supply skin over the back of the neck and scalp. The ventral rami supply skin covering the lateral and anterior portions of the neck and even extend onto the face over the angle of the mandible.

The dorsal rami of the first, sixth, seventh and eighth cervical nerves have no cutaneous distribution. From the medial branch of the dorsal ramus of the second cervical nerve comes the greater occipital nerve (10.63). This pierces the trapezius muscle close to its attachment onto the superior nuchal line of the occiput and then ascends to supply the skin over the occipital part of the scalp up to the vertex of the skull. The medial branches of the dorsal rami of the third, fourth and fifth cervical nerves also pierce trapezius to supply skin over the back of the neck in a serial manner.

The ventral rami of the second, third and fourth cervical nerves supply cutaneous branches via the cervical plexus. This plexus is located deep to sternocleidomastoid muscle and supplies both motor and sensory branches to structures in the neck (see pages 362–364). The cutaneous branches from the plexus are the lesser occipital, the great auricular, the transverse cervical, and the supraclavicular nerves. All four nerves appear from beneath the sternocleidomastoid muscle at its posterior margin.

The *lesser occipital nerve* takes fibres mainly from the second cervical nerve, although fibres from the third cervical nerve may sometimes contribute. It ascends along the posterior margin of the sternocleidomastoid muscle to supply the scalp above and behind the ear and a small area on the cranial surface of the auricle.

The *great auricular nerve* receives fibres from the second and third cervical nerves. It runs up the superficial surface of the sternocleidomastoid muscle towards the ear. It supplies the skin overlying the mastoid process (the mastoid branch), much of the auricle (auricular branches), and the parotid region and the angle of the mandible (facial branches).

The *transverse cervical nerve* also takes fibres from the second and third cervical nerves. It crosses the sternocleidomastoid muscle horizontally to supply skin overlying the anterior part of the neck from the mandible to the sternum.

The *supraclavicular nerves* receive fibres from the third and fourth cervical nerves. Initially, it is a single nerve. This passes downwards towards the clavicle where it divides into three branches – medial, intermediate and lateral supraclavicular nerves. These nerves supply skin at the root of the neck and over the upper part of the thorax.

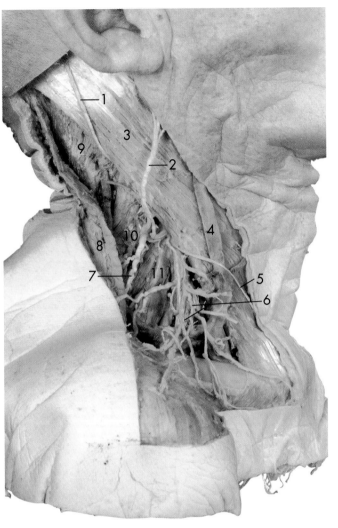

10.2 Lateral view of the neck showing the cutaneous innervation from the cervical plexus

1	Lesser occipital nerve
2	Greater auricular nerve
3	Sternocleidomastoid muscle
4	External jugular vein
5	Transverse cervical nerve
6	Supraclavicular nerves
7	Spinal accessory nerve
8	Trapezius muscle
9	Splenius capitis muscle
10	Levator scapulae muscle
11	Scalenus medius muscle

10.3 Cutaneous innervation of the neck

1	Supraclavicular nerves
2	Cervical spinal nerves (dorsi rami C3 to C5)
3	Lesser occipital nerve
4	Greater occipital nerve
5	Greater auricular nerve
6	Transverse cervical nerve

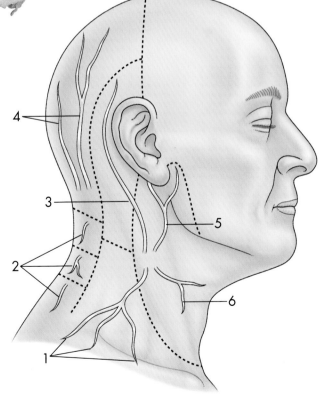

SUPERFICIAL DISSECTION OF THE NECK

Immediately beneath the skin of the neck lie the investing layer of deep cervical fascia (see page 332) and the platysma muscle.

THE PLATYSMA MUSCLE (10.4)

This muscle belongs to the group of muscles comprising 'the muscles of facial expression' (see pages 104–113). It appears as a thin, broad sheet running up the front of the neck from the root of the neck towards the mandible. However, it varies considerably in extent and may even be absent.

Attachments: The platysma muscle arises from the superficial fascia of the upper part of the thorax. It then runs across the clavicle and up the neck to insert into the lower border of the body of the mandible, the skin of the lower part of the face, and the musculature around the angle and lower part of the mouth.

Innervation: The cervical branch of the facial nerve innervates the platysma muscle.

Vasculature: The muscle receives its blood supply from the facial artery (submental branch) and the thyrocervical trunk (the suprascapular artery).

Actions: Platysma is said to be the muscle associated with the expression of horror or surprise. It wrinkles the skin of the neck in an oblique direction, it draws down the lower lip and angle of the mouth, and slightly depresses the mandible. The muscle is also active during deep sudden inspiration.

Just visible beneath the platysma muscle are the external jugular and anterior jugular veins (see page 348).

On removing the platysma muscle, the prominent structure seen is the sternocleidomastoid muscle.

THE STERNOCLEIDOMASTOID MUSCLE (10.5, 10.6)

The sternocleidomastoid muscle lies on the side of the neck. It is enclosed by the investing layer of deep cervical fascia which splits to pass round it. The muscle is an important landmark in the neck because many of the structures seen in both superficial and deep dissections can be directly related to it.

The sternocleidomastoid muscle forms the boundary demarcating regions termed the anterior and posterior triangles of the neck. On its superficial surface lie the external jugular vein, the superficial cervical chain of lymph nodes and, emerging from behind its posterior margin, the cutaneous nerves from the cervical plexus. At the root of the neck, sternocleidomastoid is covered by the platysma muscle. Near its insertion, it is covered by the parotid gland. Beneath the sternocleidomastoid muscle are the great vessels of the neck (accompanied by the vagus nerve) within the carotid sheath. The deep cervical chain of lymph nodes, the cervical plexus, the ansa cervicalis, the upper part of the brachial plexus, and the phrenic nerve are also located beneath the muscle. Near its origin, the sternocleidomastoid muscle overlaps the infrahyoid (strap) musculature.

Attachments: The sternocleidomastoid muscle arises by two heads. The sternal head is tendinous and attached to the anterior surface of the manubrium sterni. The clavicular head is a wide muscular head arising from the upper surface of the medial third of the clavicle. The two heads merge and the muscle passes upwards, laterally and posteriorly to insert onto the lateral surface of the mastoid process of the temporal bone and the adjacent part of the superior nuchal line.

Innervation: The spinal part of the accessory nerve supplies the muscle and passes through or deep to it to emerge into the posterior triangle of the neck on its way to the trapezius muscle. The sensory innervation concerned with proprioception is associated with the cervical plexus. Indeed, even its motor supply may be derived in part from this plexus.

Vasculature: Sternocleidomastoid receives its blood supply from branches of the superior thyroid, occipital, posterior auricular and suprascapular arteries.

Actions: These vary according to whether one or both sternocleidomastoid muscles are activated. When one muscle acts, the head is tipped towards the shoulder on the same side and is rotated to direct the face towards the opposite side. When the muscles act together, the head is moved forwards. The muscles may be involved in forced expiration.

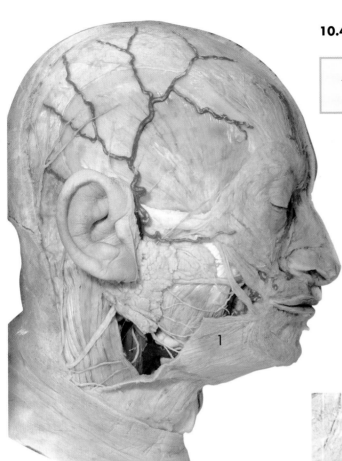

10.4 Platysma muscle

1	Platysma muscle

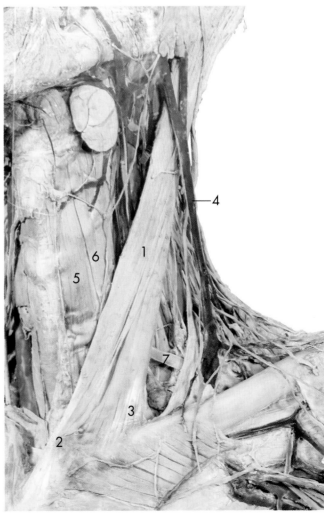

10.5 Anterior view of the neck showing the sternocleidomastoid muscle

1 Sternocleidomastoid muscle
2 Sternal head
3 Clavicular head
4 External jugular vein
5 Sternohyoid muscle
6 Omohyoid muscle (superior belly)
7 Omohyoid muscle (inferior belly)

The superficial regions of the neck anteriorly and laterally are divided for descriptive purposes into anterior and posterior triangles. The structure delineating these triangles is the sternocleidomastoid muscle. The suboccipital triangle at the back of the neck is considered with the deep dissection of the neck (see page 348).

THE ANTERIOR TRIANGLE OF THE NECK (10.6, 10.7)

This region is bounded posteriorly by the anterior margin of the sternocleidomastoid muscle, anteriorly by the median line of the neck, and superiorly by the inferior border of the mandible and the mastoid process. The sternum marks the apex of the triangle.

The anterior triangle can be subdivided in two ways. Firstly, there are the suprahyoid and infrahyoid areas above and below the hyoid bone. Secondly, the passage of the digastric and omohyoid muscles across the anterior triangle defines the digastric, submental, muscular and carotid triangles.

The *digastric triangle* is also referred to as the submandibular triangle. Indeed, the most prominent structure within it is the submandibular salivary gland. The digastric triangle is bounded by the anterior and posterior bellies of the digastric muscle and by the lower border of the mandible. Its floor is formed by the mylohyoid, hyoglossus, and middle constrictor muscles. The digastric triangle contains the submandibular gland and lymph nodes, the facial, submental and mylohyoid blood vessels, and the mylohyoid, hypoglossal and glossopharyngeal nerves. The glossopharyngeal nerve lies on the stylopharyngeus muscle. The carotid sheath and the lower part of the parotid gland just appear in the posterior region of the triangle.

The *submental triangles* lie above the hyoid bone, between the two anterior bellies of the digastric muscles as they approach the chin. The floor is formed by the mylohyoid muscle. The submental triangles contain the submental lymph nodes and the anterior jugular veins.

The structures within the digastric and submental triangles are considered later with the floor of the mouth (see Chapter 5).

The digastric muscle (10.6–10.8)

Attachments: The digastric muscle consists of an anterior belly and a posterior belly connected by an intermediate tendon. The posterior belly arises from the mastoid (or digastric) notch immediately behind the mastoid process of the temporal bone. The posterior belly passes downwards and forwards towards the hyoid bone where it becomes the digastric tendon. The tendon passes through the insertion of the stylohyoid muscle and is attached to the greater horn of the hyoid bone by a fibrous loop. The anterior belly of the digastric muscle is attached to the digastric fossa on the inferior border of the mandible beneath the chin and runs downwards and backwards to the digastric tendon.

10.6 Lateral view of the neck showing the boundaries of the anterior triangle

1 Lower border of the mandible
2 Anterior belly of digastric muscle
3 Posterior belly of the digastric muscle
4 Submandibular gland
5 Sternohyoid muscle
6 Superior belly of omohyoid muscle
7 Sternocleidomastoid muscle

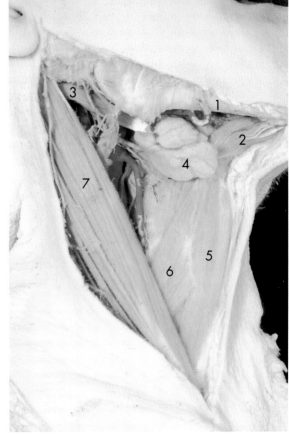

10.7 The anterior triangle between the sternocleidomastoid muscle and the midline of the neck is subdivided into the submental triangle (I), the digastric triangle (II), the muscular triangle (III), and the carotid triangle (IV). The posterior triangle between the sternocleidomastoid and trapezius muscles is subdivided into the occipital triangle (V), and the supraclavicular triangle (VI)

1 Omohyoid muscle (superior belly)
2 Digastric muscle
3 Sternocleidomastoid muscle
4 Trapezius muscle
5 Omohyoid muscle (inferior belly)

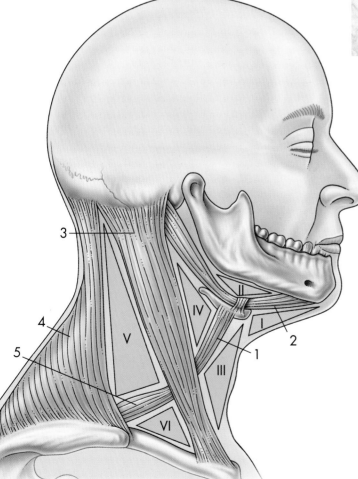

Innervation: Because the posterior belly of the digastric muscle develops from the second branchial arch of the fetus, its innervation is derived from the facial nerve (the digastric branch). The anterior belly develops from the first branchial arch and so receives its motor supply from the mandibular division of the trigeminal nerve (the mylohyoid branch).

Vasculature: The posterior belly obtains its arterial blood supply from the posterior auricular and occipital arteries. The anterior belly receives its blood supply from the facial artery (submental branch).

Actions: Although the digastric muscle helps to raise the hyoid bone and the base of the tongue and is involved in maintaining the stability of the hyoid bone, its prime function is to assist in depressing and retracting the mandible. Accompanying the posterior belly of the digastric is the stylohyoid muscle.

The stylohyoid muscle (10.8, 10.22)

Attachments: The muscle arises from the posterior surface of the base of the styloid process. It passes downwards and forwards with the posterior belly of the digastric to insert into the body of the hyoid bone at the junction with the greater horn (just above the attachment of omohyoid). Near its insertion it splits to envelop the digastric tendon.

Innervation: In common with the posterior belly of the digastric, the stylohyoid muscle develops from the second branchial arch. Consequently, it also is innervated by the facial nerve (digastric branch).

Vasculature: It receives its blood supply from the facial, posterior auricular, and occipital arteries.

Actions: It elevates and draws backwards the hyoid bone and therefore the floor of the mouth and the base of the tongue.

The digastric and stylohyoid muscles can be classified with the mylohyoid, geniohyoid, hyoglossus and genioglossus muscles as the suprahyoid musculature. These other muscles are described in relation to the floor of the mouth (see Chapter 5). The infrahyoid musculature lies within the muscular triangle of the neck.

The *muscular triangle* is bounded by the median line of the neck from the sternum to the hyoid bone, by the superior belly of the omohyoid muscle and by the anterior margin of the sternocleidomastoid muscle near its origin.

The muscular triangle contains the four infrahyoid muscles, the omohyoid, sternohyoid, sternothyroid and thyrohyoid muscles. The omohyoid and sternohyoid muscles are superficial; the sternothyroid and thyrohyoid muscles are deep. Because of their shape, these muscles are sometimes referred to as the strap muscles of the neck. As a group, they act to fix or to depress the hyoid bone and to elevate or to depress the larynx during swallowing.

The omohyoid muscle (10.9, 10.10)

Attachments: This muscle has superior and inferior bellies joined by an intermediate tendon. The superior belly of the omohyoid is attached to the lower border of the body of the hyoid bone. The inferior belly is attached to the upper border of the scapula (medial to the scapular notch). The superior belly runs down the anterior triangle of the neck whereas the inferior belly runs across the posterior triangle. Beneath the sternocleidomastoid muscle, the two bellies are connected by the intermediate tendon. Occasionally, however, there is no tendinous intersection. The intermediate tendon is attached to the clavicle and the first rib by a fibrous band which is derived from the deep cervical fascia. It is because of this fascial sling that the 'angulation' of the muscle is maintained.

Innervation: Both the superior and inferior bellies are supplied by branches from the ansa cervicalis (see page 364). However, the superior belly receives its innervation via the superior root (descendens hypoglossi) of the ansa.

Vasculature: Branches from the lingual and superior thyroid arteries supply the muscle.

Actions: The omohyoid muscle depresses the hyoid bone after it has been elevated. It also aids depression of the larynx.

10.8a Lateral view showing muscles of the neck

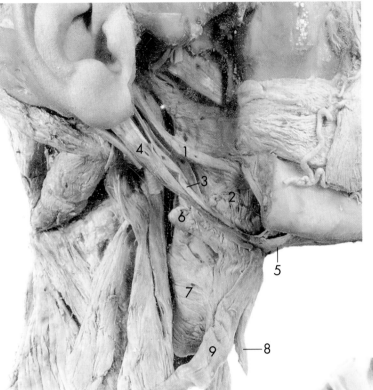

1	Styloglossus muscle
2	Hyoglossus muscle
3	Stylohyoid muscle
4	Posterior belly of digastric muscle
5	Anterior belly of digastric muscle
6	Greater horn of hyoid bone
7	Inferior constrictor muscle
8	Sternohyoid muscle (cut)
9	Superior belly omohyoid muscle
10	Inferior belly omohyoid muscle

10.8b Lateral view showing muscles of the neck

1	Posterior belly of digastric muscle
2	Tendon of digastric muscle
3	Anterior belly of digastric muscle
4	Superior belly of omohyoid muscle (reflected)
5	Sternohyoid muscle
6	Sternothyroid muscle
7	Thyrohyoid muscle
8	Superior thyroid artery
9	Common carotid artery
10	Scalenus anterior muscle
11	Phrenic nerve

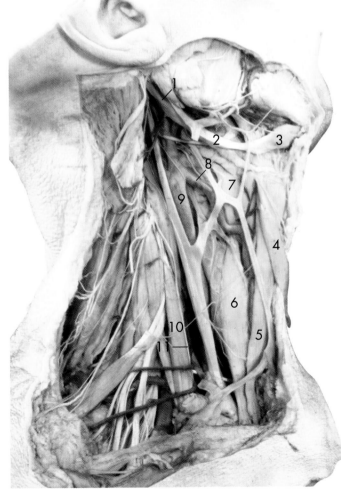

The sternohyoid muscle (10.8b, 10.9, 10.10, 10.25)

Attachments: This muscle originates mainly from the posterior surface of the manubrium sterni, but also arises from the head of the clavicle. It passes upwards and slightly medially to insert onto the inferior border of the body of the hyoid bone.

Innervation: The ansa cervicalis supplies the sternohyoid muscle.

Vasculature: Sternohyoid receives its blood supply from branches of the superior thyroid and lingual arteries.

Actions: The muscle depresses the hyoid bone after it has been elevated during swallowing.

The sternothyroid muscle (10.8b, 10.9, 10.25, 10.52b)

Attachments: Sternothyroid arises from the posterior surface of the manubrium sterni, below the attachment of the sternohyoid muscle. It passes upwards to insert onto the oblique line of the thyroid cartilage of the larynx.

Innervation: It is supplied by branches from the ansa cervicalis.

Vasculature: The blood supply of the muscle is derived from the superior thyroid artery.

Actions: From an elevated position during swallowing, the muscle depresses the larynx.

The thyrohyoid muscle (10.8b, 10.10, 10.51, 10.52)

Attachments: This muscle can be regarded as a continuation of the sternothyroid muscle. It passes upwards from the oblique line of the thyroid cartilage to the lower border of the body and the greater horn of the hyoid bone.

Innervation: Unlike the other infrahyoid muscles, the thyrohyoid muscle is not innervated by the ansa cervicalis. In common with the geniohyoid muscle, it is supplied by fibres from the first cervical nerve which pass with the hypoglossal nerve.

Vasculature: The arterial supply to the thyrohyoid muscle is derived from the superior thyroid artery.

Actions: The muscle depresses the hyoid bone or raises the larynx.

The *carotid triangle* is bounded by the upper part of the sternocleidomastoid muscle, the posterior belly of the digastric muscle and the superior belly of the omohyoid muscle. The floor of the triangle is formed by the thyrohyoid and hyoglossus muscles and by the inferior and middle constrictor muscles of the pharynx. The carotid triangle is so named because it contains the bifurcation of the common carotid artery and the superior thyroid, ascending pharyngeal, lingual, facial, and occipital branches of the external carotid artery. The veins in the triangle correspond to these branches. Also present are the hypoglossal nerve, the superior root of the ansa cervicalis (descendens hypoglossi) and the internal and external branches of the superior laryngeal nerve.

10.9 Anterior view of the neck showing strap muscles

1   Sternocleidomastoid muscle
2   Sternohyoid muscle
3   Superior belly of omohyoid muscle
4   Inferior belly of omohyoid muscle
5   Sternothyroid muscle
6   Superior thyroid artery
7   Common carotid artery
8   Thyroid cartilage
9   Anterior jugular vien
10 Trachea
11 Cricothyroid muscle

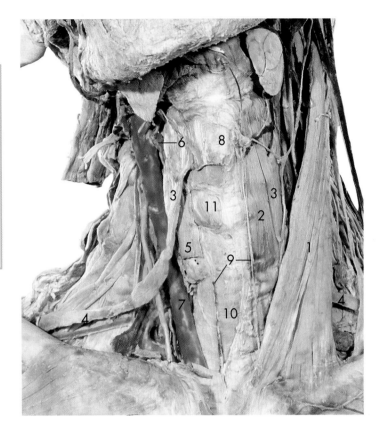

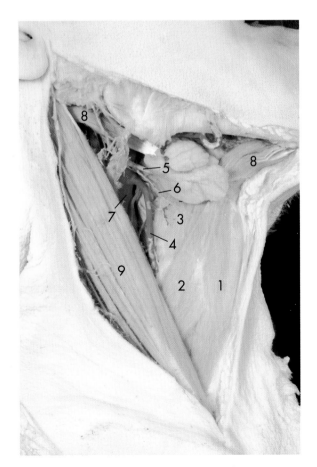

10.10 Laterial view of the neck showing strap muscles

1   Sternohyoid muscle
2   Superior belly of omohyoid muscle
3   Thyrohyoid muscle
4   Superior thyroid artery
5   Hypoglossal nerve
6   Nerve to thyrohyoid muscle
7   External carotid artery
8   Digastric muscle
9   Sternocleidomastoid muscle

THE POSTERIOR TRIANGLE OF THE NECK (10.11)

The posterior triangle is poorly named as the region lies on the lateral side of the neck. Furthermore, although diagrams of the triangle portray it as a flat region, in reality it 'spirals' around the side of the neck.

The posterior triangle is bounded in front by the posterior margin of the sternocleidomastoid muscle, behind by the anterior margin of the trapezius muscle and below by the middle third of the clavicle. The apex of the triangle is the mastoid process of the temporal bone. The floor of the triangle is formed by the prevertebral fascia which overlies semispinalis capitis, splenius capitis, levator scapulae and the scalenus posterior and medius muscles (these vertebral muscles are described on pages 376–383). The inferior belly of the omohyoid muscle crosses the posterior triangle and subdivides it into occipital and supraclavicular triangles. The roof of the posterior triangle is formed by the investing layer of deep cervical fascia.

The posterior triangle contains many important structures, particularly near its base.

The *occipital triangle* contains the occipital artery, the cutaneous branches from the cervical plexus, and the accessory nerve. The occipital artery emerges from under the splenius capitis muscle at the apex of the triangle and crosses semispinalis to penetrate the trapezius muscle. The lesser occipital nerve from the cervical plexus runs up the posterior border of the sternocleidomastoid muscle. The great auricular and transverse cervical nerves only just enter the posterior triangle, turning sharply around the posterior border of the sternocleidomastoid muscle. The supraclavicular nerves emerge from beneath the sternocleidomastoid and pass across and down the posterior triangle towards the clavicle. The accessory nerve (spinal part) also emerges from sternocleidomastoid into the posterior triangle. It runs obliquely downwards on the levator scapulae muscle to enter trapezius. The nerve is separated from levator scapulae by a distinct and dense layer of fascia.

The *supraclavicular triangle* contains the subclavian artery, part of the brachial plexus, the termination of the external jugular vein and the superficial cervical (transverse cervical) and suprascapular vessels. The subclavian artery in the posterior triangle is the third part of the artery after it has emerged from behind the scalenus anterior muscle (see page 390). The subclavian vein is not usually seen in the triangle, being behind the clavicle. The brachial plexus lies partly behind and partly above the subclavian artery. The superficial cervical and suprascapular vessels run across the superior margin of the clavicle. The external jugular vein is described on page 348.

The trapezius muscle (10.11, 10.12)

The trapezius muscle forms the posterior margin of the posterior triangle, although it is best considered as a muscle of the back. Because the trapezius shares its innervation with the sternocleidomastoid muscle, these two muscles are thought by some anatomists to be two parts of a single muscle which 'splits' to reveal the posterior triangle of the neck.

Attachments: Trapezius has an extensive origin from the midline of the back. It arises from the external occipital protuberance and the superior nuchal line at the back of the skull, and from the ligamentum nuchae, the spine of the seventh cervical vertebra and the spines of all the thoracic vertebrae. The superior fibres pass downwards, the middle fibres horizontally and the inferior fibres upwards to converge on the shoulder (the spine and acromion of the scapula) and the lateral third of the clavicle.

Innervation: It is supplied by the spinal part of the accessory nerve. It also receives branches from the cervical plexus which may be related to proprioception.

Vasculature: Its arterial supply is derived from the superficial cervical and the dorsal scapular arteries.

Actions: Trapezius is involved in controlling the position of the scapula but it can also elevate, rotate and retract the scapula when acting with other muscles. When the scapula is fixed, trapezius can move the head backwards and laterally.

10.11 Lateral view of the neck showing boundaries of the posterior triangle

1	Sternocleidomastoid muscle
2	Trapezius muscle
3	Splenius capitis muscle
4	Levator scapulae
5	Scalene muscles
6	Omohyoid muscle (inferior belly)
7	Great auricular nerve
8	Transverse cervical nerve
9	Supraclavicular nerves
10	Brachial plexus
11	Spinal accessory nerve

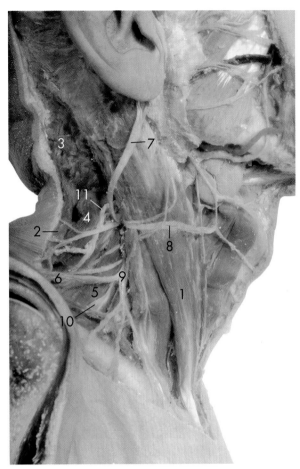

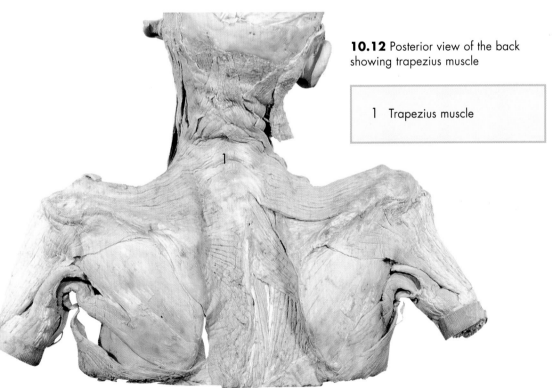

10.12 Posterior view of the back showing trapezius muscle

1	Trapezius muscle

DEEP STRUCTURES OF THE NECK (10.13)

This is a complex region which is often difficult to understand. However, it may be more easily understood by considering the disposition of structures in transverse section. This enables a division of the region into four compartments

- Two neurovascular compartments (i.e. carotid sheaths) containing many of the great vessels and nerves of the neck.

- A visceral compartment comprising the upper alimentary and respiratory passages, and some important glands.

- A musculoskeletal compartment around the cervical vertebral column.

In addition, deep dissection of the neck involves consideration of the root of the neck at the inlet of the thorax.

The four compartments comprising the deep region of the neck are related such that the musculoskeletal compartment provides a 'platform' posteriorly on which lie the neurovascular and visceral compartments. The compartments are bounded and defined by fascial layers.

THE FASCIA AND TISSUE SPACES OF THE NECK (10.13–10.19)

There has been much controversy concerning the definition of fascia. Some anatomists have applied the term to all layers of connective tissue which interconnect neighbouring structures. Others prefer to restrict the term to distinct membranous layers which can be incised and sutured. Such a definition has obvious clinical significance. Applying this definition to the fascia of the neck, three layers can be identified: the investing layer of deep cervical fascia, the prevertebral fascia and the pretracheal fascia. Nevertheless, the carotid sheath is one non-membranous layer usually described with the cervical fascia.

The investing layer of deep cervical fascia (10.13, 10.14)

This fascia is located just beneath the skin and is the most superficial of the true fascial layers of the neck. It completely encircles the neck like a surgical collar. At the front of the neck, however, the fascia is situated internal to the platysma muscles. As the fascia approaches the trapezius and sternocleidomastoid muscles, it splits to enclose them. The attachments of the investing layer of deep cervical fascia are:

- Posteriorly — the spines of the cervical vertebrae and the ligamentum nuchae.

- Superiorly — the external occipital protuberance and the superior nuchal lines at the back of the skull, the tip of the mastoid process, the lower border of the zygomatic arch, and the lower border of the mandible from the angle to the chin.

- Anteriorly — the chin, the body of the hyoid bone, and the manubrium sterni.

- Inferiorly — the sternum (where it splits into superficial and deep layers with the suprasternal space between), the clavicle (where it also splits into superficial and deep layers between the attachments of the trapezius and sternocleidomastoid muscles), and the acromion of the scapula.

Note that the attachments superiorly and inferiorly are related to the attachments of the trapezius and sternocleidomastoid muscles. Between the mastoid process and the angle of the mandible, the investing layer of deep cervical fascia splits into two layers to enclose the parotid gland, forming the parotid fascia. The superficial layer of the parotid fascia is attached to the tip of the mastoid process, the lower border of the cartilaginous part of the external acoustic meatus, and the lower border of the zygomatic arch. The deep layer extends along the base of the skull from the tip of the mastoid process towards the opening of the carotid canal where it merges with the fascia around the internal carotid artery. Part of the deep layer extends between the styloid process and the angle of the mandible as the stylomandibular ligament.

10.13 Transverse section of the neck below the hyoid bone to show the main layers of the cervical fascia

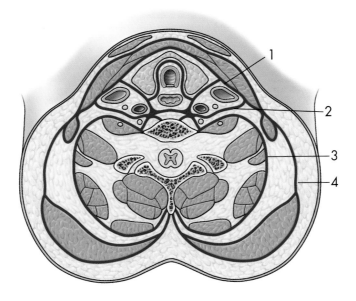

1 Petracheal fascia
2 Carotid sheath
3 Prevertebral fascia
4 Investigating layer of deep cervical fascia

The prevertebral fascia (10.13, 10.14)

This is the fascia which encloses the cervical part of the vertebral column and the prevertebral and postvertebral muscles (i.e. the musculoskeletal compartment). It is termed the prevertebral fascia because it is particularly prominent in front of the vertebral column. Indeed, here there may be two distinct layers. The prevertebral fascia forms the fascial floor of the posterior triangle of the neck. Its attachments are:

- Superiorly — the base of the skull in front of the longus capitis and rectus capitis lateralis muscles.

- Inferiorly — it extends into the thorax to merge with the anterior longitudinal ligament of the third thoracic vertebra at the lower limit of the longus cervicis muscle.

As the fascia passes around the musculoskeletal compartment of the neck, it attaches to the transverse and spinous processes of each cervical vertebra and to the ligamentum nuchae. However, the fascia becomes indistinct posteriorly and often merges with the investing layer of deep cervical fascia.

In the root of the neck, the prevertebral fascia covers the scalene muscles. As the subclavian artery and the nerves from the brachial plexus emerge from behind the scalenus anterior muscle, the prevertebral fascia forms the axillary sheath. This sheath invests the subclavian and axillary arteries but not the veins.

The prevertebral fascia provides a base upon which the pharynx, oesophagus and other cervical structures glide during swallowing and neck movements, undisturbed by movements of the prevertebral muscles.

The pretracheal fascia (10.13, 10.14)

This surrounds the viscera of the neck but is termed pretracheal because it is particularly prominent in front of the trachea. The attachments of the pretracheal fascia are:

- Superiorly — the larynx, being limited by the overlying infrahyoid musculature.

- Inferiorly — it extends into the superior mediastinum of the thorax along the great vessels to merge with the fibrous pericardium.

The pretracheal fascia merges laterally with the investing layer of deep cervical fascia and with the connective tissues comprising the carotid sheath.

The fascia forms a sheath around the thyroid gland.

The carotid sheath (10.13, 10.15)

Some anatomists recognise a distinct, but thin, fascial layer surrounding the carotid arteries (the common and internal carotids, but not the external carotid), the internal jugular vein, and the vagus nerve. The sheath is said to be attached superiorly to the base of the skull and inferiorly it merges with the connective tissue around the arch of the aorta. However, most reports suggest that the sheath may be nothing more than the merging of the adjacent investing cervical fascia, prevertebral fascia and pretracheal fascia.

The fascial layers of the neck define a number of tissue spaces. These spaces must be regarded only as 'potential spaces' and not as true anatomical entities. This is because in the healthy person the tissues are closely applied to each other or are filled with relatively loose connective tissue. Where there is pathological involvement, particularly with inflammation, this may spread through the tissue spaces, usually taking the line of least resistance. Conversely, the fascia can confine the spread of inflammation.

To aid description of the tissue spaces in the neck, we can distinguish spaces above and below the hyoid bone.

Above the hyoid bone are located the submandibular and submental spaces beneath the inferior border of the mandible, the pharyngeal spaces, and the prevertebral space near the base of the skull.

10.14 Diagram to illustrate the main laters of the cervical fascia in longitudinal section.

1 Investing layer of the deep cervical fascia
2 Petracheal fascia
3 Investing layer of the deep cervical fascia
4 Prevertebral fascia

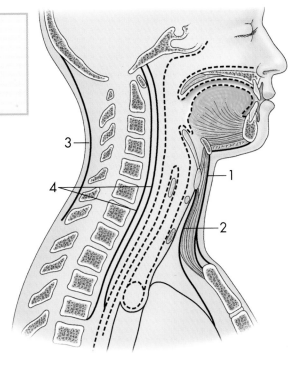

10.15 Section through the carotid sheath just below the base of the skull

I Anterior
II Lateral

1 Cervical sympathetic trunk
2 Vagus nerve
3 Internal carotid artery
4 Glossopharyngeal nerve
5 Carotid sheath
6 Accessory nerve
7 Internal jugular vein
8 Hypoglossal nerve

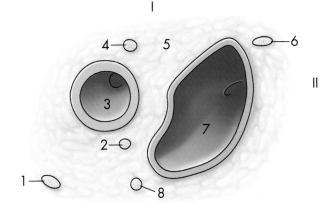

The submandibular and submental tissue spaces (10.16)

The submandibular space lies on the cervical surface of the mylohyoid muscle, between the anterior and posterior bellies of the digastric muscle. It is continuous with the sublingual tissue space in the floor of the mouth (see page 188) around the posterior free edge of the mylohyoid muscle. The submental space is situated below the chin and between the anterior bellies of the digastric muscles. There are effectively no barriers between the two submandibular spaces and the submental space. Consequently, infection can readily spread right across the neck below the inferior border of the mandible.

The pharyngeal tissue spaces (10.17–10.19)

The spaces related to the pharynx can be subdivided into the peripharyngeal and the intrapharyngeal spaces.

The anterior part of the peripharyngeal space is the submandibular and submental spaces described above. The posterior peripharyngeal space is termed the retropharyngeal space. Laterally are the parapharyngeal spaces.

The retropharyngeal space (10.49) is the area of loose connective tissue lying behind the pharynx and in front of the prevertebral fascia. It extends upwards to the base of the skull and downwards to the retrovisceral space in the infrahyoid part of the neck.

Each parapharyngeal space passes laterally around the pharynx and is continuous with the retropharyngeal space. Unlike the retropharyngeal space, however, it is a space which is retracted to the suprahyoid region. It contains loose connective tissue and is bounded medially by the pharynx and laterally by the pterygoid muscles (here being part of the infratemporal fossa) and the sheath of the parotid gland. Superiorly, it is bounded by the base of the skull. Inferiorly, it does not extend right down the neck but is limited by the suprahyoid structures, particularly the sheath of the submandibular gland. The parapharyngeal space is particularly prone to receiving infections spreading from the jaws and teeth. The subsequent spread of infection from the parapharyngeal space is into the retropharyngeal space.

An intrapharyngeal space potentially exists between the inner surface of the constrictor muscles of the pharynx and the pharyngeal mucosa. Infections at this site are either restricted locally or spread through the pharynx into the retropharyngeal or parapharyngeal spaces. An important part of the intrapharyngeal space is the peritonsillar space. This lies around the palatine tonsil between the pillars of the fauces. Infections here (quinsy) usually spread up or down the intrapharyngeal space, or through the pharynx into the parapharyngeal space.

The tissue spaces above the hyoid bone are discussed further with the spaces around the jaws (see pages 186–189). The prevertebral space is described with the tissue spaces in the infrahyoid region of the neck (see page 338).

10.16 Tissue spaces in the floor of the mouth; coronal section

1	Sublingual tissue space
2	Submandibular tissue space
3	Inferior border of mandible
4	Raphé between mylohyoid muscle
5	Anterior belly of digastric muscle
6	Mylohyoid muscle
7	Posterior free border of mylohyoid muscle (communication between the submandibular and sublingual spaces)
8	Body of the hyoid bone

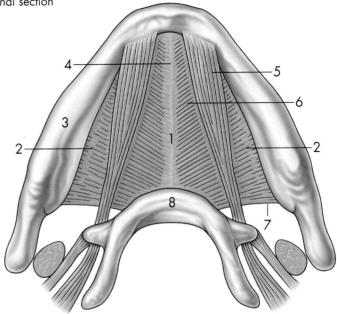

10.17 Tissue spaces in the retromandibular region

1	Fornix vestibuli
2	Peritonsillar space
3	Buccal space (filled with buccal pad of fat)
4	Submasseteric spaces
5	Pterygomandibular space
6	Parapharyngeal space
7	Parotid space
8	Buccinator muscle
9	Masseter muscle
10	Ramus of mandible
11	Superior constrictor of pharynx
12	Medial pterygoid muscle
13	Mylohyoid muscle

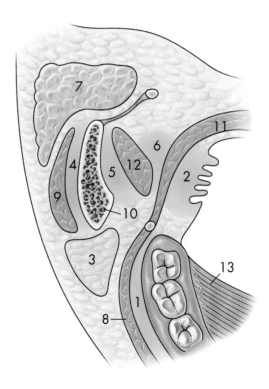

Below the hyoid bone are located the pretracheal and retrovisceral tissue spaces in the visceral compartment of the neck, the prevertebral space in front of the vertebral column, and a space associated with the carotid sheath. Although a tissue space may be expected between the pretracheal fascia and the investing layer of deep cervical fascia, the area is occupied by the infrahyoid (strap) musculature.

The pretracheal and retrovisceral tissue spaces (10.18, 10.19)

The pretracheal tissue space lies behind the pretracheal fascia and the infrahyoid (strap) muscles and in front of the anterior wall of the oesophagus. The space thus immediately surrounds the trachea. It is bounded superiorly by the attachments of the infrahyoid muscles to the thyroid cartilage of the larynx. Inferiorly, it extends down into the anterior portion of the superior mediastinum. Infection usually spreads into the pretracheal space either by perforating the anterior wall of the oesophagus or from the retrovisceral space.

The retrovisceral space is continuous superiorly with the retropharyngeal space. It is situated between the posterior wall of the oesophagus and the prevertebral fascia. Inferiorly, the retrovisceral space extends into the superior mediastinum. Should the prevertebral fascia merge with the connective tissue on the posterior surface of the oesophagus (usually at the level of the fourth thoracic vertebra), the retrovisceral space has a distinct inferior boundary.

The prevertebral tissue space (10.18, 10.19)

The prevertebral tissue space has been variously described. To some anatomists it is the potential space lying between the prevertebral fascia and the vertebral column. Others believe it to be the space between the two layers comprising the prevertebral fascia. Because the space is closed above, below and laterally, infection usually spreads into it through its fascial walls from the retrovisceral area. Inferiorly, the space extends into the posterior mediastinum.

The carotid sheath is, in reality, a layer of loose connective tissue demarcated by adjacent portions of the investing layer of deep cervical fascia, the pretracheal fascia, and the prevertebral fascia. Nevertheless, there is a potential space into which infections from the visceral spaces may track. However, it has been reported that infections around the carotid sheath are restricted because superiorly (near the hyoid bone) and inferiorly (near the root of the neck) the connective tissues adhere to the vessels.

THE GREAT VESSELS AND THE NERVES OF THE NECK

When the sternocleidomastoid muscle is removed, the major vessels and nerves in and around the carotid sheath are displayed. Within the carotid sheath are the common carotid/internal carotid arteries, the internal jugular vein, and the vagus nerve.

The carotid arteries (10.20–10.25)

There are three carotid arteries on each side of the neck, the common carotid, internal carotid, and external carotid arteries.

The carotid arteries provide the major source of blood to the head and neck. Additional arteries arise from branches of the subclavian artery in the neck — the vertebral artery, the thyrocervical trunk, and the costocervical trunk. These are described with the root of the neck (see pages 390–392).

10.18 Three of the tissue spaces of the neck seen in longitudinal section. Note that in this case the retrovisceral space is limited inferiorly by the merging of a later of prevertebral fascia with the oesophagus

1 Pretracheal space
2 Prevertebral space
3 Retrovisceral space

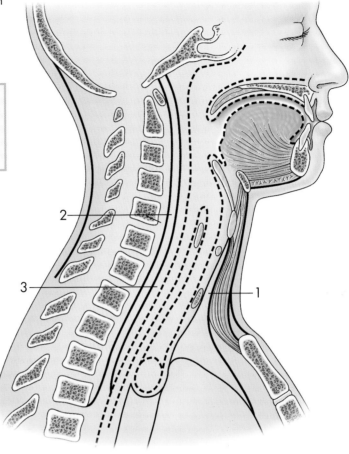

10.19 The tissue spaces of the neck below the hyoid bone, indicated by stippled regions

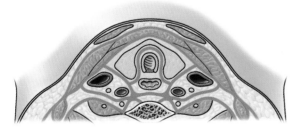

1 Pretracheal tissue space

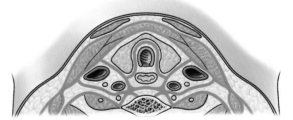

2 Retrovisceral tissue space

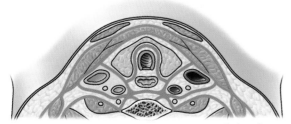

3 Tissue space associated with the carotid sheath

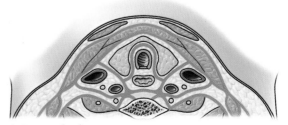

4 Prevertebral tissue space

The common carotid artery (10.20–10.23, 10.25)

The common carotid arteries differ on the right and left sides with respect to their origins. On the right, the common carotid arises from the brachiocephalic artery as it passes behind the sternoclavicular joint. On the left, the common carotid comes directly from the arch of the aorta in the superior mediastinum. The right common carotid has therefore only a cervical part whereas the left common carotid has cervical and thoracic parts. Both arteries terminate by bifurcating into the internal and external carotid arteries at the level of the upper border of the thyroid cartilage of the larynx.

The common carotid arteries usually have no branches.

Near its bifurcation, the common carotid shows two specialised organs, the carotid body and the carotid sinus. These relay information concerning the pressure and chemical composition of the arterial blood. The carotid body is a small, reddish-brown structure situated behind the bifurcation. It functions as a chemo-receptor. The carotid sinus is usually seen as a dilation of the lower end of the internal carotid. It functions as a baroreceptor. The main innervation to both the carotid body and the carotid sinus is derived from the carotid branch(es) of the glossopharyngeal nerve. The cervical sympathetic trunk and the vagus nerve also contribute.

Some of the relationships of the common carotid artery are illustrated in 10.31–10.33. In addition, the artery is crossed by the superior belly of the omohyoid, the superior and middle thyroid veins and the anterior jugular vein.

The internal carotid artery (10.21–10.24, 10.37, 10.51)

Following the bifurcation of the common carotid, the internal carotid continues up the neck within the carotid sheath. It leaves the neck by passing through the carotid canal at the base of the cranium and terminates intracranially.

Within the neck, the internal carotid artery usually has no branches. The branches of the artery within the carotid canal are the caroticotympanic and pterygoid arteries.

The external carotid artery (10.20–10.25, 10.37)

This is the component of the carotid system which lies outside the carotid sheath. From the bifurcation of the common carotid, the external carotid passes upwards, runs behind the posterior belly of the digastric muscle, crosses the styloglossus and stylopharyngeus muscles and passes into the parotid gland to divide into its terminal branches behind the condylar process of the mandible. The external carotid has eight branches:

- Superior thyroid artery
- Ascending pharyngeal artery
- Lingual artery
- Facial artery
- Occipital artery
- Posterior auricular artery
- Maxillary artery
- Superficial temporal artery

The *superior thyroid artery* is the first branch of the external carotid artery. It arises just below the greater horn of the hyoid bone. It runs downwards on the surface of the inferior constrictor muscle of the pharynx to the apex of the lobe of the thyroid gland. The external branch of the superior laryngeal nerve lies medial and usually behind the artery. Apart from its obvious supply to the upper part of the thyroid gland, the thyroid artery has branches supplying the sternocleidomastoid muscle, some of the infrahyoid (strap) muscles (infrahyoid branch) and the larynx (superior laryngeal and cricothyroid branches).

10.20 The arteries of the right side of the neck (excluding the ascending pharyngeal artery)

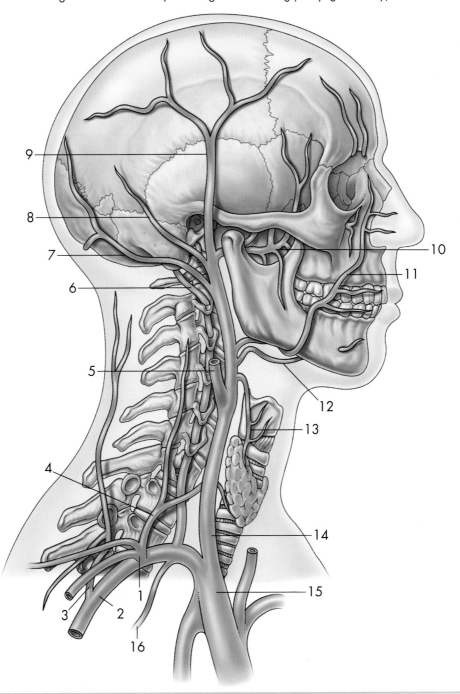

1 Thyrocervical trunk	9 Superficial temporal artery
2 Subclavian artery	10 Maxillary artery
3 Costocervical trunk	11 Facial artery
4 Inferior thyroid artery	12 Lingual artery
5 Internal carotid artery (cut)	13 Superior thyroid artery
6 Vertebral artery	14 Common carotid artery
7 Occipital artery	15 Brachiocephalic artery
8 Posterior auricular artery	16 Internal thoracic artery

10.21 Lateral view of the neck showing the course of the internal carotid artery

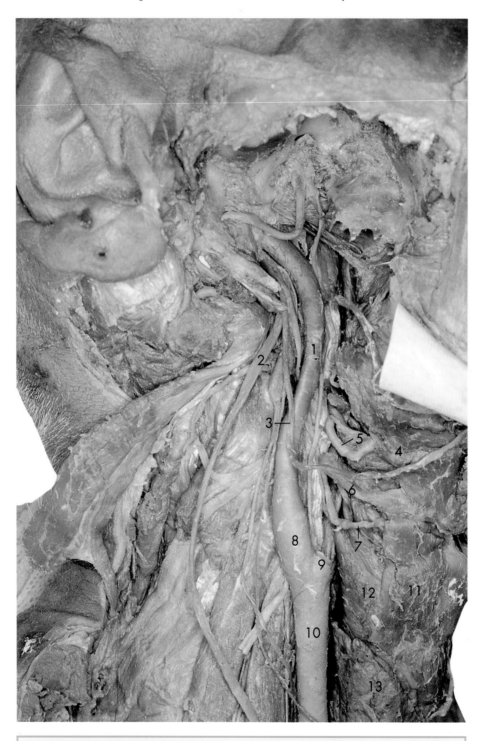

1	Internal carotid artery	8	Carotid sinus
2	Vagus nerve (displaced)	9	External carotid artery (cut end)
3	Hypoglossal nerve	10	Common carotid artery
4	Hyoglossus muscle	11	Thyrohyoid muscle
5	Lingual artery (cut end)	12	Inferior constrictor
6	Greater horn of hyoid bone	13	Thyroid gland
7	Internal laryngeal nerve		

10.22 Relations of the carotid arteries

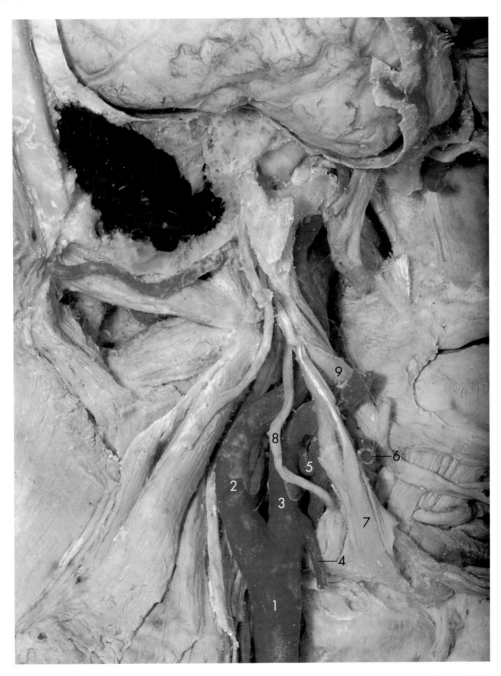

1 Common carotid artery	6 Facial artery
2 Internal carotid artery	7 Stylohyoid muscle
3 External carotid artery	8 Hypoglossal nerve
4 Superior thyroid artery	9 Styloglossus muscle
5 Lingual artery	

The *ascending pharyngeal artery* is the smallest branch of the external carotid. It arises from the posterior surface of the carotid artery, passing vertically upwards towards the pharynx. It terminates near the base of the skull. Its main branches are pharyngeal (to the muscles of the pharynx and the palate), inferior tympanic (to the middle ear), and meningeal (branches passing through the hypoglossal canal and the foramen lacerum). It also supplies some prevertebral muscles.

The *lingual artery* arises from the anterior surface of the external carotid, just above the superior thyroid artery. Near the tip of the greater horn of the hyoid bone, the artery shows a distinct loop which is related to the hypoglossal nerve. The lingual artery passes through the carotid triangle of the neck and then beneath the hyoglossus muscle to enter the tongue. Here it terminates as the deep lingual artery. Other branches are the infrahyoid artery (to the omohyoid and sternohyoid muscles) and the sublingual artery (to the sublingual gland and the floor of the mouth).

The *facial artery* also arises from the anterior surface of the external carotid. It passes forwards and upwards, deep to the digastric muscle, to enter the digastric triangle of the neck. Here, it comes into contact with the submandibular gland and weaves in and out beneath the inferior border of the mandible before crossing onto the face at the anterior edge of the masseter muscle. Its subsequent course and distribution is described in relation to the face (see page 118). In the neck, it gives off the following branches: ascending palatine artery, tonsillar artery, branches to the submandibular gland, and the submental artery to the suprahyoid muscles.

The *occipital artery* arises from the posterior surface of the external carotid, at the same level as the facial artery. It runs backwards across the carotid sheath where the hypoglossal nerve hooks around it. The occipital artery then runs upwards and backwards towards the suboccipital region of the scalp. It has branches supplying the sternocleidomastoid, digastric and stylohyoid muscles, the muscles of the suboccipital triangle, some of the prevertebral and postvertebral muscles, the mastoid air cells and the auricle. There is also a stylomastoid artery (in 66% of cases), a descending branch which anastomoses with the superficial cervical, vertebral and deep cervical arteries, and meningeal branches which pass through the jugular foramen and the condylar canal. Occipital branches are the terminal parts to the scalp.

The *posterior auricular artery* also arises from the posterior surface of the external carotid, but at the level of the upper border of the digastric muscle. It passes through the apical part of the parotid gland, along the styloid process to a groove between the auricle of the ear and the mastoid process. It gives muscular branches to the digastric, stylohyoid and sternocleidomastoid muscles, glandular branches to the parotid, a stylomastoid artery (in 33% of cases, see occipital artery above), an auricular branch and an occipital branch to the scalp.

The terminal branches of the external carotid artery, the *superficial temporal and maxillary arteries*, arise in the parotid gland. The superficial temporal artery is described in relation to the face (see page 120) and the maxillary artery in relation to the infratemporal fossa (see page 144) and nose (see page 218).

There are many important relationships of structures, particularly nerves, with the carotid arteries.

10.23 Lateral view of the neck showing distribution of the external carotid artery

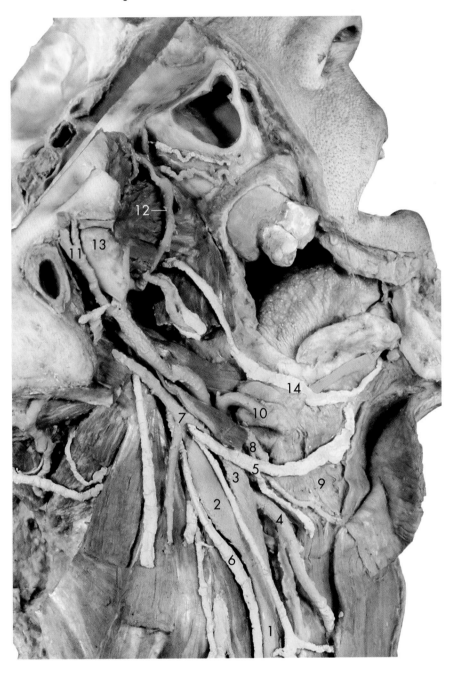

1 Common carotid artery	8 Lingual artery with branch to strap muscles
2 Internal carotid artery	9 Hyoglossus muscle
3 External carotid artery	10 Facial artery (cut end)
4 Superior thyroid gland	11 Superficial temporal artery
5 Hypoglossal nerve with branch to thyrohyoid muscle	12 Maxillary artery
6 Vagus nerve	13 Condyle of mandible
7 Occipital artery with branch to sternocleidomastoid muscle	14 Lingual nerve crossing submandibular duct (green)

The jugular veins (10.25, 10.26)

The veins in the neck show considerable variation, in terms both of size and connections. Most of the veins in the head and neck drain into the two major venous structures in the neck — the internal and external jugular veins.

The internal jugular vein (10.15, 10.25, 10.32, 10.35)

This vessel is found in the deep part of the neck, running with the carotid system of arteries in the carotid sheath. It thus lies deep to the sternocleidomastoid muscle. The vein extends from the base of the skull down to the thoracic inlet where it terminates by joining with the subclavian vein to form the brachiocephalic vein. At the base of the skull, the internal jugular vein emerges through the jugular foramen as a continuation of the sigmoid dural sinus.

Near the origin of the internal jugular vein is a dilation, the superior bulb. Another dilatation is found near its termination, the inferior bulb. Just above the inferior bulb is a pair of valves.

Tributaries include:

- Inferior petrosal dural sinus

- Facial vein

- Lingual veins

- Pharyngeal veins

- Superior and middle thyroid veins

The *inferior petrosal sinus* leaves the skull through the jugular foramen and joins the internal jugular at the superior bulb.

The *facial vein* (10.26) crosses the inferior border of the mandible where it meets the anterior branch of the retromandibular vein as it emerges from the parotid gland. Some anatomists call the vessel the common facial vein beyond this point. The vein then passes across the lingual artery, the hypoglossal nerve and the external and internal carotids to enter the internal jugular at the level of the greater horn of the hyoid bone.

The *lingual veins* are variable, but they usually follow two routes. The dorsal lingual vein drains the dorsum of the tongue and passes with the lingual artery deep to the hyoglossus muscle. It joins the internal jugular vein at the level of the greater horn of the hyoid. The deep lingual vein is seen through the mucosa of the ventral surface of the tongue. It joins the sublingual vein to become the vein accompanying the hypoglossal nerve on the hyoglossus muscle. This terminates by either joining the lingual vein or by draining directly into the internal jugular vein.

The *pharyngeal veins* arise from the pharyngeal plexus of veins. They drain generally into the internal jugular vein but may also pass into the inferior thyroid veins. Tributaries include meningeal vessels and the vein passing through the pterygoid canal.

The *superior thyroid vein* (10.25) accompanies the superior thyroid artery. It receives not only veins from the thyroid gland but also the superior laryngeal and cricothyroid veins associated with the larynx.

The *middle thyroid vein* receives blood from the lower part of the thyroid gland.

10.24 The relationships of the nerves to the internal and external carotid arteries

1 Superior thyroid artery
2 Lingual artery
3 Pharyngeal branch of vagus nerve
4 Facial artery
5 Posterior auricular artery
6 Stylopharyngeus muscle
7 External carotid artery
8 Internal carotid artery
9 Accessory nerve
10 Glossopharyngeal nerve
11 Occipital artery
12 Superior laryngeal branch of vagus nerve
13 Hypoglossal nerve
14 Ascending pharyngeal artery
15 Descendens cervicalis nerve
16 Descendens hypoglossi nerve
17 Vagus nerve

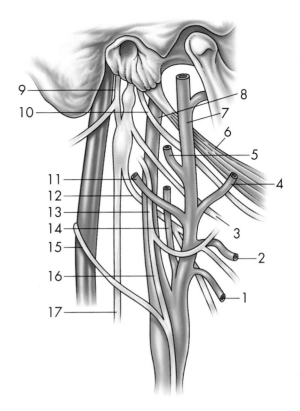

10.25 Anterior view of the neck showing the course of the internal jugular vein

1 Anterior jugular vein
2 Sternohyoid muscle
3 Superior belly of omohyoid muscle
4 Sternothyroid muscle
5 Common carotid artery
6 Superior thyroid vein
7 Descendens hypoglossi nerve
8 Internal jugular vein
9 Descendens cervicalis nerve
10 Ansa cervicalis
11 Reflected sternocleidomastoid muscle
12 Phrenic nerve on scalenus anterior muscle

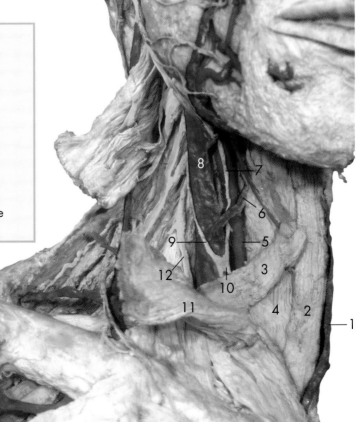

The external jugular vein (10.26)

This vein lies superficially in the neck, on the lateral surface of the sternocleidomastoid muscle. It passes from its origin near the apex of the parotid salivary gland down to its termination just in front of the scalenus anterior muscle in the posterior triangle.

The external jugular vein arises by the confluence of the posterior branch of the retromandibular vein and the posterior auricular vein. It drains into the subclavian vein as it crosses scalenus anterior. The external jugular has two sets of valves, one pair where it drains into the subclavian vein and another pair 4 cm above the clavicle. Close to its origin may be found a communicating vessel with the internal jugular vein.

On the sternocleidomastoid muscle, the external jugular lies between the investing layer of deep cervical fascia and the platysma muscle. It passes into the posterior triangle after piercing the deep cervical fascia.

Tributaries include:

- Occipital vein

- Posterior external jugular vein

- Superficial cervical vein

- Suprascapular vein

- Anterior jugular vein

The *occipital vein* is very variable. It may also be a tributary of the internal jugular vein, the posterior auricular vein, or the deep cervical and vertebral veins. It begins at the back of the scalp where it may be joined by a vein draining the diploe in the occipital bone. A parietal emissary vein links the occipital vein to the superior sagittal sinus. A mastoid emissary vein connects the occipital vein with the sigmoid sinus.

The *posterior external jugular vein* also arises in the occipital region. It drains the back of the upper part of the neck and terminates at the middle of the external jugular.

The *superficial cervical and suprascapular veins* accompany the arteries of the same name. They may drain directly into the subclavian vein (10.26).

The anterior jugular vein (10.9, 10.25, 10.26)

This vein returns blood from the front of the neck. It usually arises by the confluence of veins in the submandibular region, but may also receive veins from the retromandibular, facial or parotid veins. It passes down the neck, just to one side of the midline. Above the sternum, the two anterior jugular veins are united by the jugular arch. The anterior jugular vein then curves laterally beneath the sternocleidomastoid muscle to drain into the external jugular or subclavian veins.

The nerves of the neck

Within the carotid sheath runs the vagus nerve. Related to the carotid sheath near the base of the skull are the glossopharyngeal, accessory and hypoglossal nerves. Lying behind the carotid sheath and in front of the prevertebral fascia is the cervical sympathetic trunk. Deep to the internal jugular vein and in front of the scalenus medius and levator scapulae muscles (at the level of the first four cervical vertebrae) lies the cervical plexus of nerves. Associated with the cervical plexus is the ansa cervicalis. The brachial plexus for the arm lies in the deep part of the posterior triangle in the root of the neck. Both the cervical and brachial plexuses are derived from the ventral rami of cervical spinal nerves. The cutaneous contributions of the dorsal rami have already been described (see page 320).

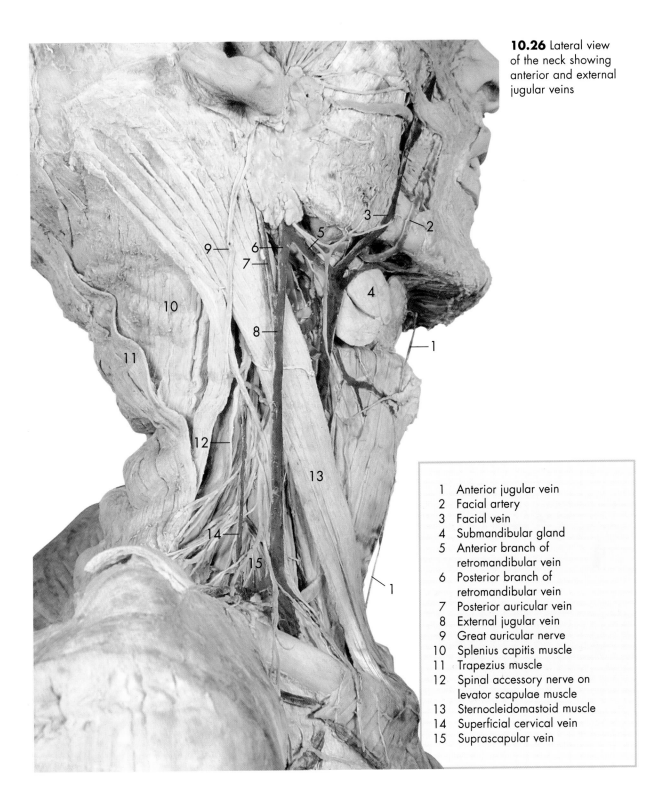

10.26 Lateral view of the neck showing anterior and external jugular veins

1	Anterior jugular vein
2	Facial artery
3	Facial vein
4	Submandibular gland
5	Anterior branch of retromandibular vein
6	Posterior branch of retromandibular vein
7	Posterior auricular vein
8	External jugular vein
9	Great auricular nerve
10	Splenius capitis muscle
11	Trapezius muscle
12	Spinal accessory nerve on levator scapulae muscle
13	Sternocleidomastoid muscle
14	Superficial cervical vein
15	Suprascapular vein

The glossopharyngeal nerve (10.27–10.29, 10.37)

This is the ninth cranial nerve. It emerges from the medulla oblongata of the brain stem as three or four rootlets. These rootlets are found in a groove between the olive and the inferior cerebellar peduncle. At this site, the glossopharyngeal nerve lies above the rootlets of the vagus nerve. The glossopharyngeal nerve has sensory, motor and parasympathetic fibres.

The glossopharyngeal nerve leaves the skull through the central part of the jugular foramen. Within the foramen, the nerve shows the superior and inferior ganglia. Below the foramen, the glossopharyngeal nerve is located anterior to the vagus and accessory nerves, passing between the internal jugular vein and the internal carotid artery. It then runs anteriorly between the internal and external carotid arteries and onto the stylopharyngeus muscle. Winding around this muscle, it passes between the superior and middle constrictor muscles of the pharynx to be distributed to the tonsil, pharynx, and tongue.

Branches include:

- Tympanic nerve

- Lesser petrosal nerve

- Carotid branch

- Pharyngeal branches

- Stylopharyngeus (muscular) branch

- Tonsillar branches

- Lingual branches

The *tympanic nerve* arises from the inferior ganglion. It passes upwards through the tympanic canaliculus to reach the middle ear cavity. Here, it contributes to the tympanic plexus which is found on the promontory of the medial wall of the tympanic cavity. This plexus provides sensory fibres to the mucosa of the tympanic cavity, the auditory tube and the mastoid air cells. From the plexus arises the lesser petrosal nerve.

The *lesser petrosal nerve* contains preganglionic parasympathetic fibres which relay through the otic ganglion to the parotid salivary gland. The nerve passes from the tympanic plexus, through the anterior wall of the tympanic cavity and onto the floor of the middle cranial fossa. It then emerges through the foramen ovale to join the otic ganglion in the infratemporal fossa (see page 142).

The *carotid branch(es)* arises just below the skull, as the glossopharyngeal crosses the internal carotid artery. It then passes between the internal and the external carotid arteries to the carotid sinus and the carotid body. During its course it is joined by the carotid branch of the vagus nerve.

The *pharyngeal branches* contribute to the pharyngeal plexus on the middle constrictor muscle (the other components of this plexus being from the sympathetic trunk and the pharyngeal branch of the vagus). The glossopharyngeal contribution to the plexus is sensory to the pharynx.

The *stylopharyngeus branch* supplies the stylopharyngeus muscle (the nerve and muscle being associated embryologically with the third branchial arch).

The *tonsillar branches* supply the palatine tonsil. They form a plexus with the lesser palatine nerve. Branches from the plexus are distributed to the soft palate.

There are two *lingual branches* of the glossopharyngeal nerve. One branch supplies the region around the sulcus terminalis of the tongue, including the circumvallate papillae. The other branch supplies the posterior third of the tongue. The lingual branches are concerned with both taste perception and general sensation.

10.27 The glosspharyngeal nerve

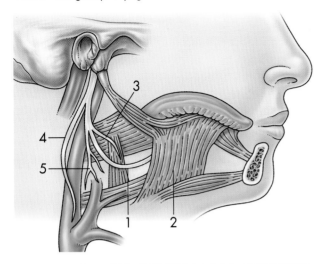

1 Branch to tongue
2 Hyoglossus muscle
3 Branch to stylopharyngeus muscle
4 Carotid branch
5 Branch to pharynx

10.28 Lateral view of the neck showing distribution of glossopharyngeal and vagus nerves

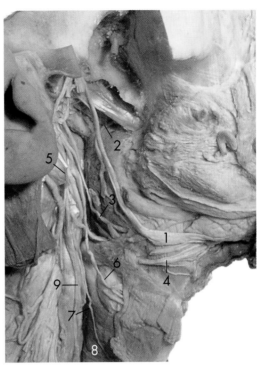

1 Lingual nerve
2 Ascending palatine artery on superior constrictor muscle
3 Glossopharyngeal nerve
4 Hypoglossal nerve
5 Superior laryngeal nerve
6 Internal laryngeal nerve
7 External laryngeal nerve
8 Inferior constrictor muscle
9 Vagus nerve

10.29 Lateral view of the neck showing glossopharyngeal nerve

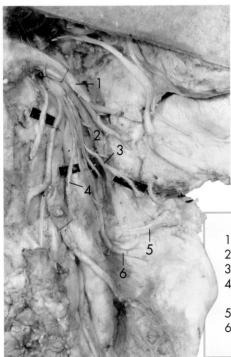

1 Styloid process
2 Stylopharyngeus muscle
3 Glossopharyngeal nerve
4 Branches of glossopharyngeal nerve to carotid body and sinus
5 Hyoid bone
6 Internal laryngeal nerve

The vagus nerve (10.28, 10.30–10.33, 10.51–10.53)
The vagus nerve is the tenth cranial nerve. It has the most extensive distribution of any of the cranial nerves and contains sensory, motor and parasympathetic fibres.

The vagus emerges from the brain stem at the medulla oblongata, between the olive and the inferior cerebellar peduncle. It exits the cranium through the jugular foramen with the glosso-pharyngeal and accessory nerves.

The vagus nerve has two ganglia, the superior and inferior ganglia. The superior ganglion lies within the jugular foramen. The inferior ganglion is situated just below.

Just below the inferior ganglion, the vagus is joined by the cranial part of the accessory nerve. The vagus then passes downwards within the carotid sheath and enters the thorax at the root of the neck.

The vagus nerves in the neck differ in one important respect, namely the origins of the recurrent laryngeal nerves.

Branches include:

- Meningeal branch

- Auricular branch

- Pharyngeal branch

- Branches to the carotid body

- Superior laryngeal nerve

- Recurrent laryngeal (right) nerve

- Cardiac branches

The *meningeal branch(es)* arises from the superior ganglion in the jugular fossa. It supplies dura in the posterior cranial fossa. There is some evidence that this nerve is not truly a branch of the vagus but is derived from upper cervical nerves and/or the superior cervical sympathetic ganglion.

The *auricular branch* also arises from the superior ganglion. It enters the temporal bone via the mastoid canaliculus on the lateral wall of the jugular fossa. It then passes out through the tympanomastoid fissure and divides into two branches. One branch joins the posterior auricular branch of the facial nerve, the other contributes to the innervation of the skin of the auricle, external acoustic meatus and tympanic membrane (see pages 294–296).

The *pharyngeal branch* is, in fact, derived from the cranial part of the accessory nerve. It runs from the inferior ganglion of the vagus, between the internal and external carotid arteries, and towards the middle constrictor of the pharynx. There it forms the pharyngeal plexus with branches from the sympathetic trunk, and the glossopharyngeal and external laryngeal nerves. The pharyngeal nerve is the main motor nerve to the muscles of the pharynx and palate.

Although the carotid body is supplied mainly by the glossopharyngeal nerve, the vagus nerve can also contribute.

The *superior laryngeal nerve* also arises from the inferior ganglion. It then passes deep to both the internal and external carotid arteries on its way to the larynx. It divides into internal and external branches. The internal branch passes between the middle and inferior constrictor muscles to supply sensation to the larynx. The external branch runs down on the inferior constrictor muscle (with the superior thyroid artery) to supply the cricothyroid muscle of the larynx.

The *right recurrent laryngeal nerve* arises in the root of the neck. It leaves the vagus in front of the subclavian artery, loops below and behind the artery and then ascends towards the larynx.

10.30 The right vagus nerve

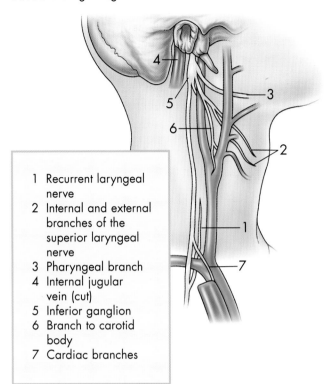

1 Recurrent laryngeal nerve
2 Internal and external branches of the superior laryngeal nerve
3 Pharyngeal branch
4 Internal jugular vein (cut)
5 Inferior ganglion
6 Branch to carotid body
7 Cardiac branches

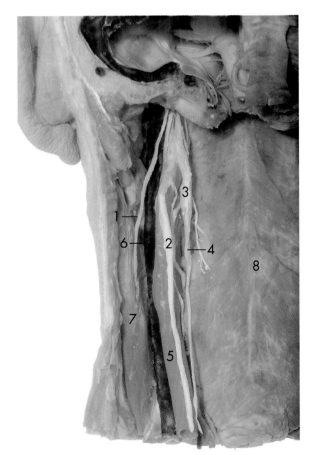

10.31 Front view of the neck showing vagus nerve

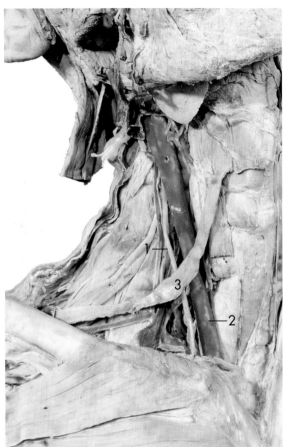

1 Vagus nerve
2 Common carotid artery
3 Omohyoid muscle

10.32 Neck viewed posteriorly showing lower cranial nerves and sympathetic trunk

1 Spinal accessory nerve
2 Vagus nerve
3 Superior sympathetic ganglion
4 Sympathetic trunk
5 Left common carotid artery
6 Internal jugular vein
7 Sternocleidomastoid muscle
8 Pharynx

The *left recurrent laryngeal nerve* arises in the thorax, as the vagus passes across the arch of the aorta. Both recurrent laryngeal nerves reach the larynx by passing upwards in grooves between the trachea and the oesophagus and they are closely related to the inferior thyroid arteries. They pass beneath the inferior borders of the inferior constrictor muscles to supply the mucosa of the larynx and most of the intrinsic muscles.

Usually two or three *cardiac branches* emanate from the vagus nerve in the neck. They run downwards and medially into the thorax, terminating at the deep part of the cardiac plexus.

The accessory nerve (10.11, 10.32, 10.34, 10.36)

This is the eleventh cranial nerve. It consists of two distinct parts, the cranial accessory and the spinal accessory nerves.

The *cranial part of the accessory nerve* is a motor nerve which emerges from the medulla oblongata between the olive and the inferior cerebellar peduncle. It joins the spinal part of the accessory at the jugular foramen. Once through the jugular foramen, the cranial and spinal parts again separate. The cranial part then joins the vagus nerve, eventually to be distributed in the pharyngeal branch of the vagus to the pharyngeal and palatine musculature. Some of its fibres also run with the recurrent laryngeal nerve and the cardiac branches of the vagus. Because of its close association with the vagus, some anatomists consider the cranial part of the accessory nerve to be a part of the vagus and not a separate cranial nerve.

The *spinal part of the accessory nerve* is also a motor nerve, although there may be some sensory fibres. It is derived from the upper five segments of the cervical spinal cord. A series of rootlets emerge from the cord between the dorsal and ventral roots of the upper cervical nerves. They join to form the main nerve trunk which passes intracranially through the foramen magnum. At the jugular foramen, the spinal and cranial parts of the accessory nerve unite but soon separate on exiting the cranium. The spinal part of the accessory nerve then crosses the internal jugular vein (usually on its lateral surface) and runs obliquely downwards and backwards to reach the upper part of the sternocleidomastoid muscle. It passes into the substance of this muscle and subsequently enters the posterior triangle of the neck. It crosses the posterior triangle on the levator scapulae muscle before entering the trapezius muscle. The spinal part of the accessory nerve provides the motor supply of the sternocleidomastoid and trapezius muscles.

10.33 Great vessels of the neck viewed posteriorly showing left recurrent laryngeal nerve

1 Inferior constrictor muscle
2 Oesophagus
3 Right common carotid artery
4 Thyroid gland
5 Right recurrent laryngeal nerve
6 Inferior thyroid artery
7 Left recurrent laryngeal nerve
8 Internal thoracic artery
9 Subclavian artery
10 Descending aorta
11 Vena azygos
12 Vagus nerve
13 Superior vena cava

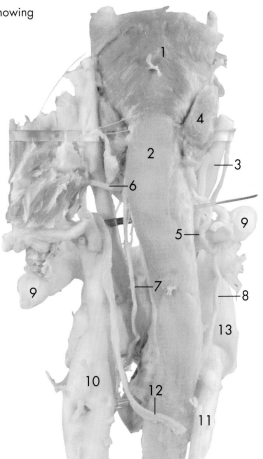

10.34 The accessory nerve. Note that its cranial root joins the inferior ganglion of the vagus nerve

1 Inferior ganglion of vagus nerve (receiving branch of accessory nerve)
2 Accessory nerve (cranial and spinal parts) emerging from jugular foramen
3 Internal jugular vein
4 Sternocleidomastoid muscle
5 Spinal part of accessory nerve
6 Trapezius muscle

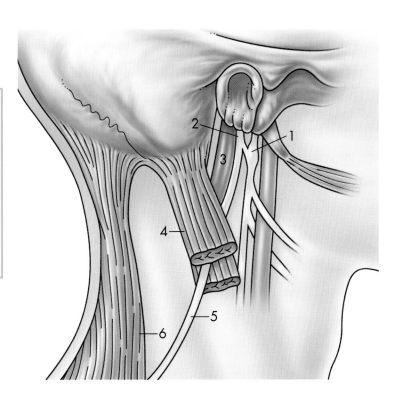

The hypoglossal nerve (5.14, 5.15, 10.35–10.37)

This is the twelfth cranial nerve and is a motor nerve supplying the musculature of the tongue. It originates as a series of rootlets on the medulla oblongata, between the pyramid and the olive.

The hypoglossal nerve runs through the hypoglossal canal of the occipital bone and emerges deep to the carotid sheath. It then passes downwards and, under cover of the posterior belly of the digastric muscle, outwards between the internal jugular vein and the internal carotid artery. Subsequently, it runs forwards across the vagus nerve and the external and internal carotid arteries. Indeed, it loops around the occipital artery near its origin (at its sternocleidomastoid branch). Continuing forwards, it passes below the submandibular salivary gland, onto the hyoglossus muscle to be distributed to the muscles of the tongue (see pages 166–168).

Like most cranial nerves, the hypoglossal nerve has connecting branches with other cranial and cervical spinal nerves and with the sympathetic system. An important connection is with the ventral ramus of the first cervical nerve.

Branches include:

- Meningeal branch

- Upper root of ansa cervicalis

- Muscular branches to thyrohyoid and geniohyoid

- Muscular branches to the tongue

The *meningeal branch* is probably derived from the upper cervical and sympathetic fibres which communicate with the hypoglossal. It appears as the hypoglossal nerve emerges through its canal in the occipital bone. It mainly supplies the dura in the posterior cranial fossa.

The *upper root of the ansa cervicalis* is also derived from the ventral ramus of the first cervical nerve. This branch first appears as the hypoglossal nerve loops around the occipital artery. It passes down on the carotid sheath covering the carotid arteries and is joined by the lower root of the ansa cervicalis from the cervical plexus to form the ansa cervicalis. The upper root of the ansa cervicalis gives a branch to the superior belly of the omohyoid muscle.

The *muscular branches supplying the thyrohyoid and geniohyoid muscles* are also derived from the first cervical spinal nerve. The nerve to thyrohyoid arises as the hypoglossal nerve reaches the hyoglossus muscle. The nerve to geniohyoid is given off in the floor of the mouth, above the mylohyoid muscle.

The *branches to the tongue musculature* are the only true branches of the hypoglossal nerve. They are distributed to the intrinsic muscles of the tongue and to the styloglossus, hyoglossus and genioglossus muscles.

10.35 The hypoglossal nerve

1 Omohyoid muscle
2 Common carotid artery
3 Internal jugular vein
4 Descendens cervicalis nerve
5 Descendens hypoglossi nerve
6 Sternocleidomastoid branch of occipital artery
7 Hypoglossal nerve
8 Digastric muscle (posterior belly)
9 Branch to geniohyoid muscle
10 Hypoglossal nerve on hyoglossus muscle
11 Branch to thyrohyoid muscle
12 Sternohyoid muscle

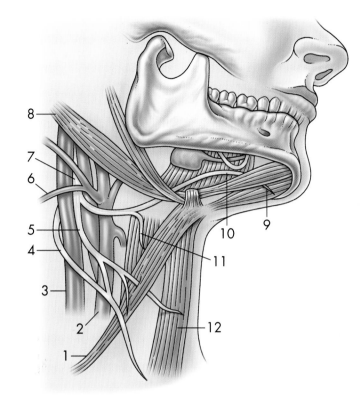

10.36 Lateral view of the face showing initial pathway of hypoglossal nerve

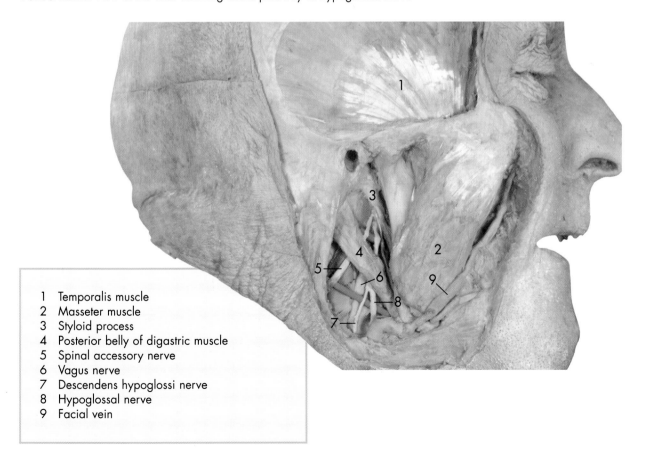

1 Temporalis muscle
2 Masseter muscle
3 Styloid process
4 Posterior belly of digastric muscle
5 Spinal accessory nerve
6 Vagus nerve
7 Descendens hypoglossi nerve
8 Hypoglossal nerve
9 Facial vein

The cervical sympathetic trunk (10.32, 10.37–10.39)

The sympathetic outflow for all parts of the body is derived principally from the thoracic spinal cord (segments T1 to L2). These preganglionic fibres then pass into the sympathetic trunk via the spinal nerves as white rami communicantes. Here, they may synapse at a ganglion or they pass up or down the sympathetic trunk to a ganglion at a different level. In this manner the cervical part of the sympathetic trunk receives its preganglionic fibres from the upper thoracic nerves.

The cervical sympathetic trunk exhibits a variable number of ganglia (usually between two and four). The ganglia are designated according to their position (superior, middle, inferior etc.).

The *superior cervical ganglion* lies at the level of the second and third cervical vertebrae. It is situated behind the carotid sheath on the longus capitis muscle (a prevertebral muscle). It is the largest of the cervical sympathetic ganglia and is believed to represent the coalescence of four ganglia which correspond with the upper four cervical spinal nerves.

The branches from the superior cervical ganglion are variable, but can be broadly classified into lateral, medial and anterior groups.

The lateral branches include the grey rami communicantes to the upper four cervical spinal nerves. In addition, there are branches which communicate with some of the cranial nerves: to the inferior ganglion of the glossopharyngeal nerve, to both ganglia of the vagus nerve, and to the hypoglossal nerve. The nerve which joins the glossopharyngeal and vagus nerves is termed the jugular nerve. The lateral branches of the superior cervical ganglion also include nerves to the superior jugular bulb and to the meninges of the posterior cranial fossa.

There are two medial branches of the superior cervical sympathetic ganglion. There is a laryngo-pharyngeal branch which supplies the carotid body and the pharyngeal plexus, and a cardiac branch.

The anterior branches pass onto the common and external carotid arteries to form plexuses. In addition to supplying the blood vessels, the plexus around the facial branch of the external carotid provides the sympathetic supply to the submandibular parasympathetic ganglion (see page 182). The plexus around the middle meningeal artery (a branch of the maxillary artery from the external carotid) serves the otic parasympathetic ganglion (see page 126).

Emerging above the superior ganglion is the internal carotid nerve. This nerve may be thought of as the cranial part of the sympathetic system. It passes with the internal carotid artery into the carotid canal. Within the canal, it forms the internal carotid plexus around the internal carotid artery.

10.37 Lateral view of the neck showing the course and relations of the cervical sympathetic chain

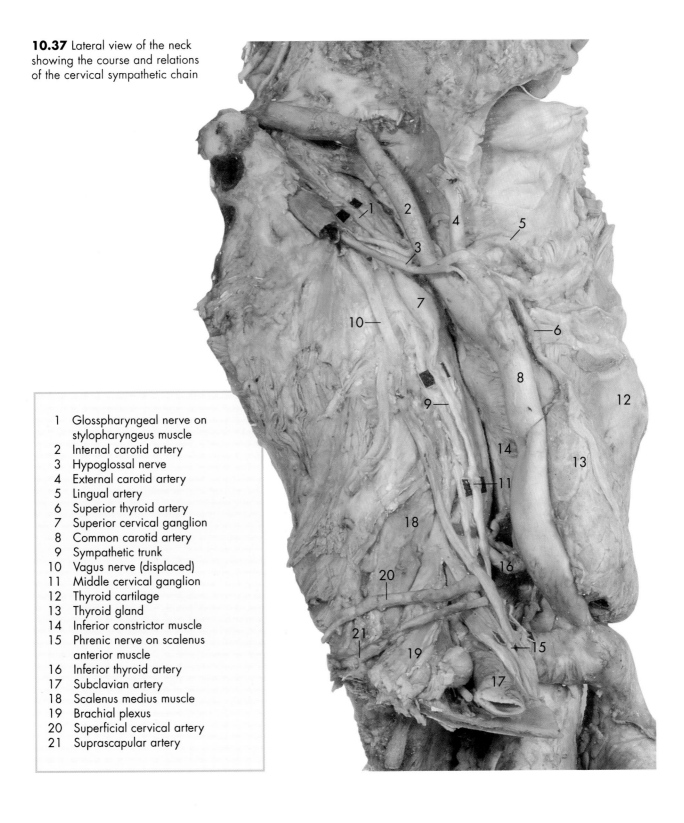

1   Glosspharyngeal nerve on stylopharyngeus muscle
2   Internal carotid artery
3   Hypoglossal nerve
4   External carotid artery
5   Lingual artery
6   Superior thyroid artery
7   Superior cervical ganglion
8   Common carotid artery
9   Sympathetic trunk
10 Vagus nerve (displaced)
11 Middle cervical ganglion
12 Thyroid cartilage
13 Thyroid gland
14 Inferior constrictor muscle
15 Phrenic nerve on scalenus anterior muscle
16 Inferior thyroid artery
17 Subclavian artery
18 Scalenus medius muscle
19 Brachial plexus
20 Superficial cervical artery
21 Suprascapular artery

The *internal carotid plexus* can be divided into two parts, lateral and medial.

The lateral part gives branches which communicate with the trigeminal and abducent cranial nerves. Superior and inferior caroticotympanic nerves traverse the posterior wall of the carotid canal to communicate with the tympanic branch of the glossopharyngeal nerve. An important branch is the deep petrosal nerve. This nerve is destined for the pterygopalatine ganglion (see page 216). It passes through the foramen lacerum and, joining the greater petrosal branch of the facial nerve, becomes the nerve of the pterygoid canal.

The medial part of the internal carotid plexus supplies the internal carotid artery itself and communicates with the oculomotor, trochlear, ophthalmic division of the trigeminal and the abducent cranial nerves. Branches also pass through the superior orbital fissure to the ciliary ganglion in the orbit (see page 260). These branches subsequently run with the short ciliary nerves to be distributed to the blood vessels of the eyeball. The fibres to the dilator pupillae travel by a different course (via the ophthalmic, nasociliary and then the long ciliary nerves). The terminal branches of the internal carotid plexus form plexuses around the ophthalmic artery and the anterior and middle cerebral arteries of the brain, passing eventually to the pia mater.

The *middle cervical ganglion* is usually situated at the level of the sixth cervical vertebra. It is the smallest cervical ganglion and is occasionally absent. It may fuse with the superior cervical ganglion. The middle ganglion lies close to the inferior thyroid artery just before it enters the gland. Some claim that it represents the coalescence of two ganglia which correspond with the fifth and sixth cervical segments.

Branches from the middle cervical ganglion communicate with the fifth and sixth cervical spinal nerves (also sometimes the fourth and seventh). Two distinct cords pass down to the inferior cervical/cervicothoracic sympathetic ganglion. The anterior cord loops in front and below the subclavian artery as the ansa subclavia. The posterior cord encloses the vertebral artery. The middle cervical ganglion also sends branches to the thyroid gland (along the inferior thyroid artery), to the heart via its cardiac branches, and to the trachea and oesophagus.

An occasional ganglion known as the vertebral ganglion may be found on the front of the vertebral artery. It can be considered as either a low middle cervical ganglion or as a detached part of the inferior ganglion. When present, it gives rise to the ansa subclavia.

The *inferior cervical ganglion* often combines with the first thoracic ganglion to form the cervicothoracic ganglion (stellate ganglion). The inferior cervical ganglion (or upper end of the cervicothoracic ganglion) is situated just posterior to the vertebral artery. The lower end of a cervicothoracic ganglion lies behind the subclavian artery on the first thoracic vertebra.

Branches from the inferior cervical ganglion pass to the seventh and eighth cervical nerves and to the first thoracic nerve. There are also cardiac branches and fibres which form plexuses around the subclavian artery and its derivatives. Around the vertebral artery is a plexus which continues up into the skull. This plexus eventually meets the plexus around the internal carotid artery. Some anatomists believe this to be the main intracranial extension of the sympathetic system.

10.38 The cervical sympathetic trunk

1 Inferior cervical ganglion
2 Vertebral ganglion
3 Middle cervical ganglion
4 Superior cervical ganglion
5 Longus colli muscle
6 Cervicothoracic ganglion

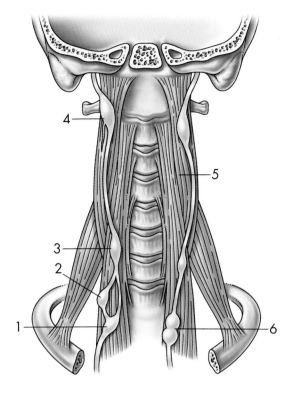

10.39 Front view of the neck showing ansa subclavia of the sympathetic trunk

1 Sternocleidomastoid muscle
2 Omohyoid muscle
3 Common carotid artery
4 Vagus nerve
5 Ansa subclavia on subclavian artery
6 Thyrocervical trunk
7 Inferior thyroid artery
8 Phrenic nerve on scalenus anterior
9 Brachial plexus

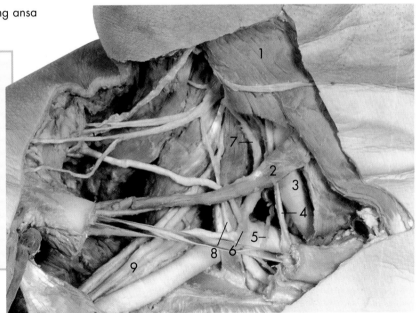

The cervical plexus (10.3, 10.40, 10.41)

This plexus lies deep to the sternocleidomastoid muscle and the internal jugular vein, and in front of the scalenus medius and levator scapulae muscles. It is formed by the ventral rami of the upper four cervical spinal nerves (i.e. C1, C2, C3, C4).

The cervical plexus contains both sensory and motor fibres. In addition, grey rami communicantes near the origins of the ventral rami of the cervical nerves supply sympathetic fibres.

Branches from the cervical plexus are distributed to some of the muscles of the neck, to the diaphragm, and to much of the skin of the back of the head, the neck, and the chest around the thoracic inlet. The cutaneous nerves are superficial, the muscular branches deep.

The cutaneous nerves from the cervical plexus are the lesser occipital (C2), great auricular (C2, C3), transverse cervical (C2, C3), and supraclavicular (C3, C4) nerves. These nerves are described on page 320.

The deep (mainly motor) branches can be subdivided into those which pass medially and those which pass laterally.

The medial branches supply the following muscles:

- Longus capitis (C1, C2, C3)
- Longus colli (C2, C3, C4)
- Rectus capitis anterior (C1, C2)
- Rectus capitis lateralis (C1)

Other medial branches are the inferior root of the ansa cervicalis (C2, C3) and the phrenic nerve (C3, C4, C5). Some branches also communicate with the hypoglossal and vagus nerves, and the sympathetic trunk.

The lateral branches supply the following muscles:

- Levator scapulae (C3, C4)
- Scalenus medius (C3, C4)
- Sternocleidomastoid (C2)
- Trapezius (C3, C4)

There is also a communicating branch to the accessory nerve (C2, C3, C4).

The *phrenic nerve* arises from the cervical plexus and usually takes fibres from the third, fourth and fifth cervical nerves (mainly from the fourth). It provides the motor nerve supply to the diaphragm.

The phrenic nerve in the neck passes downwards and medially on the superficial surface of the scalenus anterior muscle (10.39, 10.42). Here, it lies under cover of a layer of the prevertebral fascia. As it passes through the thoracic inlet, it runs behind the subclavian vein and in front of the subclavian artery and its internal thoracic branch.

Some of the roots may not join the main nerve trunk until just before leaving the neck. Such roots are called accessory phrenic nerves.

The phrenic nerve contains not only motor fibres but also proprioceptive fibres to the diaphragm and sensory fibres to the pleura and pericardium. Sympathetic fibres may join the phrenic nerve from cervical sympathetic ganglia.

The *branches to the hypoglossal nerve* from the cervical plexus arise mainly from the first cervical spinal nerve. These fibres leave the hypoglossal nerve as four distinct nerves: the meningeal branch of the hypoglossal nerve, the superior root of the ansa cervicalis, and the motor nerves to the thyrohyoid and the geniohyoid muscles. Some C1 fibres also travel with the vagus nerve, and indeed may form its meningeal branch.

10.40 The cervical plexus

1   Supraclavicular nerve (C3, C4)
2   Transverse cervical nerve (C2, C3)
3   Great auricular nerve (C2, C3)
4   Lesser occipital (C2)
5   Hypoglossal nerve
6   Nerve to thyrohyoid muscle
7   Descendens hypoglossi nerve
8   Descendens cervicalis nerve
9   Phrenic nerve

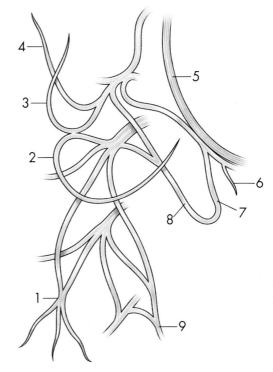

10.41 Lateral view of the neck showing the cervical plexus

1   Lesser occipital nerve
2   Great auricular nerve
3   Transverse cervical nerve
4   Supraclavicular nerves
5   Spinal accessory nerve on levator scapulae muscle

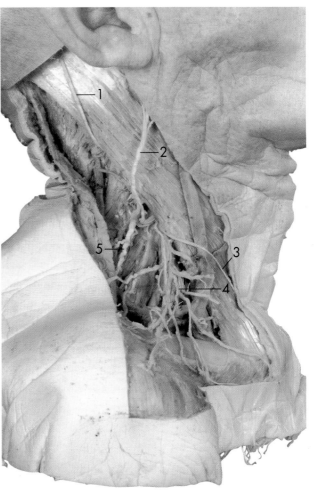

The *ansa cervicalis* is a nerve plexus located in front of the common carotid artery. It is formed by the union of two nerve trunks, the superior root of the ansa cervicalis from the hypoglossal nerve (conveying C1 fibres) and the inferior root of the ansa cervicalis from the cervical plexus (conveying C2 and C3 fibres). The superior root is also called the descendens hypoglossi, indicating its path from the hypoglossal nerve as it crosses the external carotid artery (see page 356). The inferior root may also be termed the descendens cervicalis. It usually appears lateral to the internal jugular vein, crossing the vein to join the superior root (10.25). Occasionally, the inferior root may run medial to the internal jugular vein.

The ansa cervicalis supplies all the infrahyoid muscles with the exception of the thyrohyoid muscle. The innervation of the superior belly of the omohyoid muscle is often given off from the superior root just before it reaches the ansa cervicalis.

The brachial plexus (10.39, 10.42, 10.43)
This plexus lies in the deep part of the posterior triangle of the neck, between the clavicle and the lower part of the posterior border of the sternocleido-mastoid muscle. It emerges between the scalenus anterior and scalenus medius muscles to pass between the clavicle and first rib, around the axillary artery and into the upper limb.

The brachial plexus is formed by the ventral rami of the fourth to the eighth cervical nerves and by most of the ventral ramus of the first thoracic nerve. The plexus provides the innervation for structures in the upper limb.

The branches arising from the brachial plexus above the clavicle in the neck are:

- Nerves to the scalene and longus colli muscles (C5, C6, C7, C8)

- Communicating branch to the phrenic nerve (C5)

- Dorsal scapular nerve to the rhomboid muscles (C5)

- Long thoracic nerve to serratus anterior muscle (C5, C6, C7)

- Nerve to the subclavius (C5, C6)

- Suprascapular nerve to the supraspinatus and infraspinatus muscles and to the shoulder joint (C5, C6)

Thus, the branches are mainly motor.

10.42 Front view of the neck showing the brachial plexus

1 Posterior belly of digastric muscle
2 Hypoglossal nerve
3 External carotid artery
4 Superior thyroid artery
5 Thyroid gland
6 Scalenus medius and posterior muscles
7 Spinal accessory nerve on levator scapulae muscle
8 Trapezius muscle
9 Brachial plexus
10 Phrenic nerve on scalenus anterior muscle
11 Subclavian artery
12 Internal thoracic artery (cut end)
13 Superficial cervical artery
14 Suprascapular artery
15 Trachea
16 Vagus nerve
17 Thoracic duct (cut end)

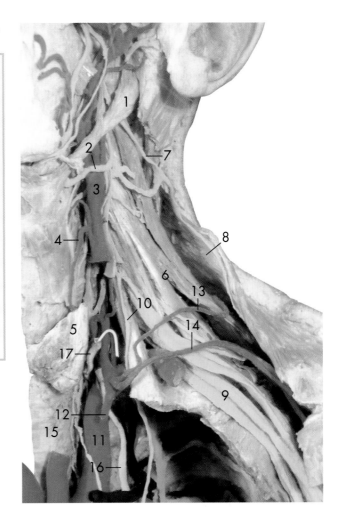

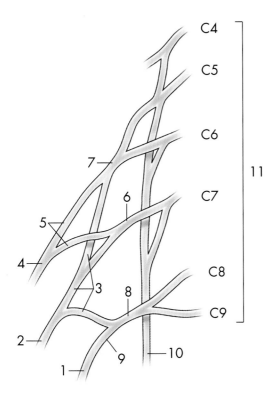

10.43 The brachial plexus

1 Medial cord
2 Posterior cord
3 Posterior divisions
4 Lateral cord
5 Anterior divisions
6 Middle trunk (C7)
7 Upper trunk (C5, C6)
8 Lower trunk (C8, T1)
9 Anterior division
10 Long thoracic nerve
11 Roots

The lymphatics of the neck (10.44)

The lymphatic system is very variable. It is composed of plexuses of small vessels, the lymph capillaries, which run into small masses of lymphoid tissue, the lymph nodes.

The lymph nodes in the neck can be categorised into superficial and deep lymph nodes. The superficial lymph nodes are the submental, submandibular, anterior cervical and superficial cervical nodes. The deep lymph nodes are the infrahyoid, prelaryngeal, pretracheal and paratracheal, retropharyngeal, and deep cervical lymph nodes.

The *submental nodes* lie beneath the chin, on the mylohyoid muscle and between the anterior bellies of the digastric muscles. They receive lymph vessels from the anterior part of the mandible, the lower lip and the tip of the tongue. Vessels from the submental nodes drain into either the jugulo-omohyoid group of the deep cervical nodes near the root of the neck or into the submandibular nodes.

The *submandibular nodes* are situated close to, or within, the submandibular salivary glands. The nodes receive vessels from many parts of the oral cavity and from the submental and, when present, the buccal and lingual nodes. Efferent vessels drain into the deep cervical nodes.

The *anterior cervical nodes* lie along the anterior jugular veins at the front of the neck. They drain lymph from the front of the neck below the hyoid bone. Vessels from the nodes pass to any of the deep lymph nodes in the neck.

The *superficial cervical nodes* are associated with the external jugular vein on the superficial surface of the sternocleidomastoid muscle. They receive vessels from around the lower part of the ear, the floor of the external acoustic meatus, the apical part of the parotid gland and the region around the angle of the mandible. The efferent vessels pass to the deep cervical nodes.

The *infrahyoid nodes* lie beneath the investing layer of deep cervical fascia on the thyrohyoid membrane.

Lymph vessels from the region of the epiglottis pass to these nodes. Vessels pass from this group to the deep cervical chain.

The *prelaryngeal nodes* lie on the anterior cricothyroid ligament and the cricovocal membrane of the larynx. The *pretracheal nodes* lie on the trachea close to the inferior thyroid veins. The *paratracheal nodes* are found in association with the recurrent laryngeal nerves, between the trachea and the oesophagus. The *retropharyngeal nodes* are situated between the back of the larynx and the prevertebral fascia. The prelaryngeal and pretracheal nodes receive vessels from the larynx below the vocal fold and from the trachea. The thyroid gland sends vessels to the prelaryngeal and tracheal nodes. The pharynx and oesophagus send vessels to the paratracheal and retropharyngeal nodes. Efferent vessels from all these nodes pass to the deep cervical chain of lymph nodes.

The *deep cervical lymph nodes* lie along the carotid sheath, deep to the sternocleidomastoid muscle. A prominent group of these nodes superiorly is located close to the digastric muscle, and is consequently designated the jugulo-digastric group of lymph nodes. Inferiorly, another prominent group lies close to the omohyoid muscle, the jugulo-omohyoid group. The upper deep cervical nodes (including the jugulo-digastric nodes) receive lymph vessels from the tongue, most of the nose, the air sinuses, the ear, the tonsil, the larynx above the vocal fold, the submandibular and parotid salivary glands, and from the retro-auricular and superficial lymph nodes. The lower deep cervical nodes receive vessels from all the other deep nodes of the neck, and from the submental, anterior and superficial cervical, and occipital lymph nodes.

From the deep cervical nodes, lymph is collected into the jugular trunk. The left jugular trunk drains into the thoracic duct (10.42, 10.71), although it may pass directly into the subclavian or internal jugular veins. The right jugular trunk drains directly into the right brachiocephalic vein at its origin or into the right lymphatic duct (this duct collects lymph from the right arm and the right half of the thorax and also drains into the right brachiocephalic vein).

10.44 The lymphatics of the neck. The nodes with the light shading are the superficial nodes; the nodes with the dark shading are deep nodes

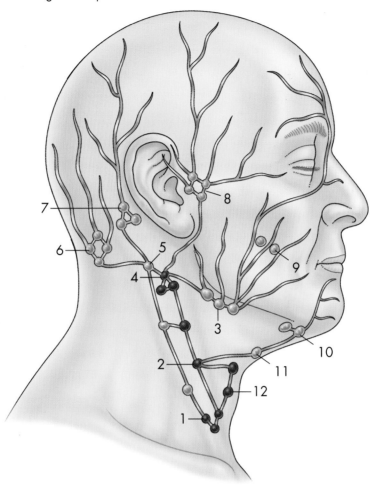

1 Jugulo-omohyoid nodes
2 Deep cervical nodes
3 Submandibular nodes
4 Jugulodigastric nodes
5 Superficial cervical nodes
6 Occipital nodes
7 Retro-auricular nodes
8 Parotid nodes
9 Buccal nodes
10 Submental nodes
11 Anterior cervical node
12 Tracheal node

THE VISCERA OF THE NECK

The visceral structures of the neck include the larynx and the trachea, the pharynx and the oesophagus, and the thyroid, parathyroid and cervical thymus glands.

The pharynx and larynx are described in Chapters 11 and 12 respectively.

The trachea (10.45–10.50, 10.65)

The trachea is part of the respiratory system and is a tube composed of cartilages and membranes.

The trachea begins at the lower border of the cricoid cartilage of the larynx, at the level of the sixth cervical vertebra. It extends down the neck along the median plane and through the thoracic inlet. It ends in the superior mediastinum by dividing into the right and left principal bronchi.

The patency of the trachea is maintained by a series of C-shaped rings of hyaline cartilage which are incomplete posteriorly. The cartilages are united by fibro-elastic membranes. Posteriorly, across the gap of each cartilage, is a thin coat of unstriated muscle (the trachealis muscle). Contraction of this muscle narrows the lumen of the trachea.

The relationships between the trachea and other cervical structures are of clinical importance, particularly as a tracheostomy is not an uncommon procedure. Anteriorly is situated the thyroid gland, the thyroid isthmus being at the level of the second to the fourth tracheal cartilages. Below the thyroid gland are the inferior thyroid veins, tracheal lymph nodes and occasionally a thyroidea ima artery. All these structures are covered by the infrahyoid muscles. Lateral to the trachea are the lobes of the thyroid gland and the carotid sheaths. Posteriorly, the trachea lies on the oesophagus. Posterolaterally are the recurrent laryngeal nerves. These lie in grooves between the sides of the trachea and the oesophagus.

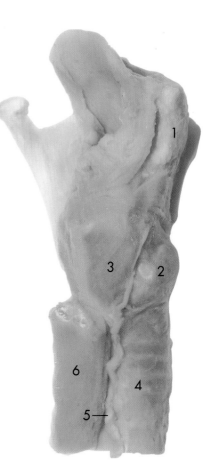

10.45 The trachea viewed laterally

1	Thyroid cartilage
2	Cricoid cartilage
3	Posterior cricoarytenoid muscle
4	Trachea
5	Recurrent laryngeal nerve
6	Oesophagus

10.46 Neck viewed anteriorly showing relations of trachea

1	Thyroid cartilage
2	Sternohyoid muscle
3	Omohyoid muscle
4	Sternothyroid muscle (cut end)
5	Cricothyroid muscle
6	Arch of cricoid cartilage
7	Common carotid artery
8	Thyroid gland remnant
9	Anterior jugular vein
10	Trachea
11	Sternocleidomastoid muscle

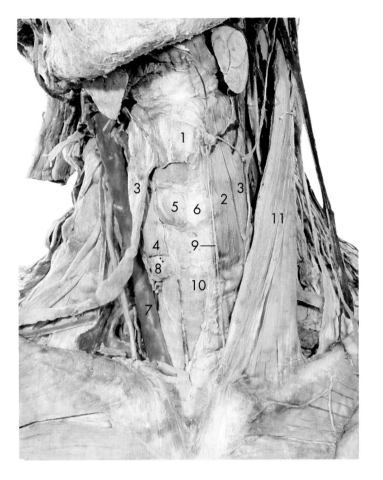

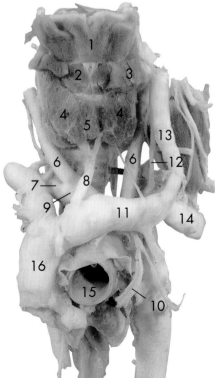

10.47 Front view showing relations of the trachea in root of the neck

1	Thyroid cartilage
2	Cricothyroid muscle
3	Insertion of sternothyroid muscle
4	Bilobed thyroid gland
5	Isthmus of thyroid gland
6	Common carotid artery
7	Subclavian artery (right)
8	Inferior thyroid vein
9	Brachiocephalic artery
10	Recurrent laryngeal nerve (left)
11	Brachiocephalic vein (left)
12	Vagus nerve (left)
13	Internal jugular vein
14	Subclavian vein
15	Aorta
16	Superior vena cava

The main blood supply to the cervical part of the trachea is derived from the inferior thyroid arteries. The veins drain into the bracheocephalic veins via the inferior thyroid plexus. Lymphatic vessels drain into the pretracheal and paratracheal nodes.

The nerve supply to the trachea arises from the vagi, recurrent laryngeal nerves, and sympathetic trunks.

The oesophagus (10.45, 10.49, 10.50, 10.65)
The oesophagus is the alimentary tube connecting the laryngopharynx to the stomach. It commences at the lower border of the cricoid cartilage. Here, the cricopharyngeal part of the inferior constrictor muscle of the pharynx acts as a sphincter.

The cervical part of the oesophagus takes a curved course down the median plane of the neck. It lies between the spine and the trachea. Anterolaterally are situated the lobes of the thyroid gland, the recurrent laryngeal nerves, the inferior thyroid arteries and the carotid sheaths.

The muscles within the cervical part of the oesophagus are arranged in inner and outer layers. The inner layer is circular and the outer layer is longitudinal. The circular musculature is continuous with the inferior constrictor of the pharynx.

The blood supply of the oesophagus in the neck is derived mainly from the inferior thyroid arteries. The veins drain into the brachiocephalic veins. Lymphatic vessels pass into retropharyngeal, paratracheal, or deep cervical lymph nodes.

The cervical part of the oesophagus is innervated by the recurrent laryngeal nerves and by the sympathetic plexus around the inferior thyroid artery.

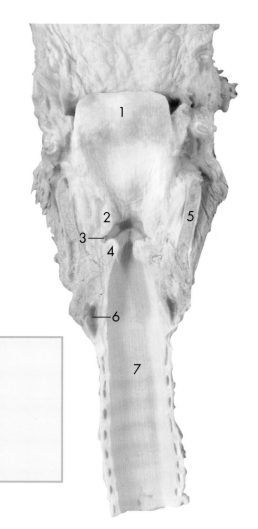

10.48 Anterior portion of the trachea

1	Epiglottis
2	Vestibular fold
3	Sinus of the larynx
4	Vocal fold
5	Lamina of thyroid cartilage
6	Arch of cricoid cartilage
7	Trachea

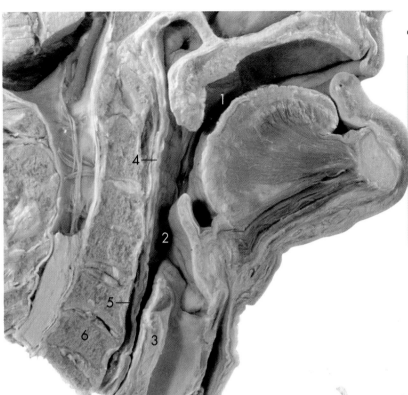

10.49 Sagittal sections of neck showing commencement of oesophagus

1 Oropharynx
2 Laryngopharynx
3 Lamina of cricoid cartilage
4 Wall of pharynx
5 Retropharyngeal space
6 Vertebral column
7 Commencement of trachea
8 Commencement of oesophagus

10.50 The oesophagus viewed posteriorly

1 Inferior constrictor muscle (thyropharyngeus)
2 Inferior constrictor muscle (cricopharyngeus)
3 Oesophagus
4 Trachea
5 Recurrent laryngeal nerve
6 Thyroid gland
7 Parathyroid glands
8 Common carotid artery
9 Inferior thyroid artery
10 Internal jugular vein

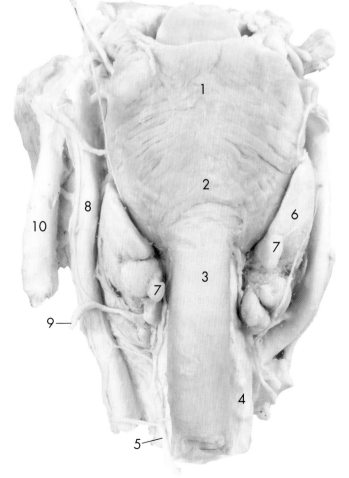

The thyroid gland (10.47, 10.50–10.54)

The thyroid gland is an endocrine gland situated in the front of the neck. It lies on the trachea and just above the thoracic inlet. The gland is closely related to the thyroid cartilage of the larynx and extends from the level of the fifth cervical vertebra to the first thoracic vertebra.

The gland consists of right and left lobes joined by an isthmus. The isthmus lies just below the cricoid cartilage on the second to the fourth tracheal rings. The isthmus is occasionally absent.

Each lobe of the thyroid gland is conical or pear-shaped and has a narrow apex and a broad base. The apex lies beneath the oblique line of the thyroid cartilage. The base lies at about the level of the fourth tracheal ring.

A process of thyroid tissue, termed the pyramidal process, often projects upwards from the isthmus. There may also be a fibrous or fibro-muscular structure called the levator glandulae thyroidae. This passes from the body of the hyoid bone to the isthmus or pyramidal process of the thyroid gland. When muscular, some anatomists believe the levator glandulae thyroidae to be a derivative of the infrahyoid musculature. It can be innervated either through the ansa cervicalis or through the vagus nerve (usually the superior laryngeal branch).

The thyroid gland is invested by a connective tissue capsule. This capsule has been variously described. Most accounts state that the gland has its own delicate perithyroid sheath which lies on the surface of the gland and which sends septa between the lobules. There is also a surrounding layer of pretracheal fascia. The gland is maintained in position by this fascia and by ligamentous bands (the lateral ligaments) which attach the gland on each side to the cricoid cartilage of the larynx.

Accessory (or ectopic) thyroid tissue can be found throughout the neck and even within the tongue. This reflects the fact that the thyroid gland develops at the tongue and migrates down the neck to its adult position.

The thyroid gland has many important relationships in the neck, and these have been described with the trachea and oesophagus (see pages 368–370). In addition, the parathyroid glands lie posteriorly.

The thyroid gland has a very rich blood supply derived from four main arteries, the two superior thyroid arteries and the two inferior thyroid arteries. There are considerable anastomoses between these vessels both ipsilaterally and contralaterally. The superior thyroid artery is the first branch of the external carotid artery. It descends to the apex of the lobe of the thyroid gland with the external branch of the superior laryngeal nerve. The superior thyroid artery pierces the thyroid fascia and then divides into anterior and posterior branches. The anterior branch supplies the anterior surface of the gland, the posterior branch supplies the lateral and medial surfaces. The inferior thyroid artery arises from the thyrocervical trunk of the subclavian artery in the root of the neck. As it approaches the base of the thyroid gland, the artery divides into superior (ascending) and inferior thyroid branches. These supply the inferior and posterior surfaces of the gland. The superior branch also supplies the parathyroid glands. The relationship between the inferior thyroid artery and the recurrent laryngeal nerve has clinical importance. The nerve initially lies in front of the artery but, near the thyroid gland, it usually passes behind the left inferior thyroid artery but may remain in front of the right inferior thyroid artery. An occasional artery to the thyroid gland is the thyroidea ima artery. This may arise either from the brachiocephalic artery, the right common carotid, or the arch of the aorta.

Figure 10.52a (opposite)
1 Epiglottis
2 Greater horn of hyoid bone
3 Lesser horn of hyoid bone
4 Body of hyoid bone
5 Thyrohyoid muscle
6 Cricothyroid muscle
7 Lobe of thyroid gland
8 Isthmus of thyroid gland
9 Levator glandulae thyroidea
10 Trachea

10.51 Lateral view of the neck showing some relations of the thyroid gland

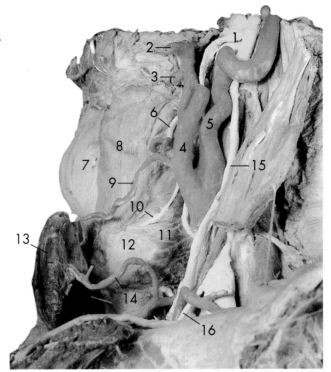

1	Superior laryngeal nerve
2	Facial artery
3	Lingual artery
4	External carotid artery
5	Internal carotid artery
6	Internal laryngeal nerve and laryngeal branch of superior thyroid artery
7	Thyroid cartilage
8	Thyrohyoid muscle
9	Superior thyroid artery
10	External laryngeal nerve
11	Inferior constrictor muscle
12	Cricothyroid muscle
13	Thyroid gland
14	Inferior thyroid artery
15	Vagus nerve
16	Phrenic nerve on scalenus anterior muscle

10.52a The thyroid gland viewed anteriorly

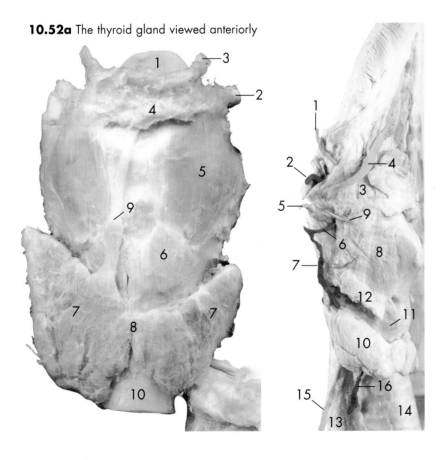

10.52b The thyroid gland veiwed laterally showing associated nerves and vessels

1	Glossopharyngeal nerve
2	Lingual artery (cut end)
3	Hyoglossus muscle
4	Hypoglossal nerve
5	Internal laryngeal nerve
6	Laryngeal branch of superior thyroid artery
7	Superior thyroid artery
8	Thyrohyoid muscle
9	Nerve to thyrohyoid muscle
10	Thyroid gland
11	Cricothyroid muscle
12	Sternothyroid muscle (cut end)
13	Trachea
14	Oesophagus
15	Recurrent laryngeal nerve
16	Laryngeal branch of inferior thyroid artery

The venous drainage of the thyroid gland is usually via superior, middle, and inferior thyroid veins. The superior thyroid vein emerges from the upper part of the gland and runs with the superior thyroid artery towards the carotid sheath. It drains into the internal jugular vein. The middle thyroid vein collects blood from the lower part of the gland. It emerges from the lateral surface of the gland and drains into the internal jugular vein. The inferior thyroid vein forms a plexus with the vein on the opposite side. This plexus is located below the thyroid gland and in front of the trachea. From the plexus, the left vein descends into the thorax to terminate at the left brachiocephalic vein. The right inferior thyroid vein drains into the right brachiocephalic vein. Alternatively, there may be a common trunk draining into the left brachiocephalic vein.

The lymphatics from the gland usually pass to the prelaryngeal and the tracheal nodes. They may also pass directly into the deep cervical nodes or into the thoracic duct or the right lymph duct.

The innervation of the thyroid gland is derived from the cervical sympathetic trunk.

The parathyroid glands (10.54)
There are usually four parathyroid glands, two on each side. They are small, spherical endocrine glands which are situated at the back of the thyroid gland. To indicate their relative positions, the glands are designated the superior and inferior parathyroid glands. Alternatively, they have been called parathyroid 3 and parathyroid 4 to indicate their embryological origins from the branchial pouches. The superior parathyroid glands are derived from the fourth pouches, the inferior glands from the third pouches.

The superior parathyroid glands are said to lie near the middle of the lobes of the thyroid gland. The positions of the inferior parathyroid glands are more variable. Indeed, evidence from dissection and surgery suggests that both sets of glands are so variable in location that a meaningful description of site is not possible. This also means that their relationship to the fascia surrounding the thyroid gland is variable. Nevertheless, the parathyroid glands are usually described as lying between the posterior surface of the thyroid gland and the thin capsule of the perithyroid sheath (lying within the pretracheal fascia).

The parathyroid glands receive a rich blood supply, usually from the inferior thyroid arteries. The veins drain into the thyroid veins. The lymphatic vessels pass with those from the thyroid gland. The nerve supply is derived from the cervical sympathetic trunks.

The thymus gland
This gland has an important role in the development of the lymphoid system. It is situated mainly in the thorax, although there are cervical extensions which may reach up in the midline as far as the base of the thyroid gland. The thymus gland has a flattened, bilobed appearance. Its size varies considerably with age. It increases in size until puberty but progressively diminishes thereafter to be eventually replaced by fat.

Accessory thymus tissue may be found in the neck. The inferior parathyroid glands may connect with the thymus by means of prominent strands of connective tissue. This may reflect the fact that both the thymus and the inferior parathyroid glands develop from the third branchial pouch.

The blood supply to the thymus gland is derived from the internal thoracic and inferior thyroid arteries. The venous drainage is via the internal thoracic, inferior thyroid, and left brachiocephalic veins. The lymphatic vessels drain into nodes within the thorax. The innervation of the thymus gland arises from the sympathetic system and the vagus nerves.

10.53 Lateral view of the thyroid gland showing part of the innervation and vasculature

1 Hypoglossal nerve
2 Lingual artery
3 Internal laryngeal nerve
4 External laryngeal nerve
5 Superior thyroid artery
6 Laryngeal branch of superior thyroid artery

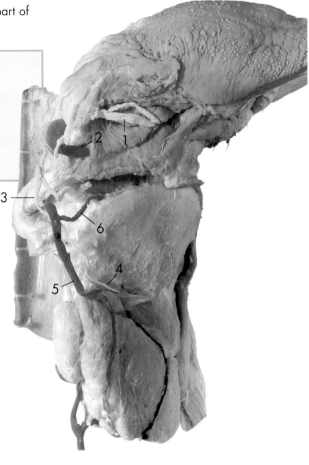

10.54 Posterior view of the thyroid gland showing parathyroid glands

1 Inferior constrictor muscle
2 Oesophagus
3 Trachea
4 Thyroid gland
5 Superior parathyroid gland
6 Inferior parathyroid gland

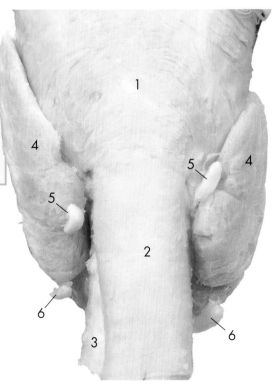

THE MUSCULOSKELETAL COMPARTMENT OF THE NECK

This compartment is composed of the cervical vertebral column (see Chapter 2) and the prevertebral muscles and postvertebral muscles. The region is ensheathed by layers of the prevertebral fascia (see page 334).

The prevertebral muscles

These muscles lie in front of the bodies of the cervical vertebrae and deep to the prevertebral fascia. All are essentially flexors of the head and neck. The anterior prevertebral muscles are longus colli, longus capitis, rectus capitis anterior and rectus capitis lateralis. The lateral prevertebral muscles are the scalene muscles (anterior, medius, posterior, and minimus) and levator scapulae.

Longus colli (10.55)

This muscle lies on the anterior surface of the vertebral column and extends from the first cervical vertebra to the third thoracic vertebra. It has three parts, superior oblique, inferior oblique and vertical parts.

Attachments: The superior oblique part arises from the transverse processes (anterior tubercles) of the third to the fifth cervical vertebrae. It passes upwards and medially to insert onto the anterior arch (anterior tubercle) of the first cervical vertebra.

The inferior oblique part originates from the bodies of the first to the third thoracic vertebrae. It passes up to the transverse processes (anterior tubercles) of the fifth and sixth cervical vertebrae.

The vertical part arises from the bodies of the upper three thoracic vertebrae and the lower three cervical vertebrae. It inserts onto the bodies of the second to the fourth cervical vertebrae.

Innervation: The motor supply of longus colli is derived from the ventral rami of the second to the eighth cervical spinal nerves.

Vasculature: Its arterial blood supply is derived from the ascending pharyngeal, inferior thyroid (ascending cervical branch) and vertebral arteries.

Actions: The longus colli muscles flex and assist in rotating the head and neck. Acting singly, the cervical vertebral column is flexed laterally.

Longus capitis

Attachments: This muscle arises from the transverse processes (anterior tubercles) of the third to the sixth cervical vertebrae. It inserts onto the basilar part of the occipital bone at the cranial base.

Innervation: Its motor innervation comes from the ventral rami of the first to the third cervical spinal nerves.

Vasculature: The blood supply to longus capitis is similar to that of longus colli, coming from the ascending pharyngeal, inferior thyroid and vertebral arteries.

Actions: It flexes the head.

Rectus capitis anterior (10.55)

Attachments: This muscle lies behind longus capitis. It originates from the lateral mass of the first cervical vertebra and inserts onto the basilar part of the occipital bone.

Innervation: It is supplied by the ventral rami of the first and second cervical spinal nerves.

Vasculature: Its blood supply is derived from the vertebral and ascending pharyngeal arteries.

Actions: Rectus capitis anterior flexes the head.

10.55 The prevertebral muscles

1 Scalenus anterior muscle
2 Scalenus medius muscle
3 Scalenus posterior muscle
4 Levator scapulae muscle
5 Longus capitis muscle
6 Rectus capitis lateralis muscle
7 Rectus capitis anterior muscle
8 Longus colli muscle (upper part)
9 Longus colli muscle (lower part)

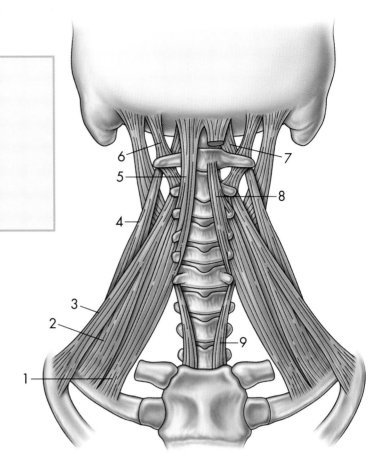

10.56 The deep postvertebral muscles

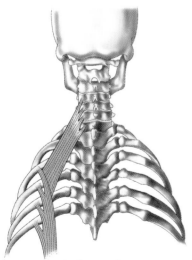

1 Iliocostalis

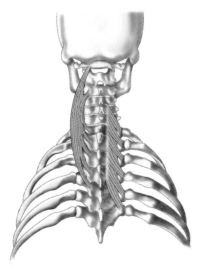

2 Longissimus cervicis (left) and
   semispinalis cervicis (right)

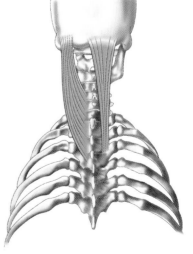

3 Longissimus capitis (left) and
   semispinalis capitis (right)

Rectus capitis lateralis (10.55)

Attachments: This muscle passes from the upper surface of the transverse process of the first cervical vertebra to the inferior surface of the jugular process of the occipital bone.

Innervation: Its motor supply is derived from the ventral rami of the first and second cervical spinal nerves.

Vasculature: The vertebral, occipital and ascending pharyngeal arteries contribute to the muscle's blood supply.

Actions: It flexes the head laterally.

The scalene muscles are flexors and rotators of the vertebral column. They extend obliquely from the transverse processes of the cervical vertebrae to the ribs. They provide important landmarks in the root of the neck (see page 386).

Scalenus anterior (10.39, 10.42, 10.55, 10.57, 10.58)

Attachments: Scalenus anterior lies behind the sternocleidomastoid muscle. It arises from the transverse processes (anterior tubercles) of the third to the sixth cervical vertebrae. It descends almost vertically to insert onto the scalene tubercle and ridge on the upper surface of the first rib.

Innervation: The muscle is innervated by the ventral rami of the fourth to the sixth cervical spinal nerves.

Vasculature: The ascending cervical branch of the inferior thyroid artery is the main source of the muscle's blood supply.

Actions: Acting from above, scalenus anterior elevates the first rib. Acting from below, it flexes the cervical part of the vertebral column anteriorly and laterally and also rotates the vertebral column.

Scalenus medius (10.37, 10.55–10.57)

Attachments: This is the largest of the scalene muscles. It arises from the transverse processes (posterior tubercles) of the lower six cervical vertebrae. It inserts onto the upper surface of the first rib, behind the groove for the subclavian artery.

Innervation: It receives its motor supply from the ventral rami of the third to the eighth cervical spinal nerves.

Vasculature: Scalenus medius receives its blood supply from the inferior thyroid artery (ascending cervical branch).

Actions: Acting from above, it elevates the first rib. Acting from below, it flexes the cervical vertebral column to the same side.

Scalenus posterior (10.55, 10.63)

Attachments: This is the smallest of the scalene muscles. It is also the deepest and forms part of the floor of the posterior triangle with scalenus medius. It is often difficult to separate from scalenus medius, and is consequently sometimes considered as part of this muscle. Scalenus posterior arises from the transverse processes (posterior tubercles) of the fourth to the sixth cervical vertebrae. It inserts onto the outer surface of the second rib, behind the attachment of the serratus anterior muscle.

Innervation: The motor innervation comes from branches of the ventral rami of the lower three cervical spinal nerves.

Vasculature: Both the ascending cervical branch of the inferior thyroid artery and the superficial cervical artery supply scalenus posterior.

Actions: Acting from above, it elevates the second rib. Acting from below, it flexes the lower part of the cervical vertebral column to the same side.

10.57 Anterior view of the root of the neck showing scalene muscles

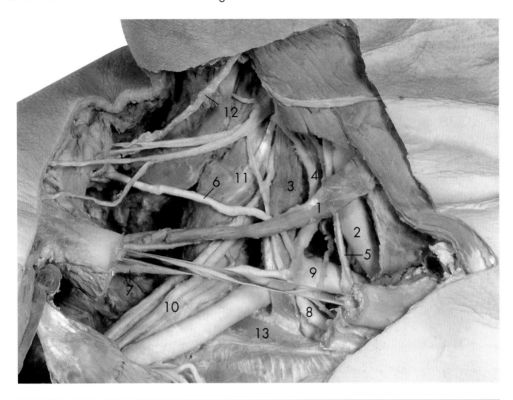

1	Omohyoid muscle	8	Internal thoracic artery
2	Common carotid artery	9	Subclavian artery
3	Scalenus anterior muscle	10	Brachial plexus
4	Inferior thyroid artery	11	Scalenus medius and posterior muscles
5	Vagus nerve	12	Accessory nerve on levator scapulae muscle
6	Superficial cervical artery		
7	Suprascapular artery	13	First rib

10.58 Upper surface of first rib showing attachments of scalene muscles

3	Scalenus medius muscle
4	Scalenus anterior muscle

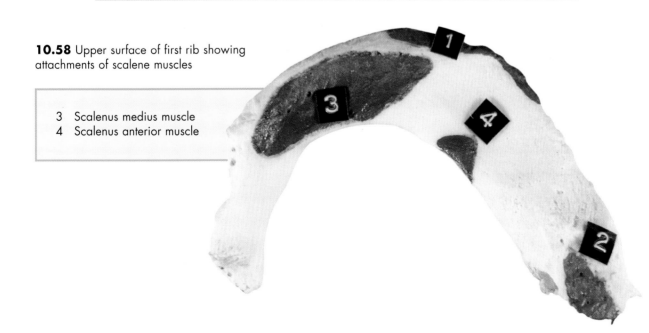

Scalenus minimus

This muscle is found in about 66% of cases. It arises from the anterior tubercle of the sixth or seventh cervical vertebra. It inserts onto the first rib and into the supraplural membrane which covers the apex of the lung in the root of the neck.

Levator scapulae (10.11, 10.26, 10.55, 10.59, 10.63)

Attachments: The muscle takes origin from the transverse processes (posterior tubercles) of the first to the fourth cervical vertebrae. It descends obliquely across the floor of the posterior triangle of the neck to insert onto the medial edge of the scapula (between the superior angle and the root of the spine).

Innervation: The innervation is derived partly from the third and fourth cervical nerves directly and partly from the fifth cervical nerve indirectly through the dorsal scapular nerve.

Vasculature: The blood supply comes mainly from the superficial cervical and inferior thyroid (ascending cervical) arteries. Near the attachments to the cervical vertebral column, it is supplied by branches from the vertebral artery.

Actions: As its name suggests, the levator scapulae elevates the scapula. This is accomplished when acting with the trapezius muscle. Levator scapulae also acts in association with other muscles to control the position of the scapula when the upper limb is in active use. Should the scapula be fixed, the muscle can incline the neck to the same side.

The postvertebral muscles

These muscles lie deep to the trapezius muscle at the back of the head and neck and behind the vertebral column. They can be subdivided into three layers, a superficial layer, a middle layer, and a deep layer.

The superficial layer consists of the splenius cervicis and capitis muscles. The middle layer comprises parts of erector spinae (iliocostalis cervicis, longissimus cervicis and capitis, spinalis cervicis and capitis). The deep layer incorporates the semispinalis cervicis and capitis muscles, and some deep slips of muscles belonging to the multifidus, rotatores, interspinalis and intertransversarii groups. The fibres in the superficial layer pass upwards and outwards. The fibres in the middle layer run parallel to the vertebral column. Most of the deep muscles lie in the groove between the spines and the transverse processes of the cervical vertebrae.

Behind the first and second cervical vertebrae are the muscles comprising the suboccipital triangle.

Splenius cervicis and capitis (10.26, 10.59, 10.63)

Attachments: Splenius cervicis takes origin from the spines of the third to the sixth thoracic vertebrae. It inserts into the transverse processes (posterior tubercles) of the upper three or four cervical vertebrae. Splenius capitis passes over splenius cervicis. It arises from the ligamentum nuchae and spines of the seventh cervical and upper three or four thoracic vertebrae. The muscle inserts into the mastoid process and superior nuchal line on the cranium.

Innervation: The nerve supply is from lateral branches of the dorsal rami of the middle cervical spinal nerves.

Vasculature: The blood supply is derived from the occipital and superficial cervical arteries.

Actions: Acting on both sides, they extend the head backwards. Acting on one side only, they pull the head to one side with slight rotation.

10.59 Muscles of the posterior triangle

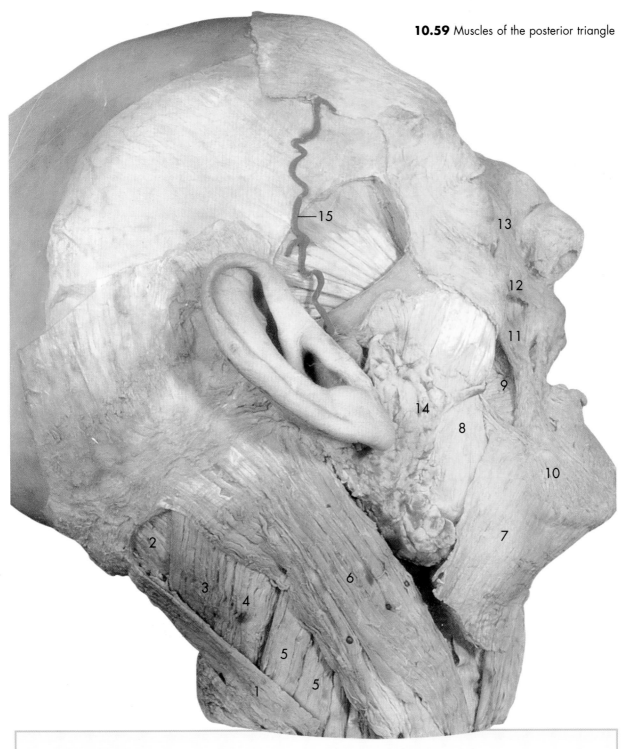

1	Trapezius muscle	9	Buccinator muscle
2	Semispinalis capitis muscle	10	Depressor anguli oris muscle
3	Splenius capitis muscle	11	Levator anguli oris muscle
4	Levator scapulae muscle	12	Levator labii superioris muscle
5	Scalene muscle block	13	Levator labii superioris alaeque nasi muscle
6	Sternocleidomastoid muscle	14	Parotid gland with duct
7	Platysma muscle	15	Superficial temporal artery on temporalis muscle
8	Masseter muscle		

The erector spinae group of muscles (10.56)

In the neck the group can be subdivided into a lateral layer (iliocostalis cervicis), an intermediate layer (longissimus cervicis and capitis), and a medial layer (spinalis cervicis and capitis).

Attachments: Iliocostalis cervicis extends from the angles of the third to the sixth ribs up to the transverse processes (posterior tubercles) of the fourth to the sixth cervical vertebrae.

Longissimus cervicis arises from the transverse processes of the upper four thoracic vertebrae. The insertion is into the transverse processes (posterior tubercles) of the second to the sixth cervical vertebrae. Longissimus capitis extends from transverse processes of the upper four thoracic vertebrae and the articular processes of the lower four cervical vertebrae to the posterior margin of the mastoid process of the temporal bone.

Spinalis cervicis takes origin from the spines of the first and second thoracic and of the seventh cervical vertebrae. It inserts onto the spine of the second cervical vertebra. Spinalis capitis arises from the transverse processes of the seventh cervical to the seventh thoracic vertebrae and from the articular processes of the fourth to the sixth cervical vertebrae. The muscle passes upwards to insert on the occipital bone between the superior and inferior nuchal lines. Near its insertion it blends with the semispinalis capitis muscle.

Innervation: The muscles of erector spinae are innervated by dorsal rami of spinal nerves.

Vasculature: They receive their blood supply from the occipital artery, costocervical trunk, and intercostal arteries.

Actions: The muscles are involved in extension, lateral flexion, and rotation of the head and neck.

Semispinalis cervicis and capitis (10.56, 10.59, 10.60, 10.63)

Attachments: Semispinalis cervicis takes origin from the transverse processes of the upper six thoracic vertebrae and from the articular processes of the lower four cervical vertebrae. It passes upwards and medially to insert onto the spines of the second to the fifth cervical vertebrae. Semispinalis capitis arises from the transverse processes of the upper six thoracic vertebrae and the seventh cervical vertebra, and also from the articular processes of the fourth to the sixth cervical vertebrae. It passes upwards to insert onto the occipital bone, between the superior and inferior nuchal lines.

Innervation: The muscles are supplied by dorsal rami of the cervical spinal nerves.

Vasculature: The arterial blood supply is derived from the occipital artery, deep cervical branch of the costocervical trunk and from muscular branches of posterior intercostal arteries.

Actions: Semispinalis cervicis extends and rotates the cervical region of the vertebral column. Semispinalis capitis extends the head and turns the face towards the opposite side.

The *multifidus, rotatores, interspinales and intertransversarii muscles* are small slips of muscle which link adjacent vertebra. They are involved in extension, lateral flexion and rotation of the vertebral column (10.61).

10.60 Muscles are the back of the neck

1 Trapezius muscle
2 Semispinalis capitis muscle
3 Splenius capitis muscle
4 Levator scapulae muscle
5 Sternocleidomastoid muscle

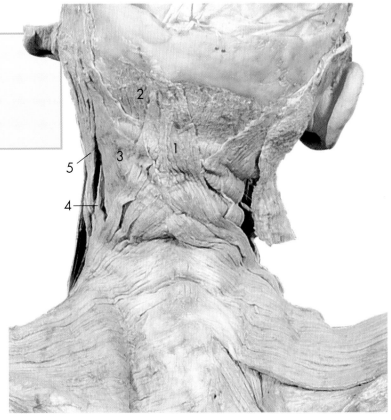

10.61 The multifidus, rotatores, interspinales and intertransversarii muscles at the back of the vertebral column

1 Multifidus muscle
2 Rotatores muscles
3 Interspinalis muscle
4 Intertransversarii muscle

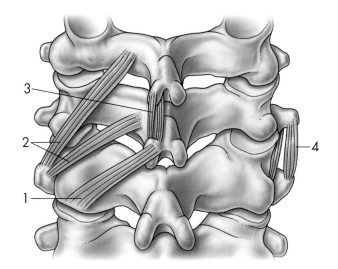

The suboccipital triangle (10.62, 10.63)

This is a region at the back of the neck which is immediately related to the first cervical vertebra. It lies under cover of the trapezius, splenius capitis, semispinalis capitis and longissimus capitis muscles.

The suboccipital triangle is bounded by the following muscles: rectus capitis posterior major (above and medially), obliquus capitis superior (above and laterally), and obliquus capitis inferior (below and laterally).

The floor of the triangle is formed by the posterior arch of the first cervical vertebra and by the posterior atlanto-occipital membrane of the atlanto-occipital joint.

Running across the floor of the triangle are the vertebral artery and the dorsal ramus of the first cervical spinal nerve (the suboccipital nerve). The artery passes horizontally behind the lateral mass of the atlas and then upwards and inwards to enter the cranial cavity through the foramen magnum (2.22, 2.23). The suboccipital nerve runs between the artery and the posterior arch of the atlas to supply the suboccipital muscles.

Within the roof of the triangle are the medial branch of the dorsal ramus of the second cervical spinal nerve (the greater occipital nerve), and the occipital artery. The greater occipital nerve pierces the trapezius muscle close to its attachment onto the superior nuchal line of the occiput. It then ascends to supply the skin over the occipital part of the scalp up to the vertex of the skull. The occipital artery runs with the greater occipital nerve, passing deep and then medial to the nerve.

Rectus capitis posterior major
Attachments: This muscle extends from the spine of the second cervical vertebra to the occipital bone below the inferior nuchal line.

Innervation: The motor supply comes from the suboccipital nerve.

Vasculature: The arterial blood supply is derived from the vertebral and the occipital arteries.

Actions: The muscle is involved in extension, lateral flexion and rotation of the head.

Obliquus capitis superior (superior oblique)
Attachments: It originates from the transverse process of the first cervical vertebra and inserts at the occipital bone between the superior and inferior nuchal lines.

Innervation: It is innervated by the suboccipital nerve.

Vasculature: The blood supply comes from the vertebral and occipital arteries.

Actions: The superior oblique muscle is involved in extension, and lateral rotation of the head.

Obliquus capitis inferior (inferior oblique)
Attachments: The muscle passes upwards and laterally from the spine of the second cervical vertebra to the transverse process of the first cervical vertebra.

Innervation: It is supplied by branches from the dorsal rami of the first and second cervical spinal nerves.

Vasculature: The arteries supplying the muscle are branches of the vertebral and occipital arteries.

Actions: The muscle rotates the first cervical vertebra and the skull around the dens of the second cervical vertebra.

Between the two rectus capitis posterior major muscles lie the rectus capitis posterior minor muscles.

Rectus capitis posterior minor
Attachments: This muscle takes origin from the tubercle on the posterior arch of the first cervical vertebra. It passes upwards to insert onto the occipital bone, below the inferior nuchal line and close to the midline.

Innervation: Its motor supply comes from the suboccipital nerve.

Vasculature: Both the vertebral and occipital arteries send branches to supply this muscle.

Actions: It extends the head.

10.62 The suboccipital triangle

1 Tubercle on posterior arch of the atlas vertebra
2 Rectus capitis posterior minor muscle
3 Rectus capitis posterior major muscle
4 Superior oblique muscle
5 Transverse process of the atlas vertebra
6 Inferior oblique muscle
7 Spine of the axis vertebra

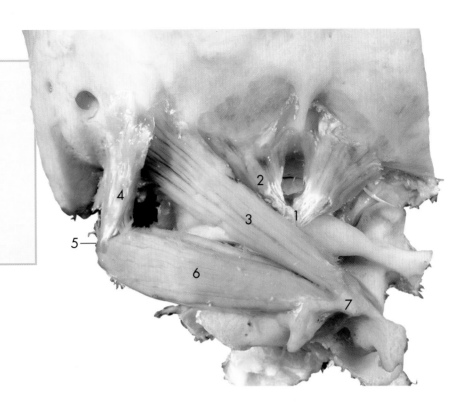

10.63 The suboccipital triangle

1 Sternocleidomastoid muscle
2 Lesser occipital nerve
3 Greater auricular nerve
4 Occipital artery
5 Greater occipital nerve
6 Rectus capitis posterior minor muscle
7 Rectus capitis posterior major muscle
8 Inferior oblique muscle
9 Superior oblique muscle
10 Vertebral artery
11 Scalenus posterior muscle
12 Levator scapulae muscle
13 Trapezius muscle (reflected)
14 Splenius capitis muscle (reflected)
15 Semispinalis capitis muscle (reflected)

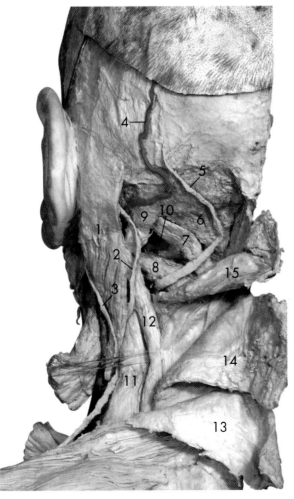

THE ROOT OF THE NECK (10.64, 10.71)

The root of the neck is the junctional region between the neck and the thorax.

The thoracic inlet itself is narrow, and is bounded anteriorly by the manubrium sterni, posteriorly by the first thoracic vertebra, and laterally by the first ribs and their costal cartilages. The apices of the lungs occupy the lateral parts of the thoracic inlet. The major structures passing between the neck and thorax lie in the mid-region between the lungs.

The contents of the root of the neck include:

- The brachiocephalic artery and the brachiocephalic veins

- The internal jugular veins

- The common carotid arteries

- The subclavian arteries and veins

- The thoracic and right lymphatic ducts

- The vagus, recurrent laryngeal and phrenic nerves

- The sympathetic trunks

- The brachial plexuses

- The oesophagus and trachea

A key landmark in the root of the neck is the scalenus anterior muscle which attaches onto the first rib (10.58). Below and in front of scalenus anterior lies the subclavian vein as it runs across the first rib and into the upper limb. Passing down the superficial surface of the muscle is the phrenic nerve (see page 362). Occasionally, the roots of the phrenic nerve may be separate and are referred to as accessory phrenic nerves. Also in front of scalenus anterior is the lateral part of the internal jugular vein, and the inferior thyroid, superficial cervical and suprascapular vessels. The vagus nerve and the common carotid artery lie between the scalenus anterior muscle and the trachea. Behind the scalenus anterior muscle are the subclavian artery, the ventral rami of the nerves comprising the brachial plexus, and the apex of the lung.

The brachiocephalic artery (10.65, 10.66, 10.68)

The major arteries passing from the thorax into the neck show differences according to side. On the right, the major artery is the brachiocephalic artery. This divides behind the right sternoclavicular joint into the right subclavian and the right common carotid arteries. On the left, however, the left subclavian and the left common carotid arteries originate directly from the arch of the aorta in the superior mediastinum of the thorax. The brachiocephalic artery occasionally provides a thyroidea ima branch to the thyroid gland.

10.64 The frontal view showing the root of the neck

1	Vertebral artery
2	Common carotid artery (cut end)
3	Cervical vertebra
4	Subclavian artery
5	Thyrocervical trunk
6	Vertebral vein
7	Subclavian vein
8	Vagus nerve
9	Spinal nerves (cervical)
10	Trachea (cut end)
11	Oesophagus (cut end)
12	Internal thoracic artery
13	Brachiocephalic vein

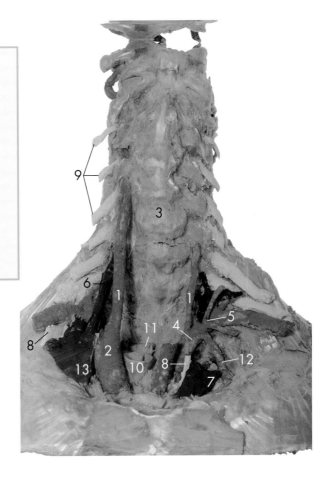

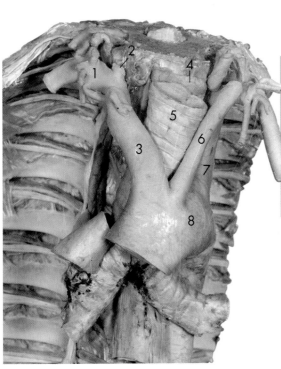

10.65 The root of the neck

1	Right subclavian artery
2	Right common carotid artery (cut end)
3	Brachiocephalic artery
4	Oesophagus
5	Trachea
6	Left common carotid artery
7	Left subclavian artery
8	Arch of the aorta

The brachiocephalic veins (10.66)

These major veins lie anteriorly in the root of the neck. Each brachiocephalic vein is formed behind the medial end of the clavicle by the union of the subclavian and internal jugular veins. The subsequent course of each brachiocephalic vein varies. The right brachiocephalic vein passes vertically downwards into the mediastinum and is located anterolateral to the brachiocephalic artery. The left brachiocephalic vein runs obliquely across the midline, behind the manubrium sterni, to join the right brachiocephalic vein on the right side of the superior mediastinum. In its course, the left brachiocephalic vein crosses the left subclavian artery, the left common carotid artery, and the brachiocephalic artery.

Tributaries include:

• Vertebral vein

• Accessory vertebral vein

• Internal thoracic vein

• Inferior thyroid vein

• First posterior intercostal vein

In addition, the left brachiocephalic vein receives the left superior intercostal vein.

The *vertebral vein* arises in the suboccipital triangle at the back of the head. It initially appears as a plexus formed by the confluence of vessels from the internal vertebral plexuses (see page 94) and from the deep muscles of the upper part of the neck. This plexus descends around the vertebral artery in the foramina transversaria of the upper five cervical vertebrae. A single vein is formed which passes through the foramen transversarium of the sixth cervical vertebra. This vein runs down in front of the vertebral artery to open into the brachiocephalic vein (10.64).

The vertebral vein communicates with the sigmoid sinus (through the condylar canal) and with the occipital vein. Its tributaries are the anterior vertebral vein, the deep cervical vein and sometimes the first posterior intercostal vein (10.64).

The anterior vertebral vein originates from a plexus around the transverse processes of the upper cervical vertebrae. The vein accompanies the ascending cervical artery, lying between the longus capitis and scalenus anterior muscles. The anterior vertebral vein drains into the vertebral vein close to its termination into the brachiocephalic vein.

The deep cervical vein accompanies the deep cervical artery. Like the vertebral vein, it commences from the venous plexus in the suboccipital region. The deep cervical vein passes down between the transverse process of the seventh cervical vertebra and the neck of the first rib and ends in the vertebral vein (or in the brachiocephalic vein).

The *accessory vertebral vein* also arises from the plexus around the vertebral artery. It passes through the foramen transversarium of the seventh cervical vertebra to terminate at the brachiocephalic vein.

The *internal thoracic vein* drains the anterior wall of the thorax. It appears in the root of the neck from behind the first rib (just lateral to the sternum). The vein crosses the apex of the lung for a short distance to drain into the brachiocephalic vein.

The *inferior thyroid vein* initially arises as a plexus from the lower part of the thyroid gland. From this plexus, right and left inferior thyroid veins pass downwards to drain separately into their respective brachiocephalic vein. Alternatively, they may unite to form a common vein which enters the left brachiocephalic vein (10.47, 10.66).

The *first posterior intercostal vein* drains the posterior part of the first intercostal space. It is a tributary of either the brachiocephalic vein or the vertebral vein.

The *left superior intercostal vein* receives the second and third (sometimes fourth) posterior intercostal veins from the left side of the body. It passes between the left vagus and phrenic nerves to reach the left brachiocephalic vein. The right superior intercostal vein drains into the azygos vein in the thorax.

10.66 The brachiocephalic veins

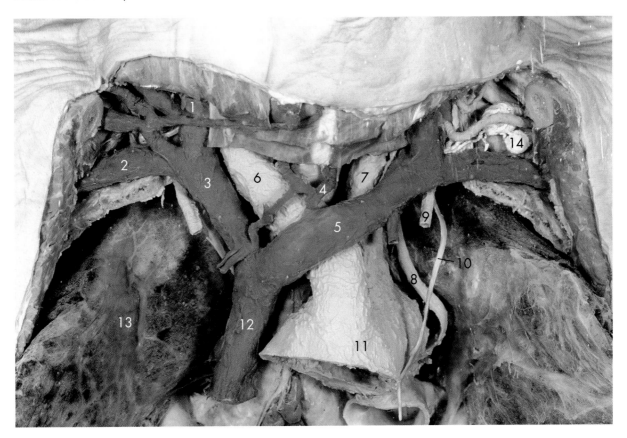

1	Internal jugular vein
2	Subclavian vein
3	Right brachiocephalic vein
4	Inferior thyroid vein
5	Left brachiocephalic vein
6	Brachiocephalic artery
7	Left common carotid artery
8	Vagus nerve
9	Internal thoracic artery
10	Left phrenic nerve
11	Aorta
12	Superior vena cava
13	Lung
14	Lymph node

The subclavian artery (10.64, 10.67–10.69)

The subclavian artery is one of the principal features in the root of the neck. As mentioned earlier, its origin differs according to side. The subclavian artery runs into the root of the neck by the side of the trachea and then passes behind the scalenus anterior muscle. The artery then continues across the apex of the lung, onto the first rib (between the rib and the clavicle), and runs into the upper limb as the axillary artery. Its branches are widely distributed — to the neck, head and brain, to the upper limb, and to the thorax. The subclavian artery can be divided into three parts according to its relationship to the scalenus anterior muscle: proximal (first part), deep (second part), and distal (third part) to the muscle.

Concerning the relationships of the subclavian artery, the first part lies behind the carotid sheath and is crossed by a loop of the sympathetic trunk (the ansa subclavia). Behind the artery lies the apex of the lung. Below and in front is the subclavian vein. On the right side, the vagus nerve gives off the recurrent laryngeal nerve which then passes up beneath the artery. On the left, the thoracic duct crosses in front of the subclavian artery. The third part of the subclavian artery is related to the brachial plexus.

Branches include:

- Vertebral artery

- Internal thoracic artery

- Thyrocervical trunk:
    Inferior thyroid artery
    Superficial cervical artery
    Suprascapular artery

- Costocervical trunk:
    Deep cervical artery
    Superior intercostal artery

Most of the branches of the subclavian artery arise from its first part. However, the left costocervical trunk arises from the second part of the left subclavian artery.

The *vertebral artery* arises from the upper surface of the subclavian artery. It passes upwards, medially and backwards to reach the foramen transversarium of the sixth cervical vertebra (N.B. the foramen for the seventh cervical vertebra does not transmit the vertebral artery). In this part of its course, the artery lies behind the common carotid and inferior thyroid arteries, and the vertebral vein. The left vertebral artery is also crossed by the thoracic duct. The vertebral artery then passes upwards through the foramina transversaria of the remaining cervical vertebrae (in front of the spinal nerves) to reach the lateral mass of the atlas. Here, it arches around the posterior surface of the lateral mass within the suboccipital triangle. Indeed, the artery lies within a groove on the upper surface of the posterior arch of the atlas, accompanied by the suboccipital nerve.

The vertebral artery then pierces the meninges and runs upwards through the foramen magnum. On the ventral surface of the medulla oblongata, the vertebral arteries join to form the basilar artery.

Extracranially, the vertebral artery gives off spinal and muscular branches. The spinal branches are arranged segmentally and supply the spinal cord (plus meningeal layers) and the cervical vertebrae. The muscular branches are found primarily in the suboccipital region.

10.67 Frontal view of the root of the neck showing the subclavian artery

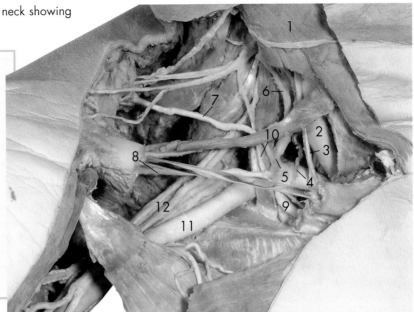

1	Sternocleidomastoid muscle
2	Common carotid artery
3	Vagus nerve
4	Ansa subclavia
5	Thyrocervical trunk
6	Inferior thyroid artery
7	Superficial cervical artery
8	Suprascapular artery
9	Internal thoracic artery
10	Phrenic nerve on the scalenus anterior muscle
11	Axillary artery
12	Brachial plexus

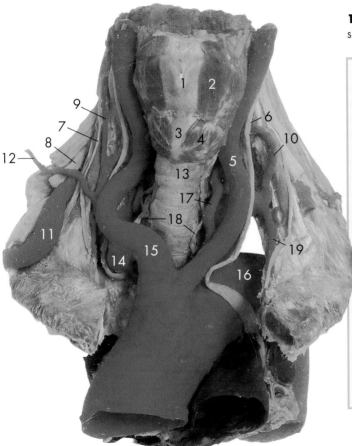

10.68 Frontal view of the root of the neck showing the subclavian artery

1	Thyroid cartilage
2	Thyrohyoid muscle
3	Arch of cricoid cartilage
4	Cricothyroid muscle
5	Common carotid artery
6	Vagus nerve
7	Phrenic nerve on scalenus anterior muscle
8	Brachial plexus
9	Ascending cervical branch of the inferior thyroid artery
10	Inferior thyroid artery
11	Continuation of subclavian artery as axillary artery
12	Superficial cervical artery
13	Trachea
14	Subclavian artery
15	Brachiocephalic artery
16	Arch of the aorta
17	Vertebral artery
18	Recurrent laryngeal nerve
19	Internal thoracic artery

The *internal thoracic artery* originates from the lower surface of the subclavian artery. It runs downwards into the thorax, behind the costal cartilages. The artery provides branches to the intercostal muscles. It has no branches in the neck.

The *thyrocervical trunk* is short and lies close to the scalenus anterior muscle. It gives rise to three branches: the inferior thyroid, superficial cervical and suprascapular arteries.

The *inferior thyroid artery* runs upwards on the medial surface of the scalenus anterior muscle. It then passes medially between the carotid sheath and the vertebral artery, finally descending to reach the inferior part of the thyroid gland where its glandular branches supply the inferior and posterior surfaces. Near the thyroid gland, the inferior thyroid artery is related to the recurrent laryngeal nerve (see page 430). The artery has branches which supply the oesophagus, trachea and the lower part of the pharynx. Branches also supply prevertebral and infrahyoid muscles.

An ascending cervical branch arises from the upper part of the inferior thyroid artery and passes up the neck close to the transverse processes of the cervical vertebrae. It supplies adjacent muscles, gives branches to the spinal cord, and anastomoses with branches from neighbouring vessels (e.g. vertebral, occipital, and ascending pharyngeal arteries).

The internal laryngeal branch of the inferior thyroid artery passes upwards (with the recurrent laryngeal nerve) beneath the inferior constrictor muscle of the pharynx to supply structures within the larynx.

The *suprascapular artery* runs downwards and laterally across the phrenic nerve, the brachial plexus and the third part of the subclavian artery, before passing to the upper border of the scapula. In the neck, it gives branches supplying the sternocleidomastoid and platysma muscles.

The *superficial cervical artery* crosses the posterior triangle to supply the trapezius muscle. To reach this muscle, the artery crosses the phrenic nerve, brachial plexus, and suprascapular artery downwards and laterally, across the phrenic nerve, the brachial plexus and the third part of the subclavian artery before passing to the upper border of the scapula. In the neck, it gives branches supplying the sternocleidomastoid and platysma muscles.

The *costocervical trunk* originates from the back of the subclavian artery. It passes backwards towards the neck of the first rib where it branches into the deep cervical and superior intercostal arteries.

The *deep cervical artery* runs upwards within the postvertebral muscles (between semispinalis cervicis and semispinalis capitis). It contributes to the blood supply of the postvertebral musculature.

The *superior intercostal artery* ascends into the thorax to give rise to the first posterior intercostal artery.

Variations in the origin and branches of the superficial cervical and suprascapular arteries are common. Furthermore, a branch termed dorsal scapular artery arises from the third part of the subclavian artery. It passes deep to levator scapulae to reach the shoulder where it contributes to the supply of the trapezius muscle.

10.69 Frontal view of the root of the neck showing the subclavian artery

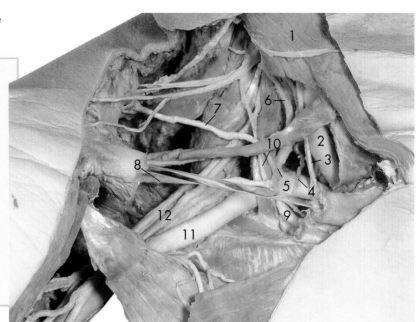

1 Sternocleidomastoid muscle
2 Common carotid artery
3 Vagus nerve
4 Ansa subclavia
5 Thyrocervical trunk
6 Inferior thyroid artery
7 Superficial cervical artery
8 Suprascapular artery
9 Internal thoracic artery
10 Phrenic nerve on the scalenus anterior muscle
11 Axillary artery
12 Brachial plexus

10.70 The root of the neck showing the subclavian veins

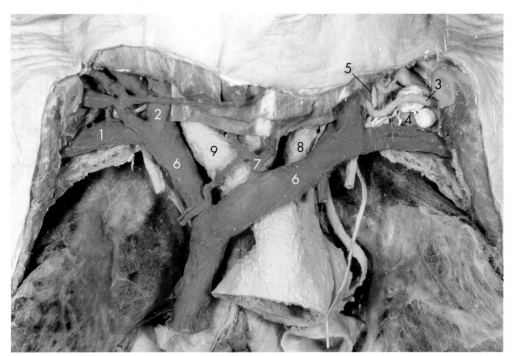

1 Subclavian vein
2 Internal jugular vein
3 Suprascapular artery
4 Subclavian artery
5 Phrenic nerve on scalenus anterior muscle
6 Brachiocephalic vein
7 Inferior thyroid vein
8 Left common carotid artery
9 Brachiocephalic artery

The subclavian vein (10.64, 10.70, 10.71)

The subclavian vein begins at the outer border of the first rib as a continuation of the axillary vein from the upper limb. It runs across the upper surface of the first rib, within a groove. Here, the vein lies below and in front of the scalenus anterior muscle and the subclavian artery. Behind the subclavian vein is the apex of the lung. The vein passes behind the sterno-clavicular joint where it meets the internal jugular vein to form the brachiocephalic vein. The external jugular vein drains into the subclavian vein just lateral to the scalenus anterior muscle. The right subclavian vein receives the right lymphatic duct near its junction with the right internal jugular vein. The left subclavian vein receives the thoracic duct.

The thoracic duct (10.42, 10.71)

This is the main collecting duct for the lymphatics of the body. It is associated with all regions excepting the right side of the head, neck, thorax and arm. The thoracic duct enters the neck through the thoracic inlet, between the oesophagus and the left pleura and behind the left common carotid artery and the left vagus nerve. It then runs between the left common carotid and left subclavian arteries, and in front of the left vertebral artery and thyrocervical trunk, to enter the left subclavian vein. The thoracic duct in the root of the neck receives the left jugular trunk (draining the left side of the head and neck) and the left subclavian trunk (draining the left arm). Valves guard the entrance of the thoracic duct into the subclavian vein.

The right lymphatic duct

This duct receives the right jugular trunk (draining the right side of the head and neck) and the right subclavian trunk (draining the right arm and right side of the thorax). It passes near the medial border of the scalenus anterior muscle to drain into the right subclavian vein. Valves are found where the right lymphatic duct joins the subclavian vein.

The vagus, recurrent laryngeal and phrenic nerves, the sympathetic trunk, and the brachial plexus are described between pages 352–365. The trachea and the oesophagus are described with the viscera of the neck (see pages 368–370).

The apex of the lung and the suprapleural membrane

The apex of the lung is rounded and extends into the root of the neck to a level about 1 cm above the medial third of the clavicle. It is covered by the cervical pleura and the suprapleural membrane. The lung apex is crossed by the subclavian vessels. Laterally, it is related to the scalenus medius muscle. Behind is the sympathetic trunk and the cervico-thoracic ganglion, whilst medially lie the great vessels and the trachea and oesophagus. The suprapleural membrane is a thin fascial sheet which covers the apex of the lung, thereby strengthening the cervical pleura. Anteriorly, the suprapleural membrane is attached to the inner border of the first rib. Posteriorly, it is attached to the transverse process of the seventh cervical vertebra.

10.71 Lateral view of the left root of the necking showing termination of thoracic duct

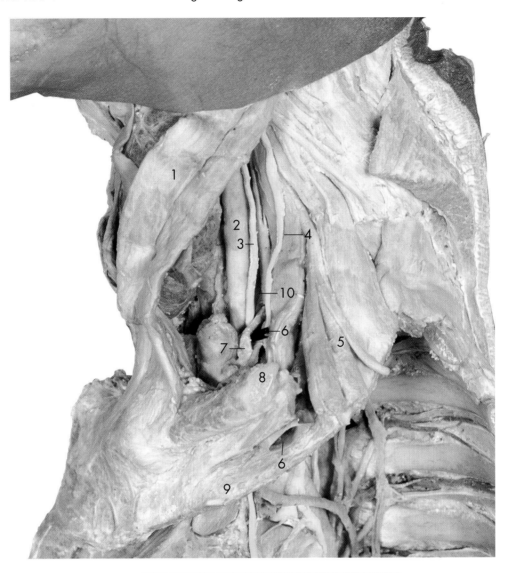

1	Sternocleidomastoid muscle
2	Common carotid artery
3	Vagus nerve
4	Phrenic nerve on scalenus anterior muscle
5	Brachial plexus
6	Subclavian vein (cut end)
7	Thoracic duct
8	Clavicle (cut end)
9	First rib
10	Internal jugular vein

chapter 11
THE PHARYNX

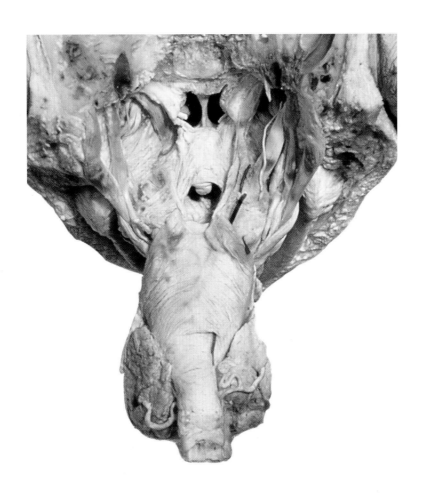

Chapter 11 THE PHARYNX

The pharynx is a common passage for the alimentary and respiratory systems. It links the oral cavity to the oesophagus, and the posterior apertures of the nasal cavity to the inlet of the larynx. During swallowing, the airway is temporarily closed by elevation of the soft palate and of the inlet of the larynx beneath the base of the tongue.

The pharynx is a fibromuscular tube situated in front of the vertebral column. It extends from the base of the skull to the lower border of the cricoid cartilage of the larynx. It is widest above and narrows at its junction with the oesophagus below. The principal muscles of the pharynx (the constrictor muscles) arise from structures at the sides of the head and neck and pass posteriorly to insert into a midline fibrous band called the pharyngeal raphe. The pharynx is thus not a complete tube, being semicircular in cross-section, with communications anteriorly with the nasal cavity, the oral cavity and the laryngeal cavity. Indeed, the pharynx is subdivided into three regions according to the cavity with which it is continuous, i.e. the nasopharynx, the oropharynx and the laryngopharynx.

The pharynx also communicates with the middle ear by way of an auditory tube.

THE NASOPHARYNX (11.1, 11.2)

The nasopharynx is the uppermost part of the pharynx and lies above the soft palate. Anteriorly, it begins at the posterior nasal apertures (choanae). Posteriorly and inferiorly, it ends at the pharyngeal isthmus (i.e. the opening between the back of the soft palate and the posterior wall of the pharynx).

The roof and posterior wall of the nasopharynx lie against the base of the skull (primarily the basilar part of the occipital bone). Its sloping floor is the upper surface of the soft palate. With the exception of the soft palate, the nasopharynx is rigid and thus contributes to the patency of the airway.

The most prominent feature on each side of the nasopharynx is a triangular elevation with rounded margins called the *tubal elevation*. This is related to the underlying cartilaginous end of the auditory tube. Within the margins of the tubal elevation lies the opening of the auditory tube. Below this opening, the mucosa bulges because of the underlying levator veli palatini muscle. A fold of mucosa runs vertically downwards from the posterior margin of the tubal elevation. This is called the salpingopharyngeal fold because it overlies the salpingopharyngeus muscle. A smaller fold named the salpingopalatine fold may be present at the anterior margin of the tubal elevation. Lymphatic material comprising the tubal tonsil is found around the opening of the auditory tube. Behind the auditory tube is a small depression called the pharyngeal recess.

The *auditory tube* has also been called the eustachian tube and the pharyngotympanic tube. It links the lateral wall of the nasopharynx to the anterior wall of the tympanic cavity. In its course from the ear to the pharynx, it passes downwards, forwards and medially (at approximately 30° to the horizontal plane and 45° to the sagittal plane). There is a bony part near the ear and a cartilaginous part near the pharynx. The cartilaginous part is twice as long as the bony part. (This relationship is the converse of that pertaining for the external acoustic meatus: see page 294.) The bony part of the auditory tube gradually narrows as it passes from the tympanic cavity. It ends as an isthmus, which is the junction of the squamous and petrous portions of the temporal bone. The isthmus has a jagged margin for the attachment of the cartilaginous part of the auditory tube. The bony and cartilaginous parts meet at an obtuse angle. The cartilaginous part is formed by a triangular plate of cartilage which is fixed to the base of the skull in the groove between the petrous part of the temporal bone and the greater wing of the sphenoid bone. The cartilaginous part widens as it passes from the isthmus to the pharyngeal orifice. The pharyngeal orifice produces the tubal elevation in the nasopharynx and is directed downwards and backwards. The auditory tube has two functions. First, it permits the passage of air into the tympanic cavity to enable equalisation of pressure on either side of the ear drum (tympanic membrane). Second, it allows drainage of mucus from the middle ear and mastoid air cells. The mucosa lining the auditory tube has a ciliated columnar epithelium.

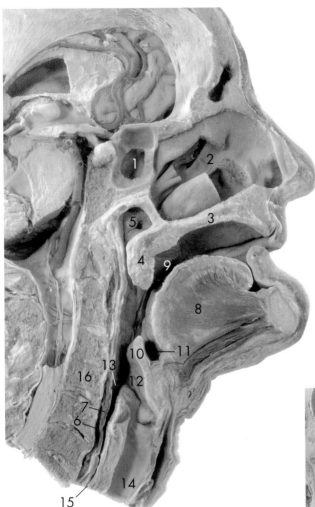

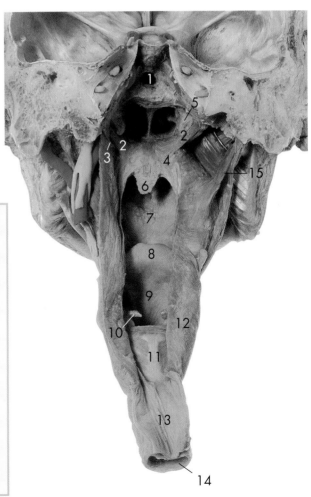

11.1 The pharynx seen in a sagittal section of the head

1	Sphenoidal air sinus
2	Nasal cavity
3	Hard palate
4	Soft palate
5	Opening of auditory tube in nasopharynx
6	Retropharyngeal space
7	Posterior wall of pharynx
8	Tongue
9	Oropharynx
10	Epiglottis
11	Vallecula
12	Laryngeal inlet
13	Laryngopharynx
14	Trachea
15	Oesophagus
16	Cervical vertebral column

11.2 Posterior view of the pharynx

1	Sphenoidal air sinus
2	Levator veli palatini muscle
3	Tensor palati muscle
4	Palatopharyngeus muscle
5	Tubal elevation in the lateral wall of nasopharynx
6	Uvula
7	Posterior third of tongue in floor of oropharynx
8	Epiglottis
9	Inlet of the larynx in laryngopharynx
10	Arytenoid cartilage
11	Lamina of cricoid cartilage
12	Reflected fibres of inferior constrictor muscle
13	Oesophagus
14	Trachea
15	Stylopharyngeus muscle

The cartilaginous part of the auditory tube gives attachment to the tensor veli palatini, the levator veli palatini and the salpingopharyngeus muscles. The tensor veli palatini intervenes between the tube and the mandibular nerve, the otic ganglion, the chorda tympani nerve and the middle meningeal artery. The bony part of the tube lies below the canal for the tensor tympani muscle. Below and medially lies the carotid canal.

The innervation of the auditory tube is derived from the pharyngeal branch of the maxillary nerve (via the pterygopalatine ganglion) and the tympanic plexus of the middle ear (see page 306). The arteries supplying the tube arise from the ascending pharyngeal branch of the external carotid artery and from the maxillary artery (middle meningeal branch, artery of the pterygoid canal). The veins drain into the pterygoid venous plexus of the infratemporal fossa.

Variable amounts of lymphatic tissue are scattered within the posterior wall of the nasopharynx. Such tissue is particularly evident in children where it forms a mass called the *pharyngeal tonsil (adenoids)*. The prominence of the pharyngeal tonsil lies close to the nasal septum and displays a median recess called the pharyngeal bursa. The tonsil may become so enlarged that it interferes with nasal respiration.

In the roof of the nasopharynx may be found a small collection of glandular tissue related to the adeno-hypophysis of the pituitary gland. This is called the *pharyngeal hypophysis*. It is thought to be a remnant of Rathke's pouch, and can secrete hormones.

Where the nasopharynx meets the soft palate, a ridge called *Passavant's ridge* becomes evident during swallowing. This contains Passavant's muscle (see page 404).

THE OROPHARYNX (11.1–11.5)

The oropharynx is the middle part of the pharynx which lies below the soft palate. It is delineated from the oral cavity proper by the palatoglossal arches (the anterior pillars of the fauces). The region between the palatoglossal arches is called the oropharyngeal isthmus.

The roof of the oropharynx is the under surface of the soft palate. The floor of the oropharynx is formed by the root of the tongue and extends back to the tip of the epiglottis. The posterior wall of the oropharynx lies adjacent to the second and third cervical vertebrae.

The root of the tongue in the floor of the oropharynx shows numerous lingual follicles. These contain lymphatic tissue and collectively form the lingual tonsil. The anterior surface of the epiglottis is joined to the tongue by three folds of mucosa called the median and lateral glosso-epiglottic folds. Between these folds are two depressions called valleculae.

The lateral wall of the oropharynx presents two prominent folds designated the pillars of the fauces. These folds diverge inferiorly and bound a triangular area called the tonsillar fossa or sinus. The anterior fold, or palatoglossal arch, runs from the soft palate to the side of the tongue and contains the palato-glossus muscle. The posterior fold, or palatopharyngeal arch, passes from the soft palate to merge with the lateral wall of the pharynx. It contains the palatopharyngeus muscle.

The *palatine tonsil* is a collection of lymphatic material that lies beneath the mucosa in the tonsillar fossa. Its size is variable, tending to be large in children and small in adults. It is a frequent site of infection. The medial surface of the palatine tonsil is the visible surface within the oropharynx (11.5). It exhibits several slit-like invaginations, the tonsillar crypts. One of the crypts is particularly deep and is called the intratonsillar cleft. The overall size of the palatine tonsil cannot be appreciated from a consideration of its medial surface alone. Indeed, it can extend some distance beyond the tonsillar fossa (e.g. upwards into the soft palate). The tonsillar bed that lies adjacent to the lateral surface of the palatine tonsil is formed by the palatoglossus and superior constrictor muscles. More deeply are found the styloglossus muscle and the glossopharyngeal nerve.

11.3 The oropharynx seen in sagittal section

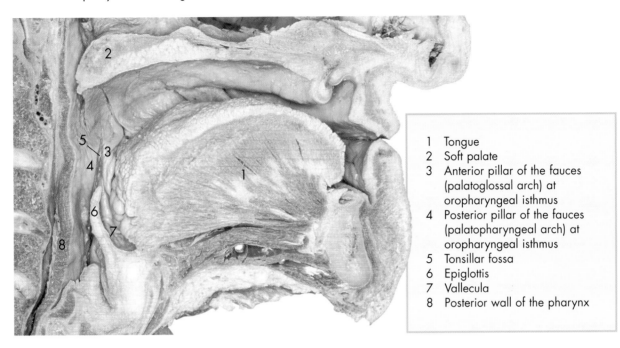

1	Tongue
2	Soft palate
3	Anterior pillar of the fauces (palatoglossal arch) at oropharyngeal isthmus
4	Posterior pillar of the fauces (palatopharyngeal arch) at oropharyngeal isthmus
5	Tonsillar fossa
6	Epiglottis
7	Vallecula
8	Posterior wall of the pharynx

11.4 Muscles of the soft palate viewed from the side of the oropharyngeal isthmus

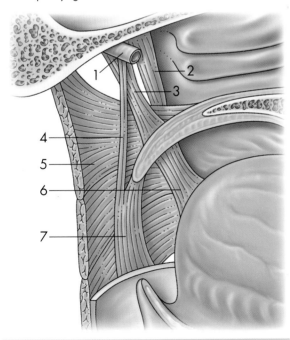

1 Auditory tube
2 Tensor veli palatini muscle
3 Levator veli palatini muscle
4 Salpingopharyngeus muscle
5 Superior constrictor muscle
6 Palatoglossus muscle
7 Palatopharyngeus muscle

11.5 The oropharyngeal isthmus seen from the mouth

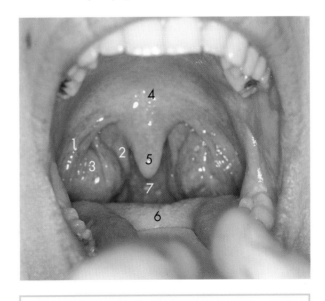

1 Anterior pillar of the fauces (palatoglossal arch) at oropharyngeal isthmus
2 Posterior pillar of the fauces (palatopharyngeal arch) at oropharyngeal isthmus
3 Palatine tonsil in the tonsillar fossa or sinus
4 Soft palate
5 Uvula
6 Dorsal surface of the tongue (pharyngeal part) with lingual follicles (lingual tonsil)
7 Posterior wall of oropharynx

THE LARYNGOPHARYNX (11.1, 11.2, 11.6)

The laryngopharynx is the lowest part of the pharynx. It extends from the upper border of the epiglottis to the lower border of the cricoid cartilage of the larynx. The laryngopharynx continues into the oesophagus. It is delineated from the oro-pharynx by the lateral glosso-epiglottic folds.

The obliquely-sloping inlet of the larynx lies in the anterior part of the laryngopharynx. This inlet is bounded above by the epiglottis, below by the arytenoid cartilages of the larynx, and laterally by the aryepiglottic folds. Below the inlet, the anterior wall of the laryngopharynx is formed by the posterior surface of the cricoid cartilage. Situated in the lateral wall of the laryngopharynx is the lamina of the thyroid cartilage of the larynx. Between the inner surface of this lamina and the outer surface of the cricoid and arytenoid cartilages is found a recess called the piriform fossa. The posterior wall of the laryngopharynx lies adjacent to the bodies of the third to the sixth cervical vertebrae.

THE WALL OF THE PHARYNX

The wall of the pharynx consists mainly of muscle. Internally, there is also a layer of mucosa and a membrane called the pharyngobasilar fascia. Externally, there is a loose connective tissue layer which is sometimes referred to as the buccopharyngeal fascia.

THE MUSCLES OF THE PHARYNX

The six pairs of muscles that comprise the pharynx can be divided into two groups. One group comprises three pairs of constrictor muscles that run transversely across the pharynx: the superior, middle, and inferior constrictors. The other group comprises three pairs of muscles that run longitudinally down the pharynx: the salpingopharyngeus, stylopharyngeus and palatopharyngeus muscles.

The constrictor muscles arise at the sides of the head and neck and insert posteriorly into the pharyngeal raphe. This raphe passes longitudinally down the back of the pharynx from the pharyngeal tubercle on the basilar part of the occipital bone. The constrictor muscles generate an ordered wave of contraction which carries the food bolus into the oesophagus. The constrictor muscles overlap each other such that the superior constrictor 'sits' within the middle constrictor and the middle constrictor 'sits' within the inferior constrictor. Important structures enter the pharynx in the intervals between the constrictors. The longitudinal muscles of the pharynx are attached onto the larynx. They elevate the pharynx and larynx during swallowing.

The superior constrictor muscle (11.7–11.12)

Attachments: The muscle originates mainly from the posterior border of the pterygomandibular raphe. This raphe provides the sites of origin for both the superior constrictor and buccinator muscles. It runs between the pterygoid hamulus of the sphenoid bone and the back of the mylohyoid line of the mandible. The superior constrictor muscle also arises from the bone adjacent to each end of the pterygomandibular raphe and from the side of the tongue. The fibres of the muscle fan out to be attached posteriorly to the pharyngeal raphe and to the pharyngeal tubercle on the occipital bone.

Innervation: The superior constrictor muscle is innervated by the cranial part of the accessory nerve.

Vasculature: The blood supply of this muscle is derived mainly from the ascending pharyngeal artery (pharyngeal branch) and facial artery (tonsillar branch).

Actions: The muscle constricts the upper part of the pharynx.

11.6 The laryngopharynx viewed posteriorly

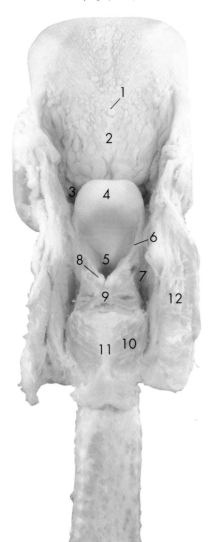

1 Foramen caecum
2 Dorsal surface of the tongue (pharyngeal part) with lingual follicles (lingual tonsil)
3 Vallecula
4 Epiglottis
5 Inlet of larynx
6 Aryepiglottic fold
7 Piriform fossa
8 Arytenoid cartilage beneath mucosa
9 Oblique and transverse arytenoid muscles
10 Posterior crico-arytenoid muscle
11 Lamina of cricoid cartilage
12 Inferior constrictor muscle

11.7 The lateral view of the constrictor muscles of the pharynx

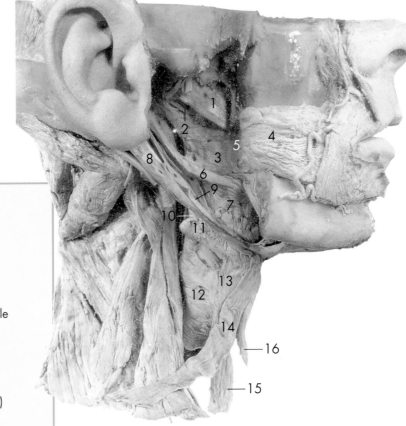

1 Tensor palati muscle
2 Levator veli palatini muscle
3 Superior constrictor muscle
4 Buccinator muscle
5 Pterygomandibular raphe
6 Styloglossus muscle
7 Hyoglossus muscle
8 Posterior belly of digaastric muscle
9 Stylohyoid muscle
10 Middle constrictor muscle
11 Greater horn of hyoid bone
12 Inferior constrictor muscle
13 Thyrohyoid muscle
14 Omohyoid muscle (superior belly)
15 Sternothyroid muscle
16 Sternohyoid muscle

The middle constrictor muscle (11.7–11.12)

Attachments: This muscle arises from the lower part of the stylohyoid ligament and from the hyoid bone (the lesser horn and the whole of the upper border of the greater horn). The fibres fan out to be inserted posteriorly into the pharyngeal raphe.

Innervation: The middle constrictor muscle is supplied by the cranial part of the accessory nerve.

Vasculature: Branches from the ascending pharyngeal artery (pharyngeal branch) and facial artery (tonsillar branch) are the chief sources of blood supply for the middle constrictor muscle.

Actions: The muscle constricts the pharynx during swallowing.

The inferior constrictor muscle (11.7–11.12)

Attachments: The inferior constrictor muscle has two main sites of origin, the thyroid and cricoid cartilages of the larynx. Indeed, the muscle consists of two parts, the thyropharyngeus and cricopharyngeus muscles.

The *thyropharyngeus muscle* arises from the oblique line on the lamina of the thyroid cartilage. Its fibres pass backwards and upwards to insert into the pharyngeal raphe.

The *cricopharyngeus muscle* arises from the lateral surface of the cricoid cartilage, just behind the origin of the cricothyroid muscle. Whereas the other constrictor muscles run backwards and upwards to insert into the pharyngeal raphe, cricopharyngeus passes only backwards to encircle the pharynx in a region lacking a pharyngeal raphe.

Between the two parts of the inferior constrictor muscle, some additional fibres arise from a tendinous cord that loops over the cricothyroid muscle.

Innervation: The muscle is supplied by the cranial part of the accessory nerve. Cricopharyngeus is also supplied by the recurrent laryngeal nerve and the internal branch of the superior laryngeal nerve.

Vasculature: The arterial supply to the muscle is derived from the ascending pharyngeal artery (pharyngeal branch) and the inferior thyroid artery (muscular branches).

Actions: The thyropharyngeus muscle constricts the lower part of the pharynx. The cricopharyngeus muscles act as a sphincter at the junction of the laryngopharynx and the oesophagus.

The palatopharyngeus muscle (11.2–11.5)

Attachments: This muscle has two heads of origin which enclose the levator veli palatini muscle. An anterior head arises from the back of the hard palate. A posterior head arises from the upper surface of the palatine aponeurosis. The palatopharyngeus muscles on each side meet in the midline at their origins in the palate.

The two heads of the palatopharyngeus muscle merge to pass down within the palatopharyngeal arch at the back of the mouth. The muscle lies on the internal surface of the constrictor muscles of the pharynx and inserts into the posterior border of the thyroid cartilage of the larynx.

Innervation: The nerve supply to the palatopharyngeus muscle is the cranial part of the accessory nerve.

Vasculature: The muscle derives its arterial supply from the facial artery (ascending palatine branch), the maxillary artery (descending palatine branch) and the ascending pharyngeal artery (pharyngeal branch).

Actions: From its superior attachments, palatopharyngeus elevates the pharynx and larynx. It can also elevate the side of the tongue, and draw together the palatopharyngeal arches to close the oropharyngeal isthmus. The muscles may depress the soft palate when acting from their inferior attachments.

Passavant's muscle is a sphincter-like muscle which encircles the pharynx at the level of the palate. Contraction of this muscle forms a ridge (Passavant's ridge) against which the soft palate is elevated. Controversy exists concerning the derivation of the muscle. Some anatomists consider Passavant's muscle to be derived from the superior constrictor and palatopharyngeus muscle. Others claim that it is a distinct palatine muscle that arises from the anterior and lateral parts of the upper surface of the palatine aponeurosis.

11.8 Posterior view showing constrictor muscles of the pharynx

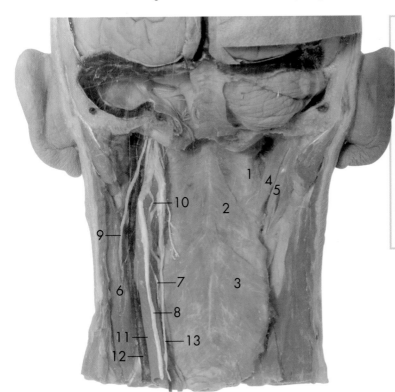

1	Superior constrictor muscle
2	Middle constrictor muscle
3	Inferior constrictor muscle
4	Stylopharyngeus muscle
5	Stylohyoid muscle
6	Sternocleidomastoid muscle
7	External laryngeal nerve
8	Vagus nerve
9	Spinal accessory nerve
10	Superior laryngeal nerve
11	Common carotid artery
12	Internal jugular vein
13	Sympathetic trunk

11.9 The relationship of the constrictor muscles to the hyoid bone and the larynx

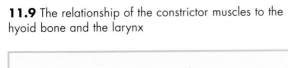

1	Digastric muscle (anterior belly)
2	Digastric muscle (posterior belly)
3	Greater horn of the hyoid bone
4	Thyroid cartilage of the larynx
5	Mylohyoid muscle
6	Middle constrictor muscle of the pharynx
7	Inferior constrictor muscle fo the pharynx
8	Thyrohyoid muscle
9	Trachea
10	Oesophagus

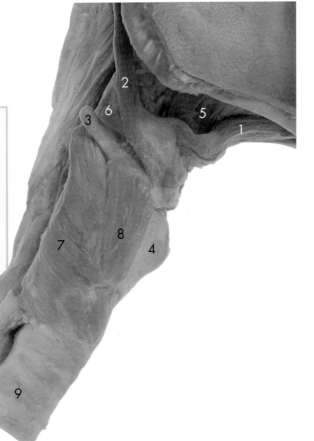

The salpingopharyngeus muscle (11.4, 11.10, 11.11)

Attachments: This muscle arises from the cartilage of the auditory tube, close to the opening in the nasopharynx. The salpingopharyngeus muscle runs down the internal surface of the pharynx, producing the salpingopharyngeal fold. It merges with the palatopharyngeus muscle.

Innervation: The nerve supply to this muscle is the cranial part of the accessory nerve.

Vasculature: The muscle derives its arterial supply from the same sources as the palatopharyngeus muscle.

Actions: The salpingopharyngeus muscle elevates the pharynx. It may also open the cartilaginous end of the auditory tube during swallowing.

The stylopharyngeus muscle (11.2, 11.8, 11.10, 11.12)

Attachments: This muscle arises from the medial surface of the base of the styloid process (temporal bone). It passes down into the pharynx between the superior and middle constrictor muscles. Some fibres merge with the constrictor muscles, others insert into the posterior border of the thyroid cartilage of the larynx.

Innervation: Unlike the other pharyngeal muscles, the stylopharyngeus muscle receives its innervation from the glossopharyngeal nerve and not from the cranial part of the accessory nerve.

Vasculature: Its arterial supply is derived from the ascending pharyngeal artery (pharyngeal branch).

Actions: The muscle elevates the pharynx and larynx.

THE MUCOSA AND FASCIA OF THE PHARYNX

The mucosa varies in different parts of the pharynx. The epithelium covering the nasopharynx is of the ciliated columnar type and therefore resembles the epithelium of the nose. The epithelium of the oropharynx and laryngopharynx is of the stratified squamous type and resembles that found in the mouth. This epithelium is tightly bound to the underlying pharyngobasilar fascia.

The mucosa of the pharynx contains aggregations of lymphatic material forming the pharyngeal and tubal tonsils in the nasopharynx and the palatine and lingual tonsils in the oropharynx. This ring of lymphoid material is referred to as Waldermeyer's ring.

The pharyngobasilar fascia is a distinct membranous fascia that lies between the mucosa and the muscle of the wall of the pharynx. It is particularly well-developed superiorly, where it extends above the free margin of the superior constrictor muscle to the base of the skull. It is attached to the basilar part of the occipital bone, the petrous part of the temporal bone in front of the carotid canal, the border of the medial pterygoid plate and to the pterygomandibular raphe. The pharyngobasilar fascia above the superior constrictor muscle is pierced by the levator veli palatini muscle, the cartilaginous end of the auditory tube and the ascending palatine artery.

The external surface of the wall of the pharynx is covered by a thin connective tissue layer, the buccopharyngeal fascia. The use of the term fascia to describe this connective tissue is debatable, as it is not a membranous layer. Indeed, a membranous layer in this site would be disadvantageous because considerable mobility of the pharynx is necessary during swallowing. On the buccopharyngeal connective tissue is found the pharyngeal venous plexus and the pharyngeal nerve plexus. The posterior part of the wall of the pharynx is separated from the prevertebral musculature and the prevertebral fascia by loose connective tissue occupying a potential tissue space called the retropharyngeal space (see page 336).

11.10 The muscles of the pharynx viewed from behind

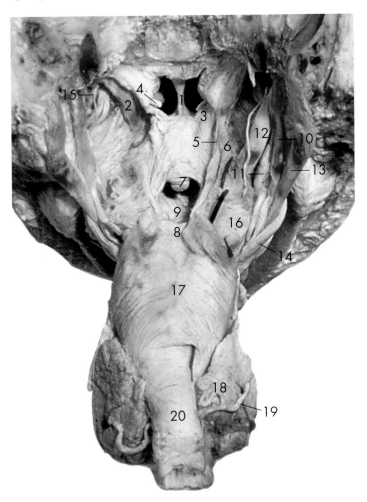

1 Nasal septum	12 Glossopharyngeal nerve on the stylopharyngeus muscle
2 Tensor palati muscle	
3 Levator veli palatini muscle	13 Posterior belly of the digastric muscle
4 Marker in the opening of the auditory tube	14 Hypoglossal nerve
5 Salpingopharyngeus muscle	15 Chorda tympani nerve joining lingual nerve
6 Superior constrictor muscle (cut end)	
7 Uvula of the soft palate	16 Middle constrictor muscle
8 Epiglottis	17 Inferior constrictor muscle
9 Back of tongue	18 Thyroid gland
10 Stylohyoid muscle	19 Inferior thyroid artery
11 Styloglossus muscle	20 Oesophagus

11.11 Internal view of the anterior wall of the pharynx

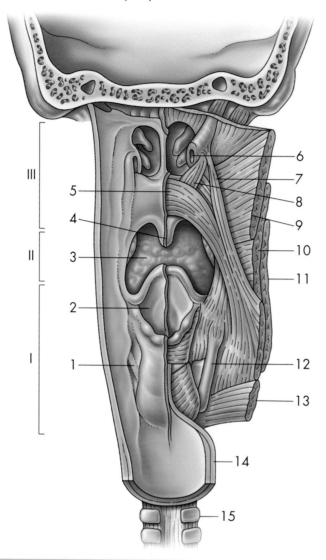

I Laryngopharynx	7 Salpingopharyngeus muscle
II Oropharynx	8 Levator veli palatini muscle
III Nasopharynx	9 Superior constrictor muscle
	10 Middle constrictor muscle
1 Piriform fossa with internal laryngeal nerve beneath mucosa	11 Thyropharyngeal part of inferior constrictor muscle
2 Inlet of larynx	12 Thyroid lamina (posterior border)
3 Tongue	13 Cricopharyngeal part of inferior constrictor muscle
4 Uvula	
5 Palatopharyngeus muscle	14 Oesophagus
6 Auditory tube	15 Trachea

11.12 The pharynx viewed from the side

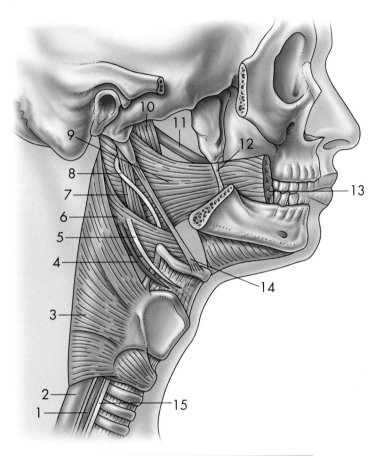

1 Inferior laryngeal artery
2 Oesophagus
3 Inferior constrictor muscle
4 Superior laryngeal artery
5 Internal laryngeal nerve
6 Middle constrictor muscle
7 Stylopharyngeus muscle
8 Glossopharyngeal nerve
9 Superior constrictor muscle
10 Levator veli palatini muscle
11 Auditory tube
12 Pterygomandibular raphe
13 Buccinator muscle
14 Stylohyoid ligament
15 Recurrent laryngeal nerve

STRUCTURES PASSING THROUGH THE WALL OF THE PHARYNX (11.12–11.14)

In the interval between the superior constrictor muscle and the base of the skull pass the levator veli palatini muscle, the cartilaginous end of the auditory tube and the ascending palatine artery.

Between the superior and middle constrictor muscles run the stylopharyngeus muscle, the glossopharyngeal nerve, the styloglossus muscle, the lingual nerve and artery, and the hypoglossal nerve.

Passing between the middle and inferior constrictor muscles are the internal branch of the superior laryngeal nerve (from the vagus nerve) and the superior laryngeal artery (a branch of the superior thyroid artery).

Underneath the lower border of the inferior constrictor muscle run the recurrent laryngeal nerve (from the vagus nerve) and the inferior laryngeal nerve (a branch of the inferior thyroid artery).

THE INNERVATION OF THE PHARYNX (11.12–11.16)

Most of the pharynx derives its sensory nerve supply from the glossopharyngeal nerve through its pharyngeal and tonsillar branches. The pharyngeal branch arises just before the glossopharyngeal nerve passes onto the posterior surface of the stylopharyngeus muscle. This branch then joins the pharyngeal branch of the vagus to reach the pharyngeal plexus. The tonsillar branch of the glossopharyngeal nerve supplies the region around the oropharyngeal isthmus.

The anterior part of the nasopharynx is not supplied by the glossopharyngeal nerve but by the pharyngeal branch of the maxillary nerve. Furthermore, the soft palate is innervated by the lesser palatine branch of the maxillary nerve. Both the pharyngeal and lesser palatine nerves are branches of the maxillary division of the trigeminal nerve via the pterygopalatine ganglion (see page 216).

The lower part of the pharynx is innervated by the superior laryngeal branch of the vagus nerve.

The muscles of the pharynx derive their innervation from the nucleus ambiguus in the brain stem. Fibres pass from this nucleus within the glossopharyngeal, vagus and cranial accessory nerves. The cranial accessory nerve, however, joins the vagus nerve shortly after emerging through the jugular foramen of the skull. These fibres, together with those already in the vagus, reach the pharyngeal plexus via the pharyngeal branch of the vagus to supply most of the muscles of the pharynx. The stylopharyngeus muscle, however, is supplied by fibres from the nucleus ambiguus that run with the glossopharyngeal nerve.

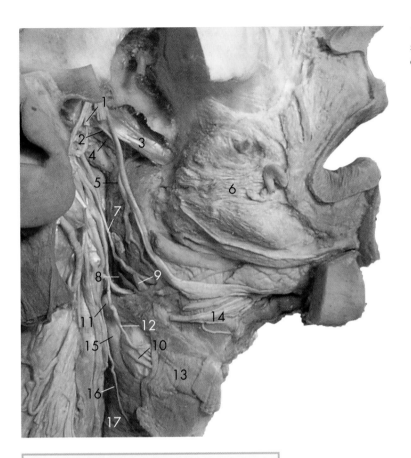

11.13 The lateral view of the pharynx showing structures passing between the constrictor muscles

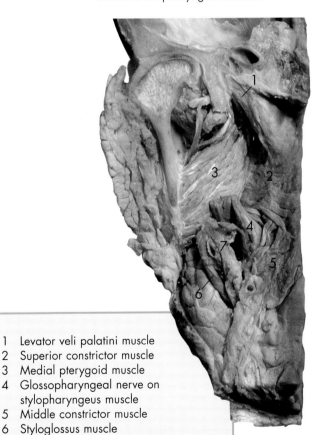

11.14 Posterior view of the pharynx showing some structures passing between the pharyngeal muscles

1   Middle meningeal artery passing between the roots of the auriculotemporal nerve
2   Chorda tympani nerve joining lingual nerve
3   Tensor palati muscle
4   Levator veli palatini muscle
5   Ascending palatine artery on superior constrictor muscle
6   Buccinator muscle
7   Glossopharyngeal nerve and cut end of stylopharyngeus muscle
8   Middle constrictor muscle
9   Lingual artery (cut end)
10 Laryngeal branch of superior thyroid artery (cut)
11 Greater horn of hyoid bone
12 Internal laryngeal nerve
13 Thyrohyoid muscle
14 Hypoglossal nerve on hyoglossus muscle
15 Superior horn of thyroid cartilage
16 External laryngeal nerve
17 Inferior constrictor muscle

1   Levator veli palatini muscle
2   Superior constrictor muscle
3   Medial pterygoid muscle
4   Glossopharyngeal nerve on stylopharyngeus muscle
5   Middle constrictor muscle
6   Styloglossus muscle
7   Stylohyoid and posterior belly of digastric muscles

The pharyngeal plexus lies on the external surface of the middle constrictor muscle. It is formed by the pharyngeal branches of the glossopharyngeal and vagus nerves, with contributions from the superior cervical sympathetic ganglion. The glossopharyngeal nerve supplies only sensory fibres to the plexus. The vagus contains motor fibres associated with the cranial part of the accessory nerve which, in addition to supplying the muscles of the pharynx, also supply the muscles of the soft palate (see pages 170–172).

THE VASCULATURE OF THE PHARYNX

The pharynx receives its blood supply from many sources, including the ascending pharyngeal artery (pharyngeal branch), the inferior thyroid artery, the facial artery (ascending palatine and tonsillar branches), maxillary artery (pharyngeal, greater palatine branches and the artery of the pterygoid canal), and the lingual artery (dorsal lingual branch).

The veins of the pharynx drain into the pharyngeal plexus. This plexus is situated on the posterior wall of the pharynx. Pharyngeal veins drain the plexus into the internal jugular or into the brachiocephalic vein (via the inferior thyroid vein). The pharyngeal plexus may communicate with other veins, including the facial vein and the pterygoid venous plexus.

The lymphatic vessels from the pharynx drain into the deep cervical lymph nodes either directly or indirectly via the paratracheal or retropharyngeal nodes. In addition, lymph from the area around the epiglottis passes into the infrahyoid nodes.

SWALLOWING

Swallowing involves an ordered sequence of reflex events which carries food (or saliva) from the mouth into the stomach. The nasopharynx during swallowing is isolated from the oropharynx by elevation of the soft palate. As this process occupies a total of only a few minutes in every day, the pharynx is normally maintained in the respiratory position.

The first stage of swallowing is voluntary and involves the passage of the bolus of food onto the tongue and towards the oropharyngeal isthmus. The airway remains patent during this phase.

When the bolus reaches the oropharyngeal isthmus during the second stage of swallowing, the process becomes involuntary. The soft palate and larynx are elevated and a wave of muscular activity of the pharyngeal constrictor muscles carries the bolus through the pharynx. This stage ends when the bolus passes into the oesophagus.

During the third stage of swallowing, the bolus passes down the oesophagus and into the stomach.

The main events during swallowing are summarised in Table 11.1.

11.15 Posterior view of the pharyngeal reqion showing some associated nerves

1 Superior constrictor muscle
2 Middle constrictor muscle
3 Inferior constrictor muscle
4 Spinal accessory nerve
5 Vagus nerve
6 Superior laryngeal nerve
7 Sympathetic chain
8 Internal jugular vein
9 Common carotid artery

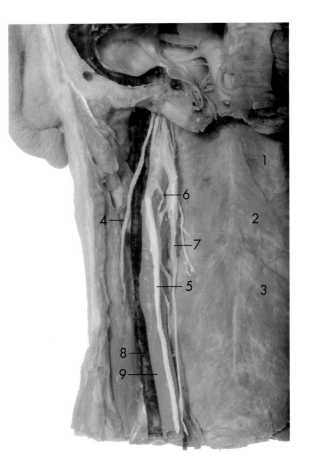

Table 11.1 Principal events during swallowing

Stage	Mechanisms associated with passage of bolus	Mechanisms associated with protecting airway
Voluntary **Bolus in mouth**	Mouth closed (temporalis, masseter, medial pterygoid) Lips closed (orbicularis oris) Tongue grooved, anterior part raised against palate (intrinsic tongue muscles, genioglossus)	**Airway open** Pillars of fauces contracted against posterior surface of tongue (palatoglossus, palatopharyngeus)
Involuntary **Bolus passes into oropharynx**	Posterior part of tongue moves upwards and backwards (styloglossus, mylohyoid) Groove in tongue flattened out (intrinsic tongue muscles) Pillars of fauces contract behind bolus	**Nasopharynx closed off** Soft palate tensed and elevated (tensor veli palatini, levator veli palatini, Passavant's muscle)
Bolus passes over epiglottis to lateral food channels	Pharynx elevated (stylopharyngeus, salpingopharyngeus, palatopharyngeus)	**Inlet of larynx closed off** Larynx elevated beneath epiglottis and posterior part of tongue (stylopharyngeus, salpingopharyngeus, palatopharyngeus, thyrohyoid) Laryngeal inlet reduced by approximation (interarytenoid, thyroarytenoid) and tension (lateral cricoarytenoid, interarytenoid) of aryepiglottic folds
Bolus passes into oesophagus	Relaxation of cricopharyngeus	**Airway re-established** Soft palate and larynx returned to original positions

chapter 12

THE LARYNX

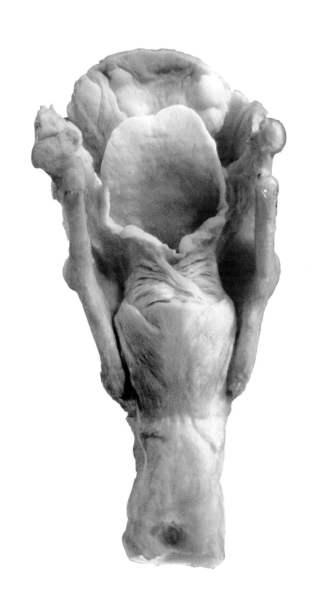

Chapter 12 THE LARYNX

The larynx is the organ responsible for speech (phonation). It is situated in the midline of the neck at the level of the third to the sixth cervical vertebrae. It extends from the laryngeal inlet near the root of the tongue to the trachea. At its inlet, the larynx communicates with the pharynx (laryngopharynx).

Not only is the larnyx an organ of speech, it is also important in maintaining the patency of the airway to allow continuous breathing. Temporary closure of the airway at the larynx can occur physiologically in three situations: swallowing, speech, and just before coughing and sneezing. The airway during swallowing is protected by the sphincter-like action of the musculature at the inlet of the larynx, by the displacement of the epiglottis over the inlet, and by the elevation of the larynx. In addition, the vocal folds within the larynx are approximated and breathing is momentarily inhibited. The vocal folds also close during speech and momentarily just before coughing and sneezing.

The larynx *in situ* shows few features externally. It is essentially a tube-like structure whose rigidity and form depends upon an underlying cartilaginous skeleton. Anteriorly, the larynx is almost completely covered by the infrahyoid (strap) muscles and the thyroid gland. The only feature usually visible is the laryngeal prominence of the thyroid cartilage (Adam's apple). From the posterior aspect, the larynx forms the anterior wall of the laryngopharynx. The inlet of the larynx (or aditus) is bounded anteriorly and superiorly by the epiglottis, posteriorly and inferiorly by the mucosa over the arytenoid cartilages, and laterally by the aryepiglottic folds. The pharynx extends along the sides of the inlet to form the piriform fossae. From above, the epiglottis and the root of the tongue are separated by depressions called the valleculae. The valleculae are bounded by the median and lateral glosso-epiglottic folds. Vestibular and vocal folds can also be seen within the larynx.

THE SKELETON OF THE LARYNX

The skeletal framework of the larynx consists of cartilages and membranes. Its function is to prevent collapse of the air passages and to give attachment to a series of muscles.

THE LARYNGEAL CARTILAGES (12.1–12.5)

The major cartilages of the larynx are the thyroid, cricoid and arytenoid cartilages. The minor cartilages are the cuneiform and corniculate cartilages. The arytenoid, cuneiform and corniculate cartilages are paired. Associated with the larynx is the epiglottic cartilage.

The epiglottic cartilage, the cuneiform cartilages, the corniculate cartilages and part of the vocal process and apex of the arytenoid cartilages are composed of elastic cartilage. The other laryngeal cartilages are hyaline cartilages and may ossify in a process commencing at about 20 years of age.

The thyroid cartilage

This is the largest and most prominent cartilage, forming most of the anterior and lateral walls of the larynx.

The overall shape of the thyroid cartilage takes the form of a shield. It consists of two flattened, quadrilateral laminae which are joined anteriorly to form the laryngeal prominence ('Adam's apple'). Above this prominence, the laminae are separated by a deep V-shaped notch called the thyroid notch. Posteriorly, the laminae project upwards and downwards as the superior and inferior horns. On the external surface of each lamina lies an oblique ridge which is the site for muscle attachments. The ridge runs downwards and forwards from the superior horn towards the lower border of the cartilage. It is bounded above and below by a tubercle. The thyroid cartilage shows sexual dimorphism: in the male, it considerably increases in size at puberty and the thyroid prominence becomes very distinct.

12.1 The larynx seen from the laryngopharynx

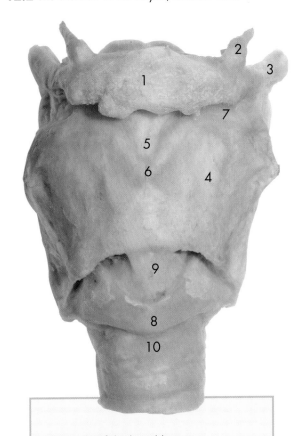

12.2 The skeleton of the larynx, anterior view

1 Dorsal surface of the tongue (pharyngeal part) with lingual follicles (lingual tonsil)
2 Foramen caecum
3 Vallecula
4 Epiglottis
5 Mucosa covering arytenoid cartilage
6 Laryngeal inlet
7 Aryepiglottic fold
8 Posterior surface (lamina) of the cricoid cartilage of larynx with posterior cricoarytenoid muscles
9 Interarytenoid muscle
10 Wall of laryngopharynx
11 Piriform fossa

1 Body of the hyoid bone
2 Lesser horn of the hyoid bone
3 Greater horn of the hyoid bone
4 Thyroid cartilage of the larynx
5 Thyroid notch
6 Laryngeal prominence
7 Thyrohyoid membrane
8 Anterior arch of cricoid cartilage of larynx
9 Anterior (median) cricothyroid ligament
10 First tracheal ring

12.3 The skeleton of the larynx, viewed internally

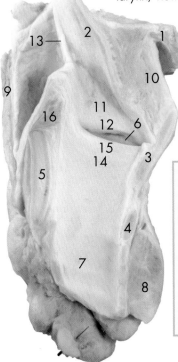

1 Hyoid bone
2 Epiglottis
3 Thyroid cartilage
4 Arch of cricoid cartilage
5 Lamina of cricoid cartilage
6 Ventricle of larynx
7 Trachea
8 Isthmus of thyroid gland
9 Muscular wall of the pharynx
10 Thyrohyoid ligament
11 Mucosa covering quadrangular membrane
12 Vestibular fold (false cord)
13 Aryepiglottic fold
14 Mucosa covering cricovocal membrane
15 Vocal fold
16 Interarytenoid muscle

The cricoid cartilage

Unlike the thyroid cartilage, the cricoid cartilage forms a complete ring. Indeed, it is the only complete cartilaginous ring in the air passages. It comprises the most inferior and posterior part of the larynx and supports the entrance to the trachea. The shape of the cricoid cartilage resembles that of a signet ring, showing a narrow arch anteriorly and a flat, quadrangular lamina posteriorly. Where the arch meets the lamina are small articular facets for the inferior horns of the thyroid cartilage. The superior edge of the lamina has sloping shoulders, and articular facets for the arytenoid cartilages. The cricoid cartilage may appear more prominent in the female.

The arytenoid cartilages

The arytenoid cartilages lie in the postero-inferior part of the larynx, on the superior edge of the lamina of the cricoid cartilage. They contribute to the margin of the inlet of the larynx. Each cartilage is pyramidal in shape, although the superior process or apex of the pyramid is really the corniculate cartilage. The base of the arytenoid cartilage presents the articulating surface with the cricoid. The arytenoid cartilage has a process anteriorly called the vocal process (for attachment of the vocal ligament), and a process laterally named the muscular process (for the attachment of some of the muscles of the larynx).

The minor cartilages of the larynx

The corniculate cartilages surmount the arytenoid cartilages, thus completing their pyramidal shapes.

The cuneiform cartilages lie within the aryepiglottic folds at the inlet of the pharynx.

Small triticeal cartilages are found in the ligaments joining the tips of the superior horns of the thyroid cartilage to the tips of the greater horns of the hyoid bone.

Articulations of the laryngeal cartilages

The inferior horn of the thyroid cartilage articulates with the cricoid cartilage by way of a synovial joint. This joint has a well-developed capsule which is strengthened posteriorly by fibrous bands. The joint permits a rotary movement with activity of the cricothyroid muscle, such that the thyroid cartilage tilts forwards and downwards with upward movement of the arch of the cricoid cartilage (12.17).

The joints between the bases of the arytenoid cartilages and the lamina of the cricoid cartilage are also synovial. The capsules of the joints are strengthened by posterior crico-arytenoid ligaments (which are primarily medial in position) which are said to limit forward movements of the arytenoids. Rotation and gliding movements of the arytenoids occur at these joints, both types of movement being responsible for opening and closing the rima glottidis. It has been postulated that the major determinant of the position taken up by the denervated vocal fold is not dependent on the musculature as is generally assumed, but on the resting position of the posterior crico-arytenoid ligament.

Synovial or cartilaginous joints link the corniculate cartilages to the arytenoids.

The epiglottis

The epiglottis consists of a thin lamina of elastic cartilage covered on all sides with mucous membrane. It is leaf-shaped, the 'stalk' providing the means of attachment to the larynx via a thyro-epiglottic ligament. A depression for this ligament lies just below the thyroid notch on the inner surface of the thyroid cartilage. The epiglottis is also anchored to the posterior surface of the body of the hyoid bone by a hyo-epiglottic ligament. The sides of the epiglottis are attached to the arytenoid cartilages by the aryepiglottic folds. Median and lateral glosso-epiglottic folds pass from the root of the tongue to the anterior surface of the epiglottis. The epiglottis projects upwards and backwards over the vestibule of the larynx and gives the appearance of a 'lid'. However, it does not seem to function as such, as its surgical removal has no adverse effects. The posterior surface of the cartilage of the epiglottis shows numerous small indentations or perforations in which lie mucous glands.

12.4 The skeleton of the larynx, lateral view

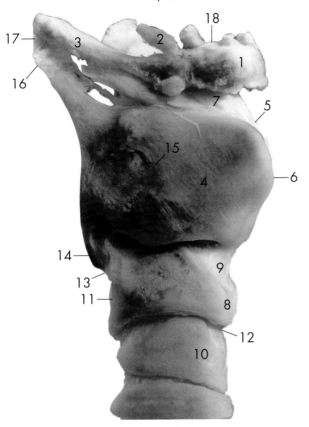

12.5 The skeleton of the larynx, posterior view

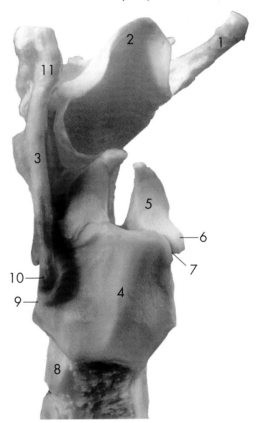

1	Body of the hyoid bone
2	Lesser horn of the hyoid bone
3	Greater horn of the hyoid bone
4	Thyroid cartilage of the larynx
5	Thyroid notch
6	Laryngeal prominence
7	Thyrohyoid membrane
8	Anterior arch of cricoid cartilage of the larynx
9	Anterior (median) cricothyroid ligament
10	First tracheal ring
11	Lamina of cricoid cartilage
12	Cricotracheal membrane
13	Capsule of cricothyroid joint
14	Inferior horn of thyroid cartilage
15	Oblique line of thyroid cartilage
16	Superior horn of thyroid cartilage
17	Lateral thyrohyoid ligament
18	Superior edge of the epiglottis

1	Greater horn of hyoid bone
2	Epiglottis
3	Thyroid cartilage of the larynx (posterior border)
4	Lamina of cricoid cartilage
5	Arytenoid cartilage (apex – minor corniculate cartilage)
6	Arytenoid cartilage (muscular process)
7	Articular surfaces of crico-arytenoid joint
8	First tracheal ring
9	Articulation between the thyroid and cricoid cartilages
10	Inferior horn of thyroid cartilage
11	Superior horn of thyroid cartilage

THE LARYNGEAL MEMBRANES (12.6–12.8)

The larynx has thyrohyoid, quadrangular and cricovocal membranes. The thyrohyoid membrane is external to the larynx, whereas the paired quadrangular and cricovocal membranes are internal. All the membranes are composed of fibro-elastic tissue. There are also two ligaments, the anterior cricothyroid ligament and the cricotracheal ligament.

The thyrohyoid membrane

This membrane extends from the upper border of the thyroid cartilage to the upper border of the inner surface of the hyoid bone (both body and greater horns). Between the membrane and the hyoid bone lies a bursa.

The thyrohyoid membrane is thickened in three places to form ligament-like structures. In the midline is found the median thyrohyoid ligament. At the lateral margins are found the lateral thyrohyoid ligaments; connecting the tips of the superior horns of the thyroid cartilage to those of the greater horns of the hyoid bone. The lateral ligaments may contain triticeal cartilages.

The thyrohyoid membrane is pierced by the superior laryngeal vessels and the internal laryngeal nerves as they course into the larynx.

The quadrangular membrane

Each quadrangular membrane passes from the lateral margin of the epiglottis to the arytenoid cartilage on its own side. It is often poorly defined. The membrane shows two free borders. The upper and posterior border forms the aryepiglottic fold. The lower border forms the ventricular fold. Within the aryepiglottic folds lie the cuneiform cartilages.

The cricovocal membrane

This membrane is more pronounced than the quadrangular membrane, and arises from the side of the larynx at the upper border of the arch of the cricoid cartilage. It passes internally, deep to the lamina of the thyroid cartilage, to become attached anteriorly to the inner surface of the thyroid cartilage close to the midline, and posteriorly to the vocal process of the arytenoid cartilage.

The cricovocal membrane has an upper free margin which passes across the larynx. This is thickened to form the vocal ligament.

The anterior (median) cricothyroid ligament

This is considered by some anatomists to be a superficial part of the cricovocal membrane. It is situated anteriorly in the midline, passing from the upper border of the cricoid cartilage to the lower border of the thyroid cartilage.

The cricotracheal ligament

This ligament joins the lower border of the cricoid cartilage to the first ring of the trachea.

Unfortunately, considerable differences in terminology are found in different textbooks with respect to the laryngeal membranes. In some the cricovocal membrane and the anterior cricothyroid ligament are collectively called the cricothyroid ligament, the cricovocal membrane being designated the lateral cricothyroid ligament. Such terminology ignores the fact that the cricovocal membrane shows a thickened ligament only where it becomes the vocal ligament. Furthermore, it is attached not only to the thyroid cartilage but also to the arytenoid cartilage. Another collective term found in the literature is conus elasticus. To add further to the confusion, some anatomists restrict the term conus elasticus to the anterior cricothyroid ligament.

12.6 The larynx viewed anteriorly to show laryngeal membranes

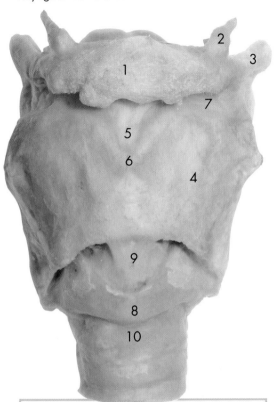

12.7 The larynx with left ala of thyroid cartilage removed, showing the internal anatomy

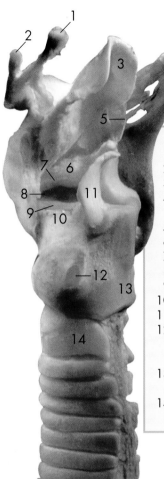

1 Greater horn of hyoid bone
2 Lesser horn of hyoid bone
3 Epiglottis
4 Superior horn of thyroid cartilage
5 Aryepiglottic fold
6 Quandrangular membrane
7 Vestibular fold
8 Ventricle of the larynx
9 Vocal fold
10 Cricovocal membrane
11 Arytenoid cartilage
12 Facet for articulation with inferior horn of the thyroid cartilage
13 Lamina of the cricoid cartilage
14 First tracheal ring

1 Body of the hyoid bone
2 Lesser horn of the hyoid bone
3 Greater horn of the hyoid bone
4 Thyroid cartilage of the larynx
5 Thyroid notch
6 Laryngeal prominence
7 Thyrohyoid membrane
8 Anterior arch of cricoid cartilage of larynx
9 Anterior (median) cricothyroid ligament
10 First tracheal ring

12.8 Sagittal section of the larynx illustrating the laryngeal membranes

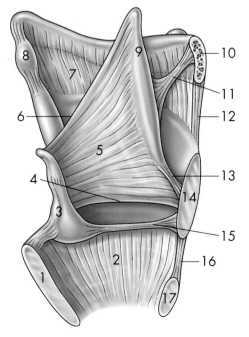

1 Lamina of cricoid cartilage
2 Cricovocal membrane
3 Arytenoid cartilage
4 Vestibular fold
5 Quadrangular membrane
6 Aryepiglottic fold
7 Thyrohyoid membrane
8 Triticeal cartilage in lateral thyrohyoid ligament
9 Epiglottis

10 Body of hyoid bone
11 Hyo-epiglottic ligament
12 Median thyrohyoid ligament
13 Thyro-epiglottic ligament
14 Thyroid cartilage
15 Vocal ligament
16 Anterior cricothyroid ligament
17 Arch of cricoid cartilage

THE INTERNAL ANATOMY OF THE LARYNX

The larynx is lined internally and on its outer, posterior surface by mucous membrane. The mucous membrane on the posterior surface also forms the anterior wall of the laryngopharynx. Internally, the mucosa lines the quadrangular and cricovocal membranes and contributes to the formation of the vestibular and vocal folds.

The interior of the larynx shows several compartments which are defined by two prominent folds, the vestibular folds above and the vocal folds below. Between the laryngeal inlet and the vestibular folds lies the vestibule. Below the vocal folds lies the infraglottic cavity. Between the vestibular and vocal folds are two slit-like spaces called the ventricles (or sinuses). A small pouch of mucosa called the saccule extends upwards from the anterior end of each ventricle between the vestibular fold and the inner surface of the thyroid cartilage. The saccule is the site of mucous glands whose secretions help to lubricate the vocal folds which themselves lack glands.

THE VESTIBULAR FOLD (12.9–12.12)

The vestibular fold has also been called the false vocal fold, the ventricular fold, or the superior vocal fold. It is a thick ridge of mucosa with a thin central layer of connective tissue which is the inferior free edge of a membrane called the quadrangular membrane.

The vestibular fold is located above and lateral to the vocal fold. This is an important relationship when viewing the internal anatomy of the larynx with a laryngoscope. With such an instrument, the vestibular fold appears simply as an inward bulge of the mucosa.

The fissure between the two vestibular folds is called the rima vestibuli.

THE VOCAL FOLD (12.9–12.12)

The anterior three-fifths of the vocal fold is formed by the vocal cord or ligament. This is the thickened free

edge of a membrane of the larynx called the cricovocal membrane. Because the mucosa covering the vocal fold in this region is firmly bound down to the vocal ligament, the fold appears pearly white in the living. The posterior two-fifths of the vocal fold is formed by the vocal process of the arytenoid cartilage.

The site where the vocal folds meet anteriorly is known as the anterior commissure. Fibres of the vocal ligament here pass through the thyroid cartilage to blend with the overlying perichondrium, forming Broyles ligament. The ligament contains blood vessels and lymphatics and is therefore a potential route for spread of malignant tumours from the larynx.

The fissure between the two vocal folds is called the rima glottidis (or glottis). That part between the vocal ligaments is called the intermembranous part. That part between the arytenoid cartilages is named the intercartilaginous part. The shape and size of the rima glottidis vary greatly during respiration and phonation. In quiet respiration, it has a triangular shape. During speech, the vocal folds are brought together. In whispering, the vocal folds are slightly separated at the intermembranous part, whereas a triangular space remains at the intercartilaginous part.

Figure 12.9 (opposite)
1 Epiglottis
2 Thyroid cartilage
3 Arch of cricoid cartilage
4 Lamina of cricoid cartilage
5 Position of arytenoid cartilage
6 Trachea
7 Thyrothyroid membrane
8 Hyoid bone
9 Vestibule of larynx
10 Quadrangular membrane
11 Vestibular fold (false cord)
12 Aryepiglottic fold
13 Cricovocal membrane
14 Vocal fold
15 Ventricle of the larynx
16 Interarytenoid muscle
17 Infraglottic cavity

12.9 The internal anatomy of the larynx, lateral view

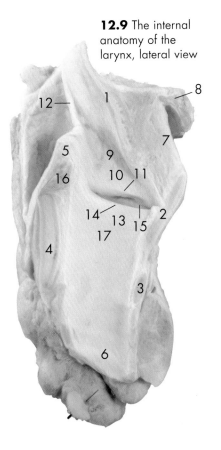

12.10 The internal anatomy of the larynx, posterior view

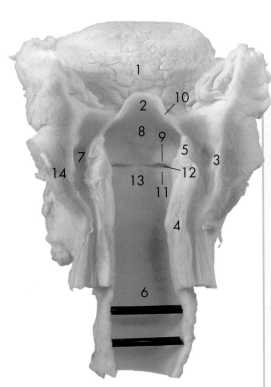

1. Dorsum of the tongue
2. Epiglottis
3. Thyroid cartilage
4. Lamina of cricoid cartilage
5. Position of an arytenoid cartilage
6. Trachea
7. Piriform fossa
8. Vestibule of larynx
9. Vestibular fold (false cord)
10. Aryepiglottic fold
11. Vocal fold
12. Ventricle of the larynx
13. Infraglottic cavity
14. Wall of the pharynx

12.11 Interior of the larynx as viewed with a laryngoscope

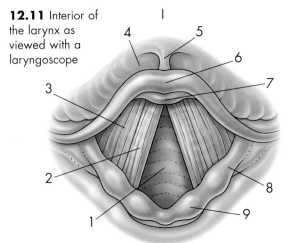

I   Anterior

1. Trachea seen through rima glottidis
2. Vocal cord
3. Vestibular fold
4. Vallecula
5. Median glosso-epiglottic fold
6. Epiglottis
7. Tubercle of epiglottis
8. Aryepiglottic fold
9. Arytenoid cartilage

12.12 The laryngeal folds seen through a laryngoscope

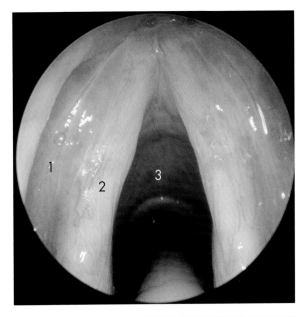

1. Vestibular fold (false cord)
2. Vocal fold
3. Rima glottidis

THE MUSCLES OF THE LARYNX (12.13–12.17)

The muscles can be categorised as extrinsic or intrinsic.

The extrinsic muscles of the larynx

These muscles have an attachment outside the larynx and include the infrahyoid (strap) muscles of the neck (see pages 328–330), and the stylopharyngeus, palatopharyngeus and inferior constrictor muscles of the pharynx (see pages 402–406).

The extrinsic muscles are responsible for movements of the whole larynx, i.e. elevation and depression during swallowing, respiration and phonation. The thyrohyoid, stylopharyngeus and palatopharyngeus muscles elevate the larynx. The omohyoid, sternohyoid and sternothyroid muscles depress the larynx. Of these latter muscles, sternothyroid is the only one that has an attachment on the larynx and which therefore depresses the larynx by direct action. The omohyoid and sternohyoid muscles can cause depression only indirectly by pressing on the larynx.

Because the larynx and the hyoid bone are connected by the thyrohyoid membrane, elevation of the larynx can occur by the actions of the suprahyoid musculature (mylohyoid, digastric, stylohyoid and geniohyoid muscles).

The intrinsic muscles of the larynx

These are confined to the larynx. Within this group are the posterior crico-arytenoid, interarytenoid, lateral crico-arytenoid, thyro-arytenoid and cricothyroid muscles. With the exception of the interarytenoid muscle, the muscles are paired.

The intrinsic muscles of the larynx are mainly concerned with the activities of the vocal folds. Subsidiary parts of the interarytenoid and thyro-arytenoid muscles (the aryepiglottic and thyro-epiglottic muscles) modify the inlet of the larynx.

Whereas most of the intrinsic muscles lie internally (under cover of the thyroid cartilage or the mucosa), the cricothyroid muscles appear on the outer aspect of the larynx.

The posterior crico-arytenoid muscle (12.13–12.15)
Attachments: This muscle arises from a broad depression on the posterior surface of the lamina of the cricoid cartilage. Passing upwards and laterally, it is inserted into the muscular process of the arytenoid cartilage.

Innervation: The recurrent laryngeal branch of the vagus nerve provides the motor supply, one branch supplying the more horizontal fibres, another branch supplying the more vertical fibres.

Vasculature: The posterior crico-arytenoid muscle receives its blood supply from the laryngeal branches of the superior and inferior thyroid arteries.

Actions: This is the only muscle that dilates the rima glottidis and it does so in two ways. First, the upper fibres, being almost horizontal, rotate the arytenoid cartilage. Second, the lower fibres, being more vertical, cause sliding of the arytenoid cartilage down the sloping superior margin of the cricoid cartilage.

The interarytenoid muscle (12.13–12.15)
Attachments: This is a single muscle in two parts, which runs posteriorly between the muscular processes of the arytenoid cartilages. Many of its fibres run transversely across the posterior surfaces of the arytenoids (the transverse arytenoid part), but some run obliquely from the muscular process of one arytenoid to the apex of the opposite cartilage (the oblique arytenoid part). The oblique fibres form two thin bands which cross to produce a distinctive X-shape. Some of the oblique fibres continue into the aryepiglottic folds as the aryepiglottic muscles.

Innervation: The muscle is innervated bilaterally by the recurrent laryngeal nerve. It also receives branches from the internal laryngeal nerve, the functional significance of which is not known.

Vasculature: The blood supply is derived from the laryngeal branches of the superior and inferior thyroid arteries.

Actions: The interarytenoid muscle closes the rima glottidis by approximating the arytenoid cartilages. This is accomplished by drawing the arytenoids upwards along the sloping shoulders of the cricoid lamina, without rotation. The aryepiglottic muscles modify the inlet of the larynx. However, their poor development limits their action as sphincters of the inlet.

12.13 Intrinsic muscles of the larynx

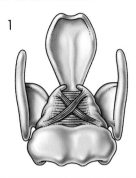

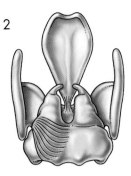

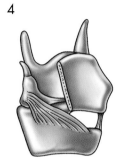

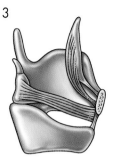

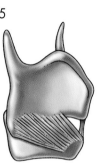

1 Interarytenoid muscle (tranverse and oblique fibres)
2 Posterior crico-arytenoid muscle
3 Thyro-arytenoid and thyro-epiglottic muscles
4 Lateral crico-arytenoid muscle
5 Cricothyroid muscle

12.14 Muscles of the larynx, posterior view

1 Epiglottis
2 Laryngeal inlet
3 Interarytenoid muscle (transverse agent)
4 Interarytenoid muscle (oblique part)
5 Posterior crico-arytenoid muscle

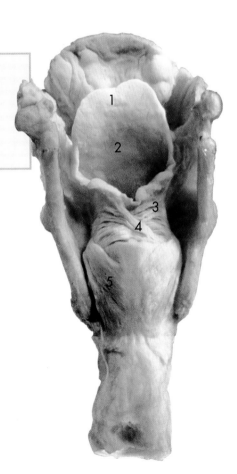

The lateral crico-arytenoid muscle (12.13, 12.15)

Attachments: This muscle originates from the lateral side of the upper border of the arch of the cricoid. It extends upwards and backwards beneath the thyroid cartilage to insert on to the muscular process of the arytenoid cartilage.

Innervation: The recurrent laryngeal nerve supplies the lateral crico-arytenoid muscle with a single main branch, suggesting the muscle acts as a 'single' unit, unlike the other intrinsic muscles of the larynx.

Vasculature: It receives its blood supply from the laryngeal branches of the superior and inferior thyroid arteries.

Actions: The lateral crico-arytenoid muscle rotates the arytenoid cartilage in a direction opposite to that of the posterior crico-arytenoid muscle, thereby closing the rima glottidis.

The thyro-arytenoid muscle (12.13, 12.15)

Attachments: This muscle lies lateral to the vocal fold. It arises on the inner surface of the thyroid cartilage in the midline. It also arises from the cricovocal membrane. The thyro-arytenoid muscle passes backwards, upwards and outwards to be inserted into the base and anterior surface of the arytenoid cartilage. The lower and deep fibres form a distinct bundle that runs parallel with, and lateral to, the vocal ligament. This bundle is sometimes referred to as the vocalis muscle and is attached to the vocal process of the arytenoid cartilage. There is doubt as to whether the fibres of vocalis are also attached to the vocal ligament. The upper fibres of the thyro-arytenoid muscle may extend into the aryepiglottic fold to form the thyro-epiglottic muscle.

Innervation: All parts of the thyro-arytenoid muscle are supplied by the recurrent laryngeal nerve. Due to its several different functional components, it possesses by far the most dense anastomotic network of nerves seen in any of the intrinsic muscles of the larynx. In addition, the muscle receives a branch from the external laryngeal nerve, the functional significance of which is not known.

Vasculature: The arterial blood supply is derived from the laryngeal branches of the superior and inferior thyroid arteries.

Actions: The primary function of the thyro-arytenoid muscle is to shorten the vocal ligament and adjust the tension within it during phonation. In addition, it can rotate the arytenoid cartilage medially and so aid closure of the rima glottidis. Relaxation of the posterior parts of the vocal ligaments by the vocalis muscles, with tension in the anterior parts of the ligaments, is responsible for raising the pitch of the voice. The thyro-epiglottic muscles widen the inlet of the larynx.

The cricothyroid muscle (12.13, 12.16)

Attachments: The cricothyroid muscle arises from the anterior and anterolateral parts of the external surface of the arch of the cricoid cartilage. Its fibres pass upwards and backwards to insert into the thyroid cartilage. Two distinct parts can be recognised. The anterior and superior fibres constitute the straight part of the cricothyroid muscle. This inserts into the lower border of the thyroid lamina. The posterior and inferior fibres constitute the oblique part of the cricothyroid muscle. This inserts into the inferior horn of the thyroid cartilage.

Innervation: Unlike the other intrinsic muscles of the larynx, the cricothyroid muscle is innervated not by the recurrent laryngeal nerve but by the external branch of the superior laryngeal nerve.

Actions: The cricothyroid muscle tenses and elongates the vocal ligaments. This is accomplished by elevating the arch of the cricoid cartilage and tilting back the upper border of its lamina. As a result, the distance between the angle of the thyroid cartilage and the vocal processes of the arytenoids is increased. A similar activity results if the muscles pull the thyroid cartilage forward. Indeed, this is thought to be the principal activity during phonation, as the lamina of the cricoid cartilage is held in position against the vertebral column by the cricopharyngeus muscles.

12.15 Muscles of the larynx, internal view

12.16 Anterior view of the larynx, showing cricothyroid muscle

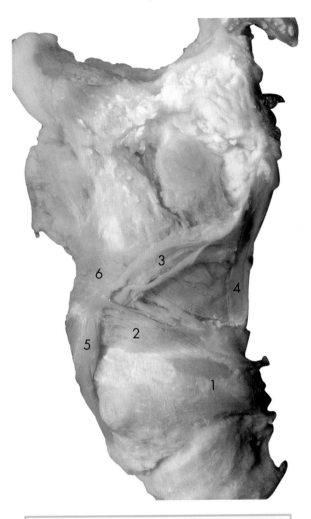

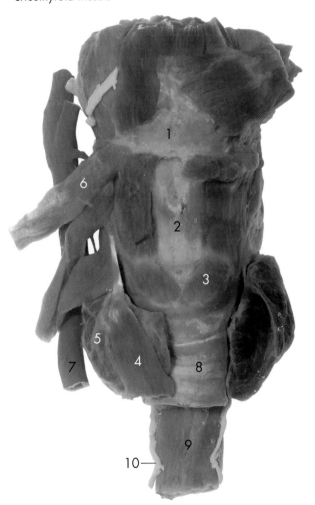

1	Arch of cricoid cartilage
2	Lateral crico-arytenoid muscle
3	Thyro-arytenoid muscle
4	Cut end of lamina of thyroid cartilage
5	Posterior crico-arytenoid muscle
6	Interarytenoid muscle

1	Hyoid bone
2	Laryngeal prominence
3	Cricothyroid muscle
4	Sternothyroid muscle covering thyroid gland
5	Thyroid gland
6	Superior belly of omohyoid
7	Common carotid artery
8	Trachea
9	Oesophagus
10	Recurrent laryngeal nerve

THE BLOOD SUPPLY OF THE LARYNX (12.18, 12.19)

The blood supply of the larynx is derived mainly from two pairs of arteries: the superior and inferior laryngeal arteries. The superior laryngeal artery supplies the larynx above the vocal folds. It is derived from the superior thyroid artery, a branch of the external carotid artery. Occasionally, it may arise directly from the external carotid artery. The superior laryngeal artery runs down towards the larynx with the internal branch of the superior laryngeal nerve. It enters the larynx by penetrating the thyrohyoid membrane. The inferior laryngeal artery supplies the larynx below the vocal folds. It is a branch of the inferior thyroid artery which itself is derived from the thyrocervical trunk of the subclavian artery. The inferior laryngeal artery runs up and into the larynx deep to the lower border of the inferior constrictor muscle. It is accompanied in its course by the recurrent laryngeal nerve. A posterior laryngeal artery of variable size has been described as an internal branch of the inferior thyroid artery.

Venous return from the larynx occurs via superior and inferior laryngeal veins. These run parallel to the laryngeal arteries. They are tributaries of the superior and inferior thyroid veins respectively.

The lymph vessels draining the larynx above the vocal folds accompany the superior laryngeal artery, pierce the thyrohyoid membrane and end in the upper deep cervical lymph nodes. Below the vocal folds, some of the lymph vessels pass through the cricovocal membrane to reach the prelaryngeal and/or pretracheal lymph nodes. Others run with the inferior laryngeal artery to join lower deep cervical nodes.

THE INNERVATION OF THE LARYNX (11.8, 12.18, 12.19)

The chief nerves supplying the larynx are the superior laryngeal and recurrent laryngeal branches of the vagus, both of which contain sensory and motor fibres. The vocal folds form a dividing line for both the sensory and the secretomotor innervation of the mucosa within the larynx. Above the vocal folds, the mucosa is innervated by the internal laryngeal branch of the superior laryngeal nerve. Below the vocal folds, the mucosa is supplied by the recurrent laryngeal nerve. However, there is evidence of overlap in the region of the vocal folds. The motor supply to the intrinsic muscles of the larynx is derived mainly from the recurrent laryngeal nerve. The cricothyroid muscle, however, is supplied by the external branch of the superior laryngeal nerve.

The *superior laryngeal nerve* leaves the trunk of the vagus at its inferior (nodose) ganglion. It curves downwards and forwards by the side of the pharynx, medial to the internal carotid artery. It divides into two branches, a smaller external branch and a larger internal branch, about 1.5 cm below the ganglion, although rarely both branches may arise from the ganglion. The superior laryngeal nerve, or its branches, receive one or more communications from the superior cervical sympathetic ganglion: most frequently, the connection is with the external laryngeal nerve.

12.17 Movements of the vocal folds. The broken outline shows the new position of the vocal folds following muscle contraction

1 Opening of the rima glottidis by rotation of the arytenoids
2 Closure of the rima glottidis by rotation of the arytenoids
3 Closure of the rima glottidis by approximation of the arytenoids without rotation
4 Tensing of the vocal folds by tilting of the anterior part of the cricoid cartilage

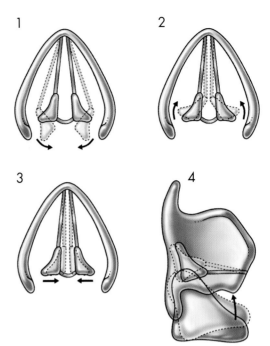

12.18 Lateral view of the larynx showing nerves and vessels

1 Internal carotid artery
2 Superior laryngeal nerve
3 Lingual artery
4 Internal laryngeal nerve and laryngeal branch of superior thyroid artery
5 External carotid artery
6 External laryngeal nerve on inferior constrictor muscle
7 Superior thyroid artery
8 Thyrohyoid muscle
9 Sternocleidomastoid muscle
10 Inferior thyroid artery
11 Recurrent laryngeal nerve
12 Brachial plexus

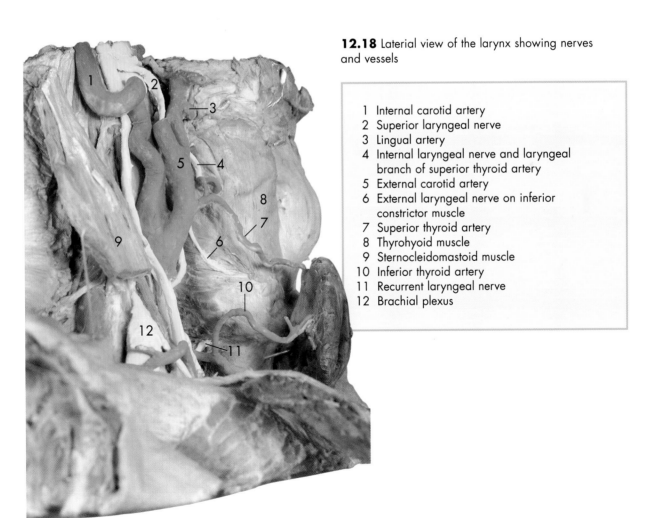

The internal laryngeal nerve descends below the level of the greater horn of the hyoid bone to pass between the middle and inferior constrictor muscles of the pharynx. It enters the larynx by piercing the thyrohyoid membrane, with the superior laryngeal artery lying below it. On entering the larynx, the nerve divides into an ascending branch (which supplies the mucosa of the piriform fossa) and a descending branch (which supplies the supraglottic mucosa). On the medial wall of the piriform fossa, descending branches give twigs to the interarytenoid muscle and there are communicating branches with the recurrent laryngeal nerve. The precise nature and function of these communicating nerves have yet to be determined.

The external branch continues downwards and forwards on the lateral surface of the inferior constrictor muscle to which it contributes some small branches. In about 30% of cases, the nerve is located within the fibres of the constrictor muscle. It passes beneath the sternothyroid muscle, below its insertion into the oblique line of the thyroid cartilage, and supplies the cricothyroid muscle. A communicating nerve continues from the posterior surface of the cricothyroid muscle, crosses the piriforma fossa, and enters the thyro-arytenoid muscle where it anastomoses with branches from the recurrent laryngeal nerve. It is suggested that such communicating branches may provide both additional motor components to the thyro-arytenoid muscle and sensory fibres to the mucosa in the region of the subglottis. Of clinical importance, when considering the external laryngeal nerve, is its close relationship to the superior thyroid artery.

The origins of the *recurrent laryngeal nerves* differ according to side. The right recurrent laryngeal nerve issues from the vagus nerve in front of the subclavian artery. It then passes below and behind the artery. The left recurrent laryngeal nerve arises in the thorax (around the arch of the aorta). Both nerves run up the neck towards the larynx in grooves between the oesophagus and trachea, giving branches to each. The considerable length of the nerves makes them particularly susceptible to damage. The upper part of the recurrent laryngeal nerve has a close and variable relationship to the inferior thyroid artery (12.18, 12.9), and it may pass in front of, behind, or parallel to the artery. The precise incidence of these relationships varies somewhat according to the particular study.

The recurrent laryngeal nerve enters the larynx either by passing deep to (in two-thirds of cases) or between (in one-third of cases) the fibres of the cricopharyngeus muscle at its attachment to the lateral aspect of the cricoid cartilage, supplying the muscle as it passes. At this point of entry, the nerve is in intimate proximity to the posteromedial aspect of the thyroid gland. The main trunk divides into two (or more) branches, generally below the lower border of the inferior constrictor muscle. However, branching may occur higher up to derive an anterior (mainly motor) branch sometimes called the inferior laryngeal nerve, and a posterior (mainly sensory) branch. The inferior laryngeal nerve passes posterior to the cricothyroid joint and its ligament. In this region it may (60%) or may not (40%) be covered by fibres of the posterior crico-arytenoid muscle.

In following the main motor branch of the recurrent laryngeal nerve, the first branch is seen to innervate the posterior crico-arytenoid muscle. The nerve continues on to innervate the interarytenoid muscle and then the lateral crico-arytenoid muscle. The nerve subsequently terminates in the thyro-arytenoid muscle.

An unusual anomaly that is of relevance to laryngeal pathology and surgery is the so-called nonrecurrent laryngeal nerve. In this condition (which has a frequency of between 0.3 and 1%), only the right side is affected and it is always associated with an abnormal origin of the right subclavian artery from the aortic arch on the left side. The right recurrent laryngeal nerve arises directly from the vagus nerve trunk high up in the neck and enters the larynx close to the inferior pole of the thyroid gland.

Parasympathetic, secretomotor fibres run with both the superior and recurrent laryngeal nerves to glands throughout the larynx. Sympathetic fibres run to the larynx with its blood supply, having their origin in the superior and middle cervical ganglia.

THE PARA-LUMENAL SPACES

The ligaments and membranes of the larynx, together with the skeletal elements, allow for the delineation of a number of potential spaces or compartments. The three most commonly considered are the pre-epiglottic, the paraglottic and the subglottic spaces. However, these spaces are not closed compartments completely separated from each other and thus the spread of tumours is possible. Knowledge of the anatomy of these spaces and of the potential pathways of the spread of tumours from them have had a major influence on the surgical approach to malignant disease in this region.

The pre-epiglottic space

The pre-epiglottic space might be expected to lie anterior to the epiglottis. In reality, it also extends beyond the lateral margins of the epiglottis, giving it the form of a horseshoe. It is primarily filled with adipose tissue and appears to contain no lymph nodes. Its upper boundary is formed by the weak hyo-epiglottic membrane, which is strengthened medially as the median hyo-epiglottic ligament. Its anterior boundary is the thyrohyoid membrane, which is strengthened medially as the median thyrohyoid ligament. Its lower boundary is the thyro-epiglottic ligament, which continues laterally with the quadrangular membrane behind. Behind, it extends beyond the margins of the epiglottis. Its upper lateral border is the greater horn of the hyoid bone. Inferolaterally, the pre-epiglottic space is in continuity with the paraglottic space (see below) and is often invaded from the latter by the laryngeal saccule. It is also in continuity with the mucosa of the laryngeal surface of the epiglottis via multiple perforations in the cartilage of the epiglottis. It is through these perforations that malignancies of the laryngeal surface of the epiglottis may invade the fat and areolar tissue of the pre-epiglottic space.

The paraglottic space

The paraglottic space is a region of adipose tissue that contains the internal laryngeal nerve. It is bounded laterally by the thyroid cartilage and thyrohyoid membrane. Superomedially, in most individuals it is continuous with the pre-epiglottic space. However, the two spaces may be partitioned by a fibrous septum. Inferomedially lies the cricovocal membrane. Posteriorly lies the mucosa of the piriform fossa. Inferiorly is the region of the lower border of the thyroid cartilage. Antero-inferiorly, however, there are deficiencies through the paramedian gap by the side of the anterior cricothyroid ligament. Postero-inferiorly, adipose tissue extends towards the cricothyroid joint. Some believe the thyro-arytenoid muscle should be excluded as a component of the paraglottic space. The paraglottic space contains the laryngeal ventricle and part, or all, of the laryngeal saccule.

The subglottic space

The subglottic space is bounded laterally by the crico-vocal membrane, medially by the mucosa of the sub-glottic region, and above by the undersurface of Broyles ligament in the midline. Below, it is continuous with the inner surface of the cricoid cartilage and its mucosa.

SPEECH

The acquisition of language is probably the most complex sensorimotor development in the individual's life. Sounds are produced initially in the larynx by the co-ordinated movements of abdominal, thoracic and laryngeal muscles. Subsequent modification of laryngeal sound to produce meaningful speech occurs principally within the pharyngeal, oral and nasal cavities.

Phonation is the term used to describe the mechanisms of voice production at the larynx. It involves vibration of the vocal folds, mainly in the horizontal plane. The vocal folds are separated during quiet respiration, but are approximated during speech. The apposed vocal folds provide a barrier to the passage of expired air. The air pressure increases until it overcomes the resistance. Consequently, air flows momentarily between the vocal folds into the pharynx. The folds return to their apposed position as a result of their elasticity and the negative pressure created by the rapid flow of air through the constricted rima glottis. The cycle is repeated with a periodicity of the order of milliseconds. In this manner, expired air escapes as a series of rapid puffs that form sound waves.

The character of a sound has three properties: intensity, pitch, and timbre. The intensity depends upon the pressure of the expired air. The pitch depends on many factors, including the length, shape and degree of tension of the vocal folds. The quality of the voice or timbre depends primarily on a series of resonators (see below).

The deeper pitch of the male voice is related to the greater length of the vocal folds (approximately 15 mm in males compared with 11 mm in females). The more rapid growth of the male larynx at puberty is responsible for the 'breaking of the voice'.

Articulation is the term used to describe the mechanism whereby laryngeal sound is modified within resonating chambers by the activity of organs such as the lips, tongue and soft palate to produce speech. This is necessary as the sound generated at the larynx carries a limited amount of speech information. Indeed, the fundamental laryngeal note has a thin reedy quality.

The resonators of the human voice are those air-filled spaces above and below the vocal folds to which sound waves have access. By a process of sympathetic vibration, the resonators act as acoustic filters, amplifying selected frequencies and attenuating others. The supraglottic resonators include the laryngeal chambers above the vocal folds, the pharynx, the oral and nasal cavities and the paranasal sinuses. It is because of the considerable alterations in both size and shape that can occur within the supraglottic resonators that the diversity of sound can be produced. For most sounds, the nasal cavity and nasopharynx are closed off by elevation of the soft palate against the posterior wall of the pharynx. The degree of elevation varies between sounds. However, for the sounds m, n and ng, resonance is produced in the nasopharynx and nasal cavities by depression of the soft palate and closure of the mouth.

12.19 Laryngopharynx viewed posteriorly, showing blood vessels and nerves

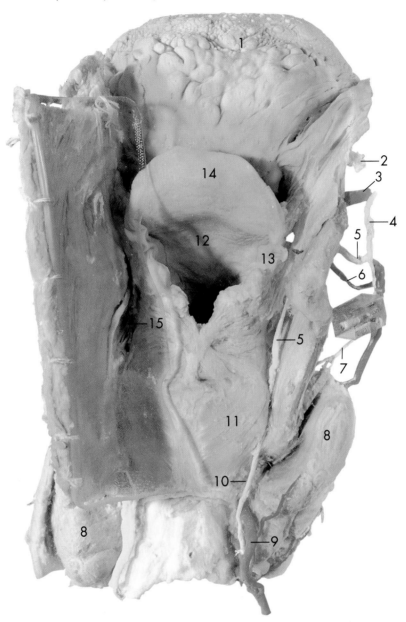

1 Dorsum of the tongue	8 Thyroid gland
2 Hypoglossal nerve	9 Inferior thyroid artery
3 Lingual artery	10 Recurrent laryngeal nerve
4 Superior laryngeal nerve	11 Posterior crico-arytenoid muscle
5 Internal laryngeal nerve	12 Inlet of larynx
6 Laryngeal branch of superior	13 Aryepiglottic fold
thyroid artery	14 Epiglottis
7 External laryngeal nerve	15 Piriform fossa

The classification of sounds

Sounds may be voiced (i.e. the vocal folds vibrate in their production) or breathed (i.e. the vocal folds do not vibrate in their production). The two main groups of speech sounds are vowels and consonants.

A vowel sound is produced when the air flow is uninterrupted. In producing different vowel sounds, air is channelled or restricted by the position of the lips and tongue. All vowels are voiced.

A consonant is produced when the air flow is impeded before it is released. Consonants may be voiced (e.g. b, d, z) or breathed (e.g. p, t, s).

Consonants may be classified in two ways: according to the place of articulation (bilabials, labiodentals, linguodentals, linguopalatals, glottals), or the manner of articulation (plosives, fricatives, affricatives, nasals, laterals, semi-vowels).

In bilabial sounds, the two lips are used. In labiodental sounds, the lower lip meets the maxillary incisors. Linguodental sounds involve the tip of the tongue contacting the maxillary incisors (and adjacent hard palate). For linguopalatal sounds, the tongue meets the palate.

In plosive sounds, there is a complete stoppage of air, while fricatives require only a partial stoppage of air. Affricatives also require a partial stoppage of air, but there is a subsequent rapid release of air. In nasal sounds, the mouth is obstructed but the nasal passages remain open. Lateral sounds require air to leave the sides of the mouth. Semi-vowels are brief vowel articulations which are followed by a true vowel articulation of longer duration.

Table 12.1 provides examples of the various categories of consonant articulations.

Although one may describe the position of articulators for a particular vowel or consonant, it must be remembered that there are no fixed positions during speech, only continuous movement. Hearing is an important monitoring system in controlling speech, but feed-back from sensory receptors in the oral cavity (particularly the tongue) also plays an important role.

Table 12.1 Examples of the categories of consonant articulations.

| Manner of articulation | Place of articulation | | | | | | |
| | | | Linguodentals | | Linguopalatals | | |
	Bilabial	Labiodental	(Dental)	(Alveolar)	(Alveolar)	(Palatal)	Glottal
Voicing	− +	− +	− +	− +	− +	− +	− +
Plosives	p b			t d		k g	
Fricatives		f v	θ δ	s z	ζ 3		h
Affricatives				tζ			
				tr dr		j	
Nasals	m			n		ng	
Laterals				l			
Semi-vowels	w						

12.20 Configurations of oral structures during consonant articulations

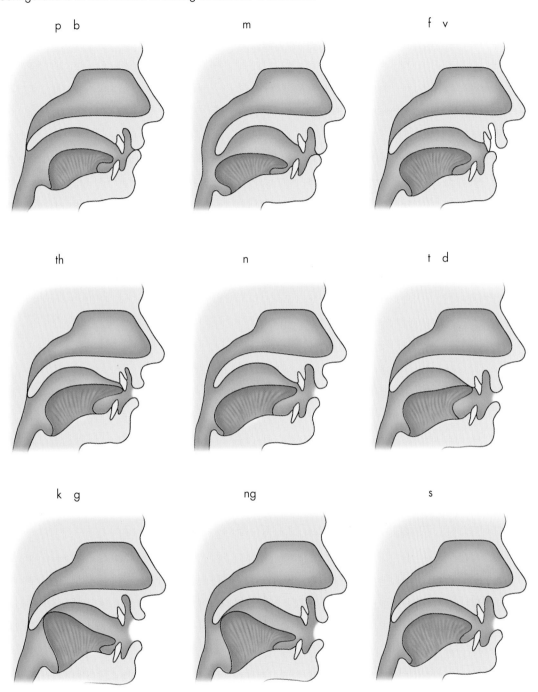

chapter 13
RADIOLOGICAL AND SECTIONAL ANATOMY

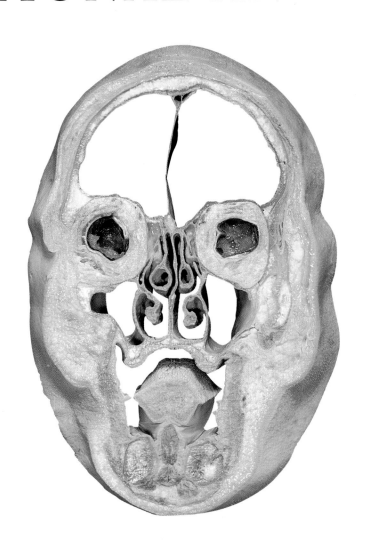

13.1 Posteroanterior radiograph of skull

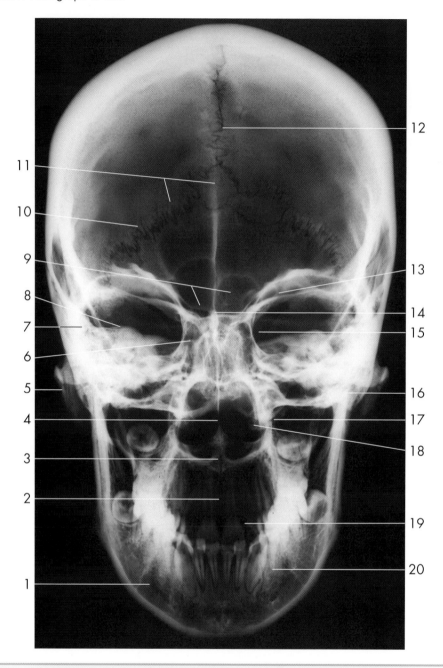

1	Mandibular canal leading to mental foramen	11	Sutural bones in region of lambda
2	Intermaxillary suture	12	Sagittal suture
3	Anterior nasal spine	13	Lesser wing of sphenoid
4	Nasal septum	14	Crista galli
5	Mastoid process	15	Superior orbital fissure
6	Ethmoidal air cells	16	Condyle of mandible
7	Orbital margin	17	Margin of maxillary sinus
8	Petrous ridge of temporal bone	18	Nasal concha
9	Frontal sinuses	19	Maxilla and teeth
10	Lambdoid suture	20	Mandible and teeth

13.2 Lateral radiograph of skull

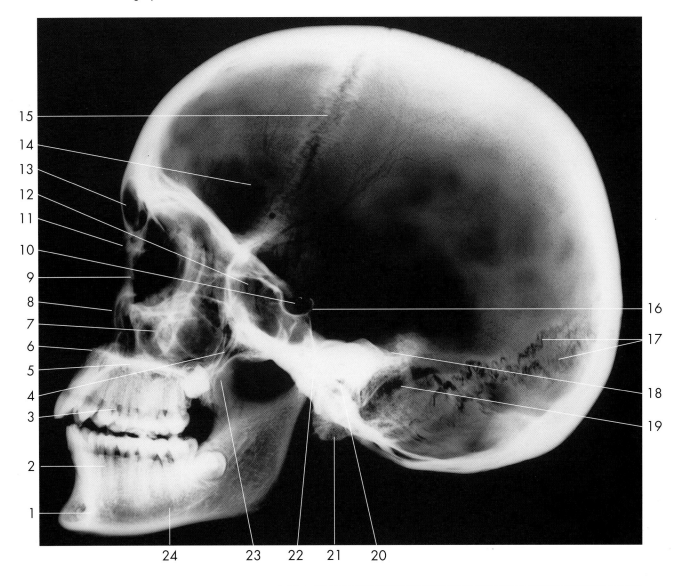

1 Mental foramen	14 Grooves for meningeal vessels
2 Mandible and teeth	15 Coronal suture
3 Maxilla and teeth	16 Dorsum sellae
4 Pterygomaxillary fissure	17 Lambdoid sutures
5 Hard palate	18 Petrous ridge
6 Anterior nasal spine	19 Groove for sigmoid sinus
7 Margin of maxillary sinus	20 External acoustic meatus
8 Anterior nasal aperture	21 Mastoid process
9 Orbital margin	22 Condyle of mandible
10 Pituitary fossa	23 Coronoid process of mandible superimposed on pterygoid plates
11 Nasal bones	
12 Sphenoid sinus	24 Mandibular canal
13 Frontal sinus	

13.3 Occipitomental radiograph of skull

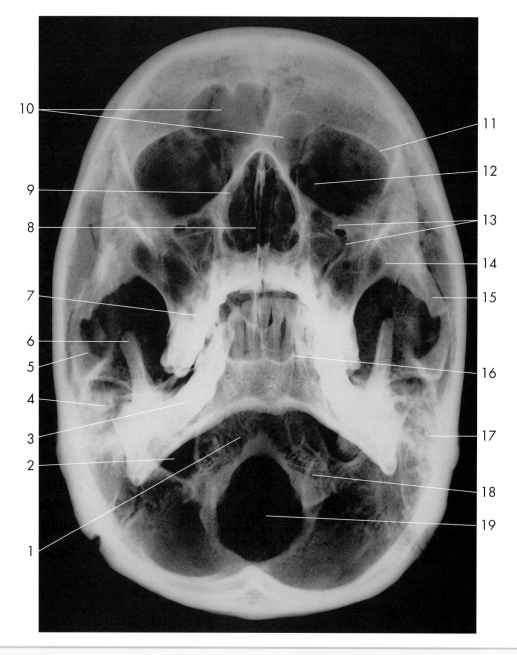

1	Basilar part of occipital bone	11	Orbital margin
2	Jugular foramen	12	Superior orbital fissure
3	Mandible and teeth	13	Infra-orbital foramen and canal
4	Condyle of mandible	14	Margin of maxillary sinus
5	Articular eminence	15	Zygomatic arch
6	Coronoid process	16	Margin of sphenoidal sinus
7	Maxilla and teeth	17	Mastoid air cells
8	Nasal septum	18	Occipital condyle
9	Ethmoidal air cells	19	Foramen magnum
10	Frontal sinuses		

13.4 Horizonal section of the head just above the mandibular condyle

1	Nasal septum
2	Nasolacrimal duct
3	Maxillary sinus
4	Zygomatic arch
5	Temporalis muscle
6	Internal carotid artery
7	Lateral pterygoid muscle
8	Mastoid air cells
9	Sigmoid sinus
10	Basilar artery
11	Middle nasal concha
12	External auditory meatus

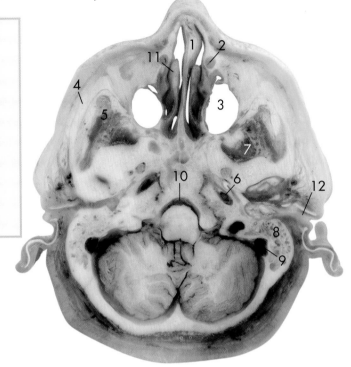

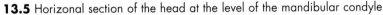

13.5 Horizonal section of the head at the level of the mandibular condyle

1	Cartilage of nasal septum
2	Maxillary sinus
3	Zygomatic arch
4	Coronoid process surrounded by temporalis muscle
5	Parotid gland
6	Lateral pterygoid muscle
7	Mandibular condyle
8	Bulb of internal jugular vein and internal carotid artery
9	Mastoid air cells
10	Jugular foramen
11	Auditory tube (cartilaginous part)
12	Sigmoid sinus
13	Trapezius muscle
14	Sternocleidomastoid muscle

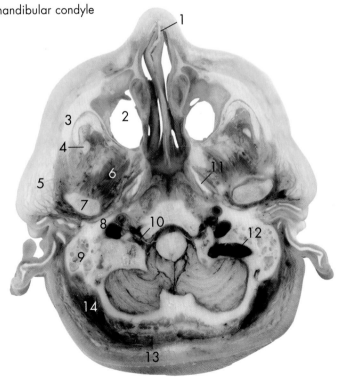

13.6 Horizonal section of the head just below the mandibular condyle

1 External naris
2 Nasal septum
3 Inferior nasal concha
4 Maxillary sinus
5 Masseter muscle
6 Ramus of mandible
7 Parotid gland
8 Superficial temporal and maxillary arteries
9 Levator veli palatini muscle
10 Medial pterygoid muscle
11 Lateral pterygoid muscle
12 Lateral pterygoid plate
13 Anterior arch of atlas
14 Dens of axis
15 Internal carotid artery, internal jugular vein and vagus nerve in carotid sheath
16 Vertebral artery
17 Sternocleidomastoid muscle
18 Retromandibular vein

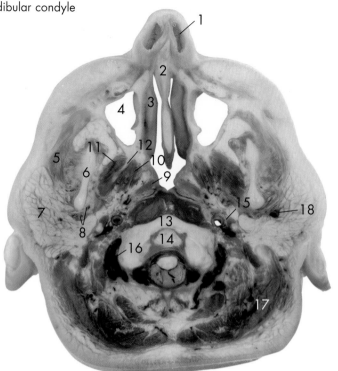

13.7 Horizontal section of the head at the level of the palate

1 Orbicularis oris muscle (upper lip)
2 Hard palate
3 Soft palate
4 Buccinator muscle
5 Masseter muscle
6 Ramus of mandible
7 Inferior alveolar nerve within mandibular canal
8 Medial pterygoid muscle
9 Parotid gland
10 Internal jugular vein
11 Internal carotid artery
12 Body of axis vertebra
13 Obliquus capitis inferior
14 Semispinalis cervicis muscle
15 Trapezius muscle
16 Semispinalis capitis muscle
17 Splenius capitis muscle
18 Sternocleidomastoid muscle
19 Styloid group of muscles
20 Nasopharynx

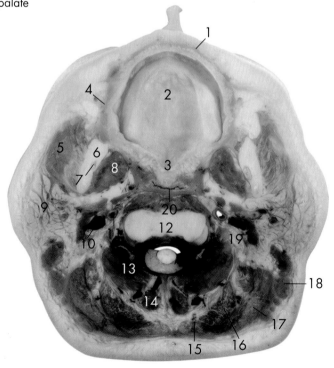

13.8 Horizontal section of the head at the level of the tongue

1   Orbicularis oris muscle (lower lip)
2   Depressor anguli oris muscle
3   Buccinator muscle
4   Masseter muscle
5   Ramus of mandible
6   Medial pterygoid muscle
7   Parotid gland
8   Sternocleidomastoid muscle
9   Trapezius muscle
10 Internal jugular vein, internal carotid
    artery and vagus nerve in carotid sheath
11 External carotid artery
12 Styloglossus muscle
13 Styloid group of muscles
14 Oropharynx
15 Nasopharynx
16 Vertebral artery

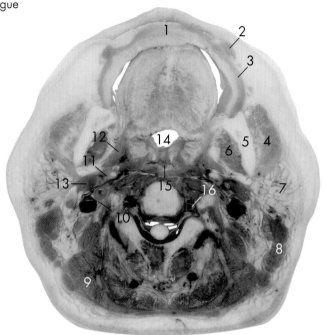

13.9 Horizontal section of the head at the level of the floor of the mouth

1   Body of mandible
2   Genioglossus muscle
3   Sublingual gland
4   Mylohyoid muscle
5   Submandibular gland
6   Hyoglossus muscle
7   Oropharynx
8   Masseter muscle
9   Platysma muscle
10 Parotid gland
11 External jugular vein
12 Sternocleidomastoid muscle
13 Internal jugular vein
14 Internal carotid artery
15 External carotid artery
16 Vertebral artery
17 Body of cervical vertebra
18 Spinal cord
19 Posterior arch of cervical vertebra
20 Spine of cervical vertebra
21 Occipital vein
22 Trapezius muscle

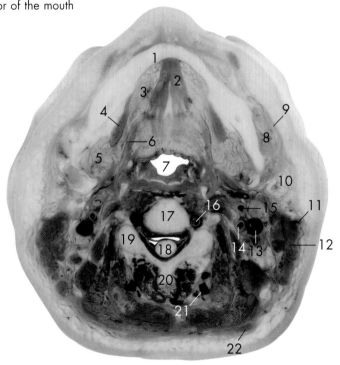

13.10 Horizontal section of the neck at the level of the hyoid bone

1	Body of mandible
2	Anterior belly of digastric muscle
3	Geniohyoid muscle
4	Hyoid bone
5	Epiglottis
6	Laryngopharynx
7	Submandibular gland
8	Platysma muscle
9	External carotid artery
10	Internal carotid artery
11	Internal jugular vein
12	Sternocleidomastoid muscle
13	Vagus nerve
14	Body of cervical vertebra
15	Vertebral artery
16	Spinal cord
17	Posteror tubercle of transverse process
18	Spine of cervical vertebra
19	Semispinalis cervicis muscle
20	Semispinalis capitis muscle
21	Splenius capitis muscle
22	Trapezius muscle

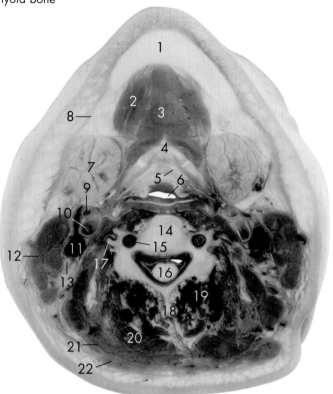

13.11 Horizontal section of the neck at the level of the thyroid cartilage

1	Platysma muscle
2	Omohyoid muscle
3	Thyrohyoid muscle
4	Sternohyoid muscle
5	Lamina of thyroid cartilage
6	Tip of arytenoid cartilage
7	Inferior constrictor muscle
8	Common carotid artery
9	Internal jugular vein
10	Sternocleidomastoid muscle
11	External jugular vein
12	Vertebral artery
13	Levator scapulae muscle
14	Trapezius muscle
15	Spine of cervical vertebra

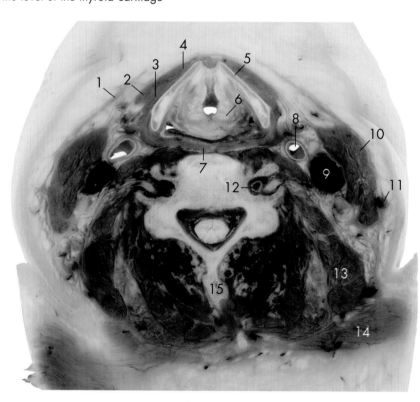

13.12 Horizontal section of the neck at the level of the cricoid cartilage

1 Sternohyoid muscle
2 Omohyoid muscle
3 Sternothyroid muscle
4 Sternocleidomastoid muscle
5 Internal jugular vein
6 Common carotid artery
7 External jugular vein
8 Inferior constrictor muscle
9 Inferior horn of thyroid cartilage
10 Cricoid cartilage
11 Cricothyroid muscle
12 Vertebral artery
13 Levator scapulae muscle
14 Trapezius muscle

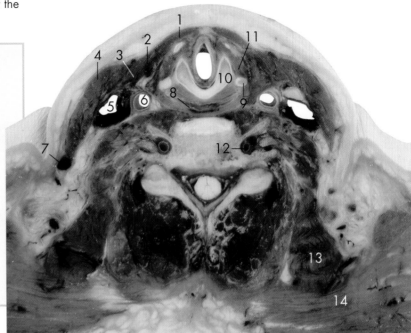

13.13 Horizontal section of the neck at the level of the trachea and thyroid gland

1 Sternohyoid muscle
2 Sternothyroid muscle
3 Omohyoid muscle
4 Sternocleidomastoid muscle
5 Thyroid gland
6 Trachea
7 Oesophagus
8 Vagus nerve
9 Common carotid artery
10 Internal jugular vein
11 Vertebral artery and vein
12 Scalene muscles
13 Trapezius
14 Transverse process of seventh cervical vertebra
15 Spine of seventh cervical vertebra

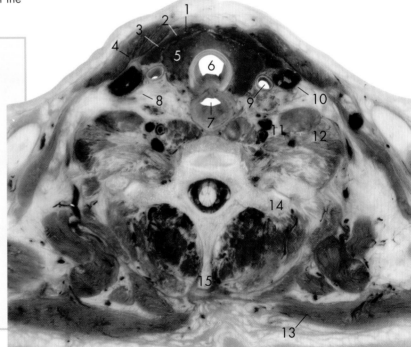

13.14 Coronal section of the head at the level of the eyeball

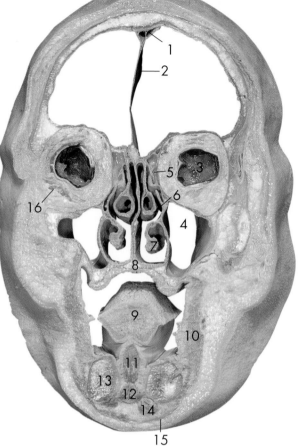

1 Superior sagittal sinus
2 Falx cerebri
3 Eyeball
4 Maxillary sinus
5 Ethmoidal sinus
6 Middle nasal concha
7 Inferior nasal concha
8 Hard palate
9 Tongue
10 Buccinator
11 Genioglossus muscle
12 Geniohyoid muscle
13 Body of mandible
14 Anterior belly of digastric muscle
15 Platysma muscle
16 Inferior oblique muscle of eye

13.15 Coronal section of the head just behind the eyeball

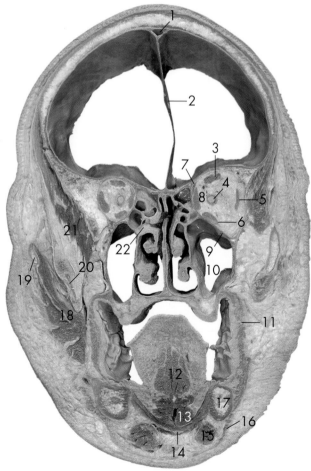

1 Superior sagittal sinus
2 Falx cerebri
3 Levator palpebrae superioris and superior rectus muscles
4 Optic nerve
5 Lateral rectus muscle
6 Inferior rectus muscle
7 Superior oblique muscle
8 Medial rectus muscle
9 Infraorbital nerve and vessels
10 Maxillary sinus
11 Buccinator muscle
12 Genioglossus muscle
13 Geniohyoid muscle
14 Mylohyoid muscle
15 Anterior belly of digastric muscle
16 Platysma muscle
17 Body of mandible
18 Masseter muscle
19 Zygomatic arch
20 Coronoid process
21 Temporalis muscle
22 Posterior ethmoid air cells draining into superior meatus

13.16 Coronal section of the head at the level of the sphenoidal sinus

1   Tentorium cerebelli
2   Temporalis muscle
3   Zygomatic arch
4   Masseter muscle
5   Mandible
6   Mylohyoid muscle
7   Submandibular gland
8   Facial artery
9   Medial pterygoid muscle
10 Lateral pterygoid muscle
11 Parotid gland
12 Mandibular condyle
13 Nasal cavity
14 Hard palate
15 Sphenoidal sinus
16 Pituitary gland
17 Internal carotid artery
18 Maxillary artery

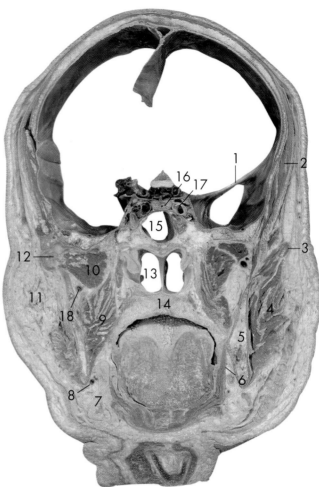

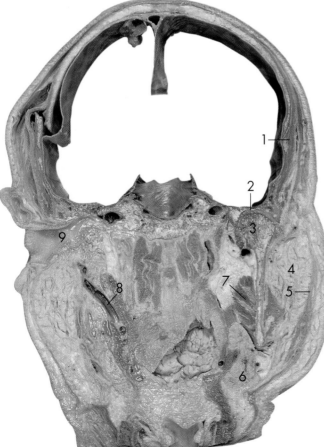

13.17 Coronal section of the head and neck at the level of the temporomandibular joint

1   Temporalis muscle
2   Intra-articular disc of temporomandibular joint
3   Mandibular condyle
4   Parotid gland
5   Platysma muscle
6   Submandibular gland
7   Medial pterygoid muscle
8   External carotid artery
9   External auditory meatus

13.18 Coronal section of the head and neck at the level of the mastoid process

1	Superior sagittal sinus
2	Falx cerebri
3	Tentorium cerebelli
4	Superior petrosal sinus
5	Mastoid air cells
6	Sigmoid sinus
7	Inferior petrosal sinus
8	Roots of hypoglossal nerve
9	Roots of glossopharyngeal, vagus and accessory nerves
10	Roots of facial and vestibulocochlear nerves
11	Cerebellum
12	Dens of axis vertebra
13	Intervertebral disc
14	Vertebral artery
15	Sternocleidomastoid muscle
16	Lateral mass of atlas
17	Parotid gland
18	Vertebral artery

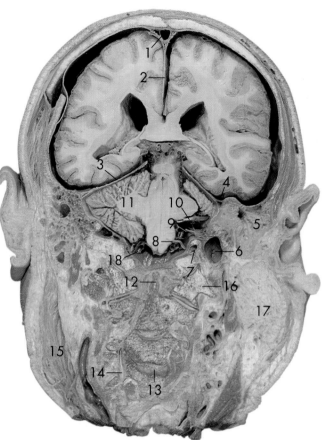

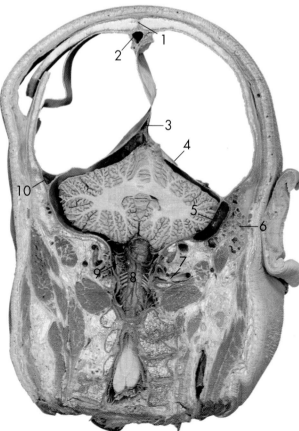

13.19 Coronal section of the head and neck at the level of the spinal cord

1	Sagittal suture
2	Superior sagittal sinus
3	Straight sinus
4	Tentorium cerebelli
5	Sigmoid sinus
6	Mastoid air cells
7	Vertebral artery
8	Spinal cord and cervical spinal nerves
9	Spinal accessory nerve
10	Transverse sinus

13.20 Orthopantomogram of adult dentition

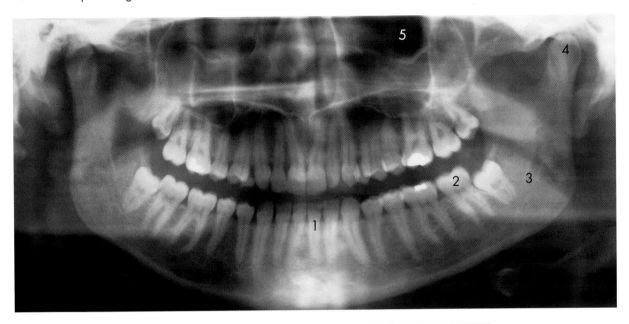

1	Mandibular first permanent incisor
2	Mandibular second permanent molar
3	Mandibular canal
4	Mandibular condyle
5	Maxillary sinus

13.21a Arteriogram of vertebral arteries

13.21b Arteriogram of vertebral arteries taken shortly after **13.21a**

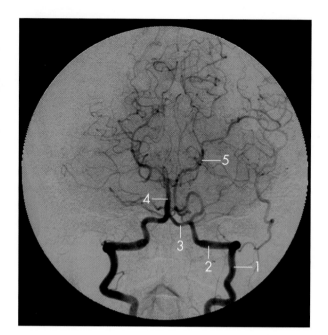

1	Vertebral artery
2	Vertebral artery winding around the lateral mass of the atlas
3	Vertebral artery in foramen magnum
4	Basilar artery
5	Posterior cerebral artery

1	Vertebral artery
2	Vertebral artery winding around the lateral mass of the atlas
3	Vertebral artery in foramen magnum
4	Basilar artery
5	Posterior cerebral artery

13.21 Arteriogram of external carotid artery

1	External carotid artery
2	Superior thyroid artery
3	Lingual artery
4	Facial artery
5	Occipital artery
6	Posterior auricular artery
7	Ascending pharyngeal artery
8	Maxillary artery
9	Superficial temporal artery

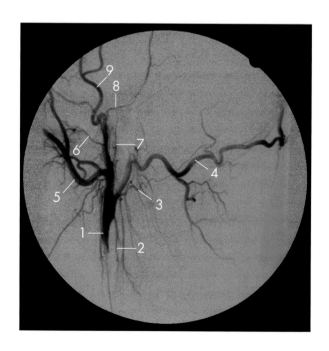

13.23a Arteriogram of the internal carotid artery

13.23b Arteriogram of the internal carotid artery taken shortly after **13.23a**

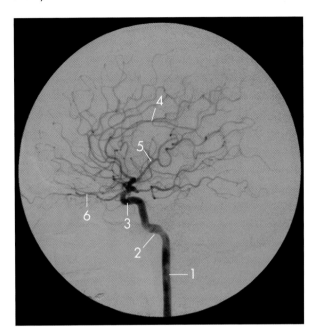

1	Internal carotid artery
2	Internal carotid artery in carotid canal
3	Internal carotid artery in cavernous sinus
4	Anterior cerebral artery
5	Middle cerebral artery
6	Ophthalmic artery

1	Internal carotid artery
2	Internal carotid artery in carotid canal
3	Internal carotid artery in cavernous sinus
4	Anterior cerebral artery
5	Middle cerebral artery
6	Ophthalmic artery

13.24c Arteriogram showing venous sinuses

1	Superior sagittal sinus
2	Inferior sagittal sinus
3	Straight sinus
4	Transverse sinus
5	Sigmoid sinus
6	Internal jugular vein

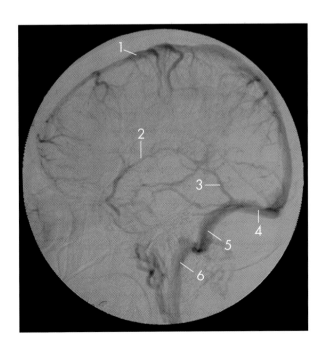

INDEX